ONCOLOGY NURSE NAVIGATION
Delivering Patient-Centered Care Across the Continuum

Edited by
Karyl D. Blaseg, RN, MSN, OCN®
Penny Daugherty, RN, MS, OCN®
Kathleen A. Gamblin, RN, BSN, OCN®

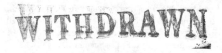

Oncology Nursing Society
Pittsburgh, Pennsylvania

KH

ONS Publications Department
Executive Director, Professional Practice and Programs: Elizabeth Wertz Evans, PhD, RN, MPM, CPHQ,
CPHIMS, FHIMSS, FACMPE
Publisher and Director of Publications: William A. Tony, BA, CQIA
Managing Editor: Lisa M. George, BA
Technical Content Editor: Angela D. Klimaszewski, RN, MSN
Assistant Managing Editor: Amy Nicoletti, BA, JD
Copy Editor: Laura Pinchot, BA
Graphic Designer: Dany Sjoen
Editorial Assistant: Judy Holmes

First printing, June 2014
Second printing, March 2015

Library of Congress Cataloging-in-Publication Data
Oncology nurse navigation : delivering patient-centered care across the continuum / edited by Karyl D. Blaseg, Penny Daugherty, and Kathleen A. Gamblin.
   p. ; cm.
Includes bibliographical references and index.
ISBN 978-1-935864-35-6 (alk. paper)
I. Blaseg, Karyl D., editor. II. Daugherty, Penny, editor. III. Gamblin, Kathleen A., editor. IV. Oncology Nursing Society, issuing body.
[DNLM: 1. Oncology Nursing–methods. 2. Nurse's Role. 3. Patient Navigation–methods. WY 156]
RC266
616.99'40231–dc23

2014011519

Publisher's Note
This book is published by the Oncology Nursing Society (ONS). ONS neither represents nor guarantees that the practices described herein will, if followed, ensure safe and effective patient care. The recommendations contained in this book reflect ONS's judgment regarding the state of general knowledge and practice in the field as of the date of publication. The recommendations may not be appropriate for use in all circumstances. Those who use this book should make their own determinations regarding specific safe and appropriate patient care practices, taking into account the personnel, equipment, and practices available at the hospital or other facility at which they are located. The editors and publisher cannot be held responsible for any liability incurred as a consequence from the use or application of any of the contents of this book. Figures and tables are used as examples only. They are not meant to be all-inclusive, nor do they represent endorsement of any particular institution by ONS. Mention of specific products and opinions related to those products do not indicate or imply endorsement by ONS. Websites mentioned are provided for information only; the hosts are responsible for their own content and availability. Unless otherwise indicated, dollar amounts reflect U.S. dollars.

ONS publications are originally published in English. Publishers wishing to translate ONS publications must contact ONS about licensing arrangements. ONS publications cannot be translated without obtaining written permission from ONS. (Individual tables and figures that are reprinted or adapted require additional permission from the original source.) Because translations from English may not always be accurate or precise, ONS disclaims any responsibility for inaccuracies in words or meaning that may occur as a result of the translation. Readers relying on precise information should check the original English version.

Printed in the United States of America

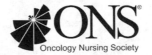

Integrity • Innovation • Stewardship • Advocacy • Excellence • Inclusiveness

2/23/16

Contributors

Editors

Karyl D. Blaseg, RN, MSN, OCN®
Manager of Cancer Programs
Billings Clinic
Billings, Montana
Chapter 2. Getting Started as a Nurse
Navigator; Chapter 6. Cancer Site–Specific
Navigation; Chapter 10. Documentation and
Patient Navigation Software; Chapter 11.
Navigation Resources

Penny Daugherty, RN, MS, OCN®
Oncology Nurse Navigator
Northside Hospital Cancer Institute
Atlanta, Georgia
Chapter 6. Cancer Site–Specific Navigation

Kathleen A. Gamblin, RN, BSN, OCN®
Coordinator, Oncology Navigation Program
Northside Hospital Cancer Institute
Atlanta, Georgia
Chapter 10. Documentation and Patient
Navigation Software; Chapter 11. Navigation
Resources

Authors

**Sharon Bartelt, RN, MSN, MBA, CPHQ,
CSSBB, OCN®**
Multidisciplinary Conference Program Manager
Hematological, Central Nervous System, and
    Cutaneous/Sarcoma Navigator
Gibbs Cancer Center and Research Institute
Spartanburg Regional Healthcare System
Spartanburg, South Carolina
Chapter 9. Program Assessment and Outcome
Metrics

Cynthia A. Cantril, RN, OCN®, MPH
Director, Oncology Service Lines/Nurse
    Navigation
Sutter Pacific Medical Foundation
Santa Rosa, California
Chapter 1. Overview of Nurse Navigation

Frank dela Rama, RN, MS, AOCNS®
Clinical Nurse Specialist, Oncology/Genomics
    and Prostate Cancer Nurse Navigator
Palo Alto Medical Foundation
Palo Alto, California
Chapter 6. Cancer Site–Specific Navigation

Barbara Francks, RN, BSN, OCN®, CBCN®
Clinical Nurse Navigator
Virtua
Marlton, New Jersey
Chapter 5. Breast Cancer Navigation

**Sharon S. Gentry, RN, MSN, AOCN®, CBCN®,
CBEC**
Breast Nurse Navigator
Novant Health Derrick L. Davis Cancer Center
Winston-Salem, North Carolina
Chapter 4. Navigation Considerations When
Working With Patients

Laura S. Hunnibell, APRN, DNP, AOCN®
Oncology Nurse Practitioner
Dayton VA Medical Center
Dayton, Ohio
*Chapter 9. Program Assessment and Outcome
Metrics*

Mary Lou Iverson, RN, MN, OCN®
Cancer Care Navigator
Billings Clinic
Billings, Montana
Chapter 5. Breast Cancer Navigation

Susan J. Keen, BSN, RN, OCN®, CTTS
Thoracic Nurse Navigator
Thomas Johns Cancer Hospital at Johnston
    Willis Hospital
Richmond, Virginia
Chapter 6. Cancer Site–Specific Navigation

Nadesda A. Mack, RN, BSN, MBA, OCN®
(at the time of this writing)
Administrator, Oncology Services
Lehigh Valley Health Network
Allentown, Pennsylvania
*Chapter 3. How to Start and Expand a Nurse
Navigation Program*

LaTonya E. Mann, FNP-BC, MSN, OCN®, CRNI
Oncology Nurse Navigator
Helen F. Graham Cancer Center at Christiana
    Care Health System
Newark, Delaware
*Chapter 8. Example of a Successful Nurse
Navigation Program*

Nicole G. Messier, RN, BSN
Upper GI and GU Nurse Navigator/Clinical
    Program Coordinator
Fletcher Allen Health Care
Burlington, Vermont
Chapter 6. Cancer Site–Specific Navigation

Jackie Miller, RN, BSN, OCN®
Clinical Nurse Navigator
Virtua
Marlton, New Jersey
Chapter 5. Breast Cancer Navigation

Elissa A. Peters, RN, MS, OCN®
Survivorship Nurse Navigator
Penrose Cancer Center
Colorado Springs, Colorado
Chapter 7. Setting-Specific Navigation

Jean B. Sellers, RN, MSN
Administrative Clinical Director
UNC Lineberger Comprehensive Cancer Center
Chapel Hill, North Carolina
*Chapter 4. Navigation Considerations When
Working With Patients*

Lisa Shalkowski, RN, BSN, MSHA
Director of Oncology Services
Virtua
Marlton, New Jersey
*Chapter 3. How to Start and Expand a Nurse
Navigation Program*

Heather Stern, RN, BSN, OCN®
Head and Neck/Neuro-Oncology Nurse Navigator
Center for Cancer Prevention and Treatment,
    St. Joseph Hospital
Orange, California
Chapter 6. Cancer Site–Specific Navigation

Patricia M. Strusowski, RN, MS
Senior Consultant
Oncology Solutions, LLC
Decatur, Georgia
*Chapter 8. Example of a Successful Nurse
Navigation Program*

Jay R. Swanson, APRN, MSN
Nurse Practitioner, Hospitalist
St. Elizabeth Regional Medical Center
Lincoln, Nebraska
*Chapter 9. Program Assessment and Outcome
Metrics*

Marguerite A. Thomas, RN, MN, AOCN®
Outreach Nurse Navigator/RN Clinic
    Coordinator, Women's Wellness Connection
Penrose Cancer Center
Colorado Springs, Colorado
Chapter 7. Setting-Specific Navigation

Disclosure

Editors and authors of books and guidelines provided by the Oncology Nursing Society are expected to disclose to the readers any significant financial interest or other relationships with the manufacturer(s) of any commercial products.

A vested interest may be considered to exist if a contributor is affiliated with or has a financial interest in commercial organizations that may have a direct or indirect interest in the subject matter. A "financial interest" may include, but is not limited to, being a shareholder in the organization; being an employee of the commercial organization; serving on an organization's speakers bureau; or receiving research from the organization. An "affiliation" may be holding a position on an advisory board or some other role of benefit to the commercial organization. Vested interest statements appear in the front matter for each publication.

Contributors are expected to disclose any unlabeled or investigational use of products discussed in their content. This information is acknowledged solely for the information of the readers.

The contributors provided the following disclosure and vested interest information:

Frank dela Rama, RN, MS, AOCNS®: Myriad Genetics, consultant or advisory role; Amgen, Myriad Genetics, honoraria

Sharon S. Gentry, RN, MSN, AOCN®, CBCN®, CBEC: Academy of Oncology Nurse and Patient Navigators and Leadership Council, consultant or advisory role; Genomic Health, Pfizer, honoraria

Susan J. Keen, BSN, RN, OCN®, CTTS: BioMedical Learning Institute, Boehringer Ingelheim, Educational Concepts Group, LLC, 3Health, honoraria

Nicole G. Messier, RN, BSN: Academy of Oncology Nurse and Patient Navigators, honoraria and other remuneration

Jean B. Sellers, RN, MSN: Academy of Oncology Nurse and Patient Navigators, honoraria

Patricia M. Strusowski, RN, MS: Oncology Solutions, LLC, consultant or advisory role; Academy of Oncology Nurse and Patient Navigators, honoraria

Contents

Foreword

Throughout American history, nurses have been the principal providers of one-on-one patient care. The concept of patient navigation, which promotes timely quality care through one-on-one guidance of a patient's journey through the healthcare continuum, is consistent with this philosophy. In recent years, oncology nurses have taken on an increasing role in the evolving field of patient navigation. This publication provides a comprehensive review of the history and current status of oncology nurse navigators.

Patient navigation had its inception in Harlem in 1990 as an intervention designed to diminish the exceedingly high breast cancer mortality rate in a population of poor Black women. The combined interventions of breast cancer screening and navigation from the point of abnormal finding to timely treatment increased the five-year survival rate from 39% to 70%. From this origin in Harlem, patient navigation has become a widely applied patient-centered healthcare service delivery model. Key markers of this progress include the signing of the Patient Navigator Outreach and Chronic Disease Prevention Act by President Bush in 2005, the designation of patient navigation as a standard of care by the American College of Surgeons Commission on Cancer, and the inclusion of patient navigation requirements in the Affordable Care Act.

The core principle of patient navigation is the elimination of barriers to timely quality care through all phases of health care including prevention, detection, diagnosis, treatment, and survivorship. Many patients, particularly the poor and the uninsured, face significant barriers to receiving timely diagnosis and timely quality care. Common barriers include financial barriers, communication barriers, and medical system barriers, as well as fear and distrust. The weight of the scientific evidence to date indicates that patient navigation, particularly when applied to vulnerable populations, can increase participation in screening and reduce the time from abnormal finding to diagnosis and treatment in breast, cervical, colon, and prostate cancers. Also, many studies show that patient navigation results in higher patient satisfaction.

It is important to make a distinction between the process of patient navigation and the role of patient navigators within the navigation process. The navigation process at a given healthcare site must be well defined. The determination of who should navigate should be based on the level of skills required in a given phase of navigation. Nurse navigators may have a significant impact in improving the quality of treatment of patients with cancer.

Patient navigation is a team effort. It is important to harness, integrate, and apply the power and energy of all patient navigators, nonprofessionals and professionals. Nurse navigators have the skills and knowledge to take on a leadership role in this team process. *Oncology Nurse Navigation: Delivering Patient-Centered Care Across the Continuum* documents the essential role played by nurse navigators in the evolving field of patient navigation.

Harold P. Freeman, MD, FACS
Founder and President
Harold P. Freeman Patient Navigation Institute

Preface

This book was originally conceived through a casual conversation at an Oncology Nursing Society (ONS) Congress in which two friends identified the need for a practical resource for nurses in the evolving specialty of navigation. While the original concept for this publication was envisioned to be a rather simple scenario-based document, as ONS further explored the growing needs of the navigation community, it became apparent that a multifaceted publication written by a diverse team of oncology nurses would be needed to depict the reality of nurse navigation.

Patient navigation is increasingly recognized as a fundamental component of comprehensive oncology care. From its early beginnings with Dr. Harold P. Freeman in Harlem, New York, to the National Cancer Institute's Patient Navigation Project and the hundreds of academic and community hospital navigation programs that have been developed thereafter, extensive efforts have been made to create meaningful and successful navigation models. As we have networked and researched various navigation programs across the country, we have come to appreciate that each navigation program is as unique and varied as the specific healthcare organization and communities served. While it has been widely acknowledged that there is no "one size fits all" when it comes to navigation programs, we believe much can be learned from the prior foundations created and successes achieved so that those new to navigation are not left to create a program from scratch.

As three oncology nurses, we have chosen to approach this book predominately from the perspective of *oncology nurse navigation*. However, we feel it is important to articulate that we readily recognize the distinct and valuable role served by others functioning as patient navigators including other members of the healthcare team, lay community members, and cancer survivors. While the title of this book and overall content is directed toward the concept of "nurse" navigation, we truly believe much of the information will resonate across the community of navigators regardless of specific position, individual background, or educational preparation.

This book is the first of its kind to provide a comprehensive resource on oncology nurse navigation. The book begins with a perspective on the historical development of navigation and then moves through the process of developing, implementing, and evaluating a navigation program. Concrete examples and tangible tools utilized by various nurse navigation models across the cancer continuum are provided, as well as a variety of community and national resources that may be of assistance to the oncology nurse navigator. While not intended to be all-inclusive, we hope this book will serve as a practical, "nuts-and-bolts" resource that navigators and program managers can use to construct and sustain a successful nurse navigation program.

As an editing team, we bring a combined 77 years of nursing experience, with 22 of those dedicated to oncology nurse navigation. During our experience with oncology nurse navigation, we have had the opportunity and great pleasure to successfully collaborate with our organizations' administrative and physician leadership teams to establish two comprehensive navigation programs that each offer a wide range of navigation services across the continuum. Additionally, chapter authors were identified and chosen to represent a variety of cancer programs, navigation models, and navigation organizations from across the country. Many of these authors have been recognized previously at the national level for their involvement in the field of patient navigation. We believe the true heart of this book is the genuine passion and commitment each author has for supporting patients with cancer and their caregivers as they traverse the daunting maze of cancer care. As you read each of their contributions, we are confident their dedication to advancing patient navigation is evident in their work.

Two popular sayings come to mind as we reflect upon our journey with this book. The first is the proverb "It takes a village to raise a child." We feel our chapter authors and our fellow navigators across the country indeed comprise "the village" committed to furthering the development of patient navigation. The second expression to mention is Margaret Mead's quote "Never doubt that a small group of thoughtful, committed people can change the world. Indeed, it is the only thing that ever has." It is our belief that oncology nurse navigators epitomize a group of thoughtful, committed people who strive to promote patient-centered, holistic cancer care.

We would like to thank all of those who have contributed to the body of knowledge that is oncology patient navigation, in particular, Dr. Harold P. Freeman for his vision and his desire to eliminate barriers to timely cancer screening, diagnosis, treatment, and supportive care. In addition, we would like to thank ONS's publishing staff for their guidance and encouragement with this project; our respective institutions for their support during the process of publishing this book and for their commitment to patient navigation and quality cancer care; and our families who have lived this book alongside of us, encouraging, reading, and believing in us.

Karyl, Penny, and Kathleen

CHAPTER 1

Overview of Nurse Navigation

Cynthia A. Cantril, RN, OCN®, MPH

Introduction

A new nursing role is only developed when there is a real or perceived need by society, the nursing profession, or the larger healthcare system. (Patten & Goudreau, 2012, p. 194)

The National Cancer Act signed by President Nixon in 1971 is considered the United States' "declaration of war on cancer." This legislation led to increased federal spending in all areas of cancer research. Over the following years, expanded knowledge increased the understanding of cancer and subsequently produced important advances in the detection, diagnosis, and treatment of cancer. Complexities of combined therapy including surgical, radiation, and medical oncology modalities have created the necessity for a comprehensive and multidisciplinary team approach to patient care. As such, a "frontline" movement emerged, transforming the care of patients with cancer.

In 1975, the Oncology Nursing Society was founded and began to define the cancer nursing specialty. Since then, specialized roles have developed to ensure that people affected by cancer will have guidance through all phases of the cancer care trajectory. Nurse navigation is a relatively new role contributing to an exciting and challenging frontier in cancer care. This chapter will review the influences on the evolution of navigation, the political and societal factors significant to the need for and development of patient navigation, and the importance of processes and role delineation of oncology nurse navigation. In addition, the overview will include comprehensive definitions of key terms within nurse navigation, and the specific nursing roles that influence and support this position, as well as the current state of the knowledge about nurse navigation programs within healthcare institutions.

Historical, Cultural, Socioeconomic, and Political Influences in Cancer Care

Cultural, socioeconomic, and legislative influences occurring during the late 1800s and throughout the 20th and 21st centuries have contributed to the introduction, evolution, and dissemination of patient navigation today. The context of the "sick poor" is hardly new but continues to underlie the concept of patient navigation. Nurse Lillian Wald, recognized as the "inventor" of public health nursing, proposed the public health nurse as "a new role for nurses who visited homes of the sick poor" (Buhler-Wilkerson, 1993, p. 1778). Wald's concept emerged from her notion that "all the responsibility of the sick poor has not been assured unless a share is taken in the problem of efficient treatment in their homes" (Wald, 1900, p. 39). She influenced the tradition of holistic nursing—care of the whole person. Wald proposed that the primary goal of public health nurses was to encourage client self-help by promoting the patient's ability to make sound health-related choices. Early public health nurses practiced autonomously to provide direct care as needed and to simultaneously organize and mobilize family and community resources (Buhler-Wilkerson, 1993).

The American Society for the Control of Cancer (ASCC), the forerunner of the American Cancer Society (ACS), was founded in 1913, advocating for patient services, research, care, and understanding of cancer among the general public and healthcare professionals. In response to public pressure and a concerted campaign by ASCC, Congress made the conquest of cancer a national goal in a unanimous vote to pass the National Cancer Act of 1937. This legislation established the National Cancer Institute and authorized annual funding for cancer research and provisions for review of all cancer research.

In 1962, President John F. Kennedy delivered a message to Congress, identifying consumers as the largest group in the U.S. economy. Consumers affect and are affected by every public and private economic decision. He outlined the following consumer rights (Kennedy, 1962).

1. The right to safety
2. The right to be informed
3. The right to choose
4. The right to be heard

The significance of this history is its application to the growing need for patients, as consumers, to realize these rights in an extremely complex and often fragmented healthcare delivery system. Healthcare systems must be able to provide these rights for patients and families.

As the consumer movement continued to grow, the concept of patient rights, with patients as consumers, was introduced. Annas and Healey (1974) defined four general patient rights applicable in a healthcare facility, which were the rights to (a) receive the whole truth, (b) maintain privacy and personal dignity, (c) retain self-determination by participation in decision making regarding one's health care, and (d) have complete access to medical records both during and after the hospitalization. In this context today, patient navigators are often the voice for patients and families traversing the healthcare system and advocating for these rights.

In 1989, ACS held seven hearings across the nation to solicit testimonies from individuals to facilitate understanding of the challenges that poor people with cancer faced and to make recommendations for change. The published report of these hearings identified the following overall findings (ACS, 1989).

- Poor people face substantial barriers in obtaining cancer care and often do not seek care if they cannot pay for it.
- Poor people and their families often make extreme personal sacrifices to obtain and pay for care.
- Fatalism about cancer is prevalent among the poor and may prevent them from seeking care.
- Cancer education programs are often insensitive and irrelevant.
- Poor people endure greater pain and suffering than other Americans.

Harold P. Freeman, MD, widely acknowledged as the founder of patient navigation, used these findings as a catalyst for the first navigation program implemented in 1990 at Harlem Hospital Center in New York City. His goal was to improve outcomes in vulnerable populations by eliminating barriers to timely diagnosis and treatment of cancer and other chronic illnesses. The primary aim of the Harlem navigation program was to decrease the high mortality rate in a population of poverty-stricken African American women, half of whom had presented with stage III and IV breast cancer (Freeman, Muth, & Kerner, 1995). Figure 1-1 outlines the general principles of navigation as established by Freeman (2013).

In his report to the president as chair of the 2001 President's Cancer Panel, Freeman identified several prevalent inequalities in access to health care: lack of health insurance, affecting 44 million people who were unable to pay out-of-pocket costs of cancer care, particularly oral medication costs; public and private health plan restrictions; physical distance from sources of care; and lack of transportation (Freeman & Reuben, 2001). Few people with cancer received full, accurate, and understandable information about their disease, either from healthcare providers or from other sources, primarily because of insufficient provider communication or knowledge and language, literacy, and cultural barriers. Moreover, bias based on cultural and racial differences far too often contributed to some providers offering less than optimal care and caused some patients to avoid accessing care because of fear or mistrust (Freeman & Reuben, 2001).

In 2005, President George W. Bush signed into law the Patient Navigator Outreach and Chronic Disease Prevention Act targeting poor and under-

---

Figure 1-1. Principles of Patient Navigation

- Patient navigation is a patient-centered healthcare service delivery model.
- The core function of patient navigation is the elimination of barriers to timely care across all segments of the healthcare continuum.
- Patient navigation may serve to virtually integrate a fragmented healthcare system for the individual patients.
- Patient navigation should be defined with a clear scope of practice that distinguishes the role and responsibilities of the navigator from that of other providers.
- Delivery of patient navigation services should be cost-effective and commensurate with the training and skills necessary to navigate an individual through a particular phase of the cancer care continuum.
- The determination of who should navigate should be determined by the level of skills required at a given phase of navigation.
- In a given system of care, there is a need to define the point at which navigation begins and the point at which it ends.
- Patient navigation can serve as a process that connects disconnected healthcare systems, such as primary and tertiary care.
- Patient navigation systems require coordination. In larger systems of patient care, this coordination is best carried out by assigning a navigation coordinator who is responsible for overseeing all phases of navigation with a given healthcare site or system.

Note. From "The History, Principles, and Future of Patient Navigation: Commentary," by H.P. Freeman, 2013, *Seminars in Oncology Nursing, 29,* p. 74. doi:10.1016/j.soncn.2013.02.002. Copyright 2013 by Elsevier. Adapted with permission.

---

served populations in need of timely access to care. This legislation authorized $25 million in grants to establish patient navigator programs in low-income and rural communities nationwide to help patients evaluate treatment options, enroll in clinical trials, obtain referrals, and apply for financial assistance.

In March 2010, President Obama signed the Patient Protection and Affordable Care Act (ACA) mandating patient navigation processes and functions as a component of health care. A brief description of the goals of patient navigation in this act included (Central Area Health Education Center, n.d.)

- A focus on overcoming individual patient–level barriers to accessing care
- Aims to reducing delays in accessing care
- Provision of navigation to individuals for a defined episode of cancer-related care
- Targeting of a defined set of health services
- A defined endpoint when services are complete.

Some challenges of implementing the ACA are clear, while others are less clear and are likely to emerge over time. The ACA fails to define navigation, leaving definition, role delineation, competencies, and reimbursement questions unaddressed. For example, most nurse navigation services are not yet recognized as billable. Furthermore, the ACA has guidelines for *BRCA* testing, yet no provision exists for financial support or reimbursement for genetic counseling. Navigators will no doubt have much to learn as the ACA continues to be implemented fully.

Interestingly, the political influences of nurse navigation can be traced back as far as 100 years ago. These notable actions and achievements have laid the foundation for the major emphasis and transformation of cancer care that has occurred over the past 20 years. Table 1-1 outlines significant milestones and initiatives that have influenced and brought navigation to its prominence in healthcare redesign.

Table 1-1. Milestones in the Emergence and Evolution of Patient Navigation

Year	Milestone
1971	President Richard Nixon signs National Cancer Act and declares "War on Cancer"
1983	The Health Care Financing Administration (HCFA, now the Centers for Medicare and Medicaid Services) implements Diagnosis Related Groups (DRGs) for the Inpatient Prospective Payment System (IPPS)
1986	Special Report on Cancer in the Economically Disadvantaged. American Cancer Society
1989	Cancer in the Poor: A Report to the Nation. American Cancer Society
1990	First navigation program launched at Harlem Hospital, New York City
1999	The Unequal Burden of Cancer. Institute of Medicine
2000	The National Cancer Program: Assessing the Past, Charting the Future (articulates the "discovery to delivery" disconnect). President's Cancer Panel Report of the Chairman, Harold P. Freeman
2001	Voices of a Broken System: Real People, Real Problems. President's Cancer Panel Report of the Chairman, Harold P. Freeman
2002	National Cancer Institute (NCI) Center to Reduce Cancer Health Disparities implements pilot project to establish Patient Navigation Research Program
2003	Unequal Treatment: Confronting Racial and Ethnic Disparities in Healthcare. Institute of Medicine
2005	Patient Navigator Outreach and Chronic Disease Act of 2005 signed into law by President George W. Bush authorizes appropriations through FY2010 to establish a competitive grant program designed to help patients access healthcare services C-Change defines Patient Navigation Program

(Continued on next page)

Table 1-1. Milestones in the Emergence and Evolution of Patient Navigation *(Continued)*	
Year	Milestone
2007	NCI Community Cancer Centers Program (NCCCP) established
2008	National Coalition of Oncology Nurse Navigators (NCONN) incorporated
	Harold P. Freeman Patient Navigation Institute launched; first Navigation Training Course
2009	Academy of Oncology Nurse Navigators (AONN) incorporated
	Association of Community Cancer Centers (ACCC) Cancer Program Guidelines, Chapter 4, Section 10, Guideline I: Patient Navigation Services
	Association of Community Cancer Centers Patient Navigation: A Call to Action
	NCONN issues Core Competencies of Oncology Nurse Navigators
2010	Oncology Nursing Society (ONS)/Association of Oncology Social Work/National Association of Social Workers Joint Position on the Role of Oncology Nursing and Oncology Social Work in Patient Navigation
	ONS Role Delineation Study begins
	Affordable Care Act (ACA) includes Patient Navigation
2011	Future of Nursing: Leading Change, Advancing Health. Institute of Medicine
2012	American College of Surgeons Commission on Cancer issues Accreditation Standard 3.1, stipulating phase-in of patient navigation process by 2015
	ONS publishes: Oncology Nurse Navigator Role Delineation Study

Note. From "Patient Navigation in the Oncology Care Setting," by C. Cantril and P.J. Haylock, 2013, *Seminars in Oncology Nursing, 29,* p. 79. doi:10.1016/j.soncn.2013.02.003. Copyright 2013 by Elsevier. Reprinted with permission.

Nursing Roles Influencing Navigation

Nurse navigation, although a relatively new concept and nursing role, has deep roots in nursing history. In 1965, Peplau described the role of the clinical nurse specialist (CNS), which originated in the 1940s and was further developed by nurse educators in efforts to decrease the fragmentation of patient care apparent after World War II (Peplau, 2003). Little (1967) defined the role of a nurse specialist as one who assumes full responsibility for the quality of nursing care provided to a patient. The specialist prescribes, organizes, and guides others in the care of a particular type of patient. Furthermore, the specialist adds unique competencies to others on the health-care team.

Theresa Christy, a preeminent nursing leader and historian, acknowl-edged the importance of the advocacy component of nursing in the early 1970s (Christy, 1973). She proposed that nurses should be a voice for indi-viduals and families traversing the complicated and confusing aspects of the American healthcare system.

Montemuro (1987) wrote that it was not until 1982 that consensus re-garding the functions of the CNS role was reached. At that point, agreement existed within the nursing community whereby the CNS was viewed as an ex-pert practitioner, educator, consultant, researcher, and change agent.

Similar to public health nursing, the case management nursing role has influenced nurse navigation. Kersbergen (1996) looked at the history of case managers coordinating care to control costs, noting that case manage-ment has been used to coordinate care for more than a century. Regardless of the setting or sophistication of the model, the overall goal of case man-agement is to coordinate complex and fragmented care to meet the needs of the patient.

The *crafting* of nurse navigation may be seen as building upon the funda-mental values, roles, and skills of nurses over the past century to address and meet the new challenges in cancer care nursing.

Nurses Supporting Patient-Centered Care

The concept of patient-centered care has been discussed in nursing since the beginning of the profession. Mitchell (2008) described the approach as characterized with meaningful interpersonal relationships between patients and providers. The patient is the center of care delivery and consequently is engaged in decision making and care planning.

In the late 1970s, a paradigm shift in health care emerged with the con-cept of patients as consumers and active participants in healthcare deci-sions. In 1978, the Planetree model of care was created and dedicated to restoring a holistic, patient-centered focus to healthcare delivery. The model includes personalized care for patients and supports individual pa-tient autonomy by allowing full participation in illness management and treatment decisions. Planetree was the first healthcare model in the coun-try to foster the support of full access to medical information, patient deci-sion making, and a comprehensive healing and holistic care environment organized first and foremost around the needs of patients (Planetree, n.d.).

Traditional and contemporary nursing requires nurses to apply critical-thinking skills and appropriate assessment and interventions while respond-ing to and advocating for patients in the dynamic healthcare environment.

Reverby (1993) observed, "Nurses, whether operating as lone public health professionals . . . or presenting position statements from large professional organizations, have offered this country vision after vision, demonstration after demonstration, of what decent, affordable, and appropriate health care could be" (p. 1663).

Definitions of Nurse Navigation

Definition of terms is essential to advancing the concept of nurse navigation. Yet, no universally accepted definition of navigator nor consensus on necessary preparation and competencies for fulfillment of the role exists. Based on the available literature, Cantril and Haylock (2013) described nurse navigation as "a function and process that shares characteristics with other clinical patient services and assistance including health education, case management, clinical nurse specialists, social workers, community health workers, patient advocates, and lay health advisors" (p. 78).

The Academy of Oncology Nurse and Patient Navigators, a nurse navigator specialty organization, defines a navigator as "a medical professional whose clinical expertise and training guides patients and their caregivers to make informed decisions, collaborating with a multidisciplinary team to allow for timely cancer screening, diagnosis, treatment, and increased supportive care across the cancer continuum" (Academy of Oncology Nurse and Patient Navigators, n.d., "Navigation" section, para. 2).

In 2010, the Oncology Nursing Society, the Association of Oncology Social Workers, and the National Association of Social Workers developed a joint position on navigation. The position adapted a definition of navigation from C-Change: "individualized assistance offered to patients, families, and caregivers to help overcome healthcare system barriers and facilitate timely access to quality health and psychosocial care . . . from prediagnosis through all phases of the cancer experience" (C-Change, n.d., "What Is Cancer Patient Navigation?" section, para. 1). The position does not differentiate nursing from social worker navigation roles but suggests that navigators' knowledge and skills extend beyond basic professional education and oncology experience to include community assessment and interventions that promote timely access to needed care and services. Navigators must possess skills to effectively collaborate with multiple providers and disciplines, excel at meeting and exceeding patient expectations, and have comprehensive knowledge of all cancer treatment modalities, side effects, and evidence-based interventions. The collaborative position stipulates that navigation processes should reflect strengths and desired outcomes related to the communities, systems, and facilities in which navigation programs reside. Figure 1-2 details the specific elements of the joint position statement.

Figure 1-2. Oncology Nursing Society, Association of Oncology Social Work, and National Association of Social Workers Joint Position on the Role of Oncology Nursing and Oncology Social Work in Patient Navigation

It is the position of the Oncology Nursing Society, Association of Oncology Social Work, and National Association of Social Workers that
• Patient navigation processes, whether provided on-site or in coordination with local agencies or facilities, are essential components of cancer care services.
• Patient outcomes are optimal when a social worker, nurse, and lay navigator (defined as a trained nonprofessional or volunteer) function as a multidisciplinary team.
• Patient navigation programs in cancer care must address underserved populations in the community.
• Patient navigation programs must lay the groundwork for their sustainability.
• Nurses and social workers in oncology who function in patient navigator roles do so based on the scope of practice for each discipline. Educational preparation and professional certification play roles in regulating the practice of both disciplines. Nationally recognized standards of practice specific to the discipline and specialty also define safe and effective practice.
• Nurses and social workers in oncology who perform navigator services should have education and knowledge in community assessment, cancer program assessment, resolution of system barriers, the cancer continuum, cancer health disparities, cultural competence, and the individualized provision of assistance to patients with cancer, their families, caregivers, and survivors at risk.
• Additional research to explore, confirm, and advance patient navigation processes, roles, and identification of appropriate evidence-based outcomes measures must be supported.
• Ongoing collaboration to identify and/or derive metrics that can be used to clarify the role, function, and desired outcomes of navigators must be supported and promoted.
• Navigation services can be delegated to trained nonprofessionals and/or volunteers and should be supervised by nurses or social workers.

Note. From "Oncology Nursing Society, the Association of Oncology Social Work, and the National Association of Social Workers Joint Position on the Role of Oncology Nursing and Oncology Social Work in Patient Navigation," by Oncology Nursing Society, Association of Oncology Social Work, and National Association of Social Workers, 2010, *Oncology Nursing Forum, 37,* pp. 251–252. Copyright 2010 by the Oncology Nursing Society. Reprinted with permission.

The common theme inherent to every description and definition of navigation is succinctly: advocating for and providing guidance and support for patients and families with cancer while they traverse the very complex cancer care environment.

State of the Knowledge Today

Despite the emerging literature regarding nurse navigation in oncology, no consensus exists concerning the scope of practice, qualifications, and competencies for navigators (McMullen, 2013). Although many training and certificate of completion programs are available for navigation, wide varia-tion exists in the entry-level educational preparation for these programs. Navigator education and preparation are further discussed in Chapter 2.

The National Coalition of Oncology Nurse Navigators in 2009 was the first organization to articulate core competencies for navigation, which are included in Chapter 2. In 2010, the Oncology Nursing Society initiated a role delineation study to identify and prioritize critical tasks, as well as essen-tial competencies of oncology nurse navigators, with findings published in 2012 (Brown et al., 2012). Data analysis clearly defined tasks and skills spe-cific to oncology nurse navigator roles (see Figure 1-3) but did not delineate the portion that are also basic oncology nursing tasks and skills or those that fall within advanced practice nursing competencies.

The Patient Navigation Research Program (PNRP) sponsored by the Na-tional Cancer Institute's Center to Reduce Cancer Health Disparities in 2005 was the first multicenter program to examine the role and benefits of patient navigation. The PNRP developed a definition of navigation and met-rics by which to assess the process and outcomes of navigation. The work-ing definition of patient navigation was support and guidance offered to vulnerable populations. Freund et al. (2008) reviewed the metrics, results, and outcomes of the project. The primary outcomes studied included time to diagnostic resolution, time to initiation of treatment, patient satisfaction with care, and cost-effectiveness for specific cancer types including breast, cervical, colorectal, and prostate cancers. Other navigation program out-come studies have been conducted with findings published in the literature. Further details on specific program metrics and outcomes are discussed in Chapter 9.

Importance of the Oncology Nurse Navigator

In 2011, the American College of Surgeons (ACoS) Commission on Can-cer (CoC) revised its accreditation standards for cancer programs and facil-ities, adding a navigation process requirement to be phased in by 2015 to address healthcare disparities and access to care (ACoS CoC, 2012). Addi-tionally, other associations and program accreditations have also designated patient navigation as a priority, such as the Association of Community Can-cer Centers and the National Accreditation Program for Breast Centers.

With regard to the new CoC program standards, community cancer cen-ters are required to assess health disparities, identify needs of patient pop-ulations, describe a patient navigation process to address those needs, and document outcomes. This standard has broad implications for cancer care in the United States, as approximately 70% of the 1.5 million newly diag-nosed patients each year are treated at CoC-accredited facilities (ACoS CoC, 2012). This standard compels CoC-accredited institutions to articulate and

---

Figure 1-3. The Top Tasks, Knowledge Areas, and Skills as Rated by Respondents to the Oncology Nursing Society's Oncology Nurse Navigator Role Delineation Study

Tasks
- Provide emotional and educational support for patients.
- Practice according to professional and legal standards.
- Advocate on behalf of the patient.
- Demonstrate ethical principles in practice.
- Orient patients to the cancer care system.
- Receive and respond to new patient referrals.
- Pursue continuing education opportunities related to oncology and navigation.
- Collaborate with physicians and other healthcare providers.
- Empower patients to self-advocate.
- Assist patients to make informed decisions.
- Provide education or referrals for coping with the diagnosis.
- Identify patients with a new diagnosis of cancer.

Knowledge Areas
- Confidentiality and informed consent
- Advocacy
- Symptom management
- Ethical principles
- Quality of life
- Goal of treatment
- Therapeutic options
- Evidence-based practice guidelines
- Professional scope of practice
- Legal and professional guidelines

Skills
- Communication
- Problem solving
- Critical thinking
- Multitasking
- Collaboration
- Time management
- Advocacy

Note. From "Oncology Nurse Navigator Role Delineation Study: An Oncology Nursing Society Report," by C.G. Brown, C. Cantril, L. McMullen, D.L. Barkley, M. Dietz, C.M. Murphy, and L.J. Fabrey, 2012, *Clinical Journal of Oncology Nursing, 16*, p. 584. doi:10.1188/12.CJON.581-585. Copyright 2012 by the Oncology Nursing Society. Reprinted with permission.

---

substantiate navigation, thereby emphasizing patient navigation programs as a key component of patient-centered care.

The evolution and emergence of navigation processes and the nurse navigator role reflect departures from the status quo of the American healthcare system and traditional nursing role boundaries. The oncology nurse navigator is one of the few roles in nursing in which an individual professional nurse is accountable for and invested in providing patient-centered care throughout an entire disease trajectory (McMullen, 2013). Patient navigation and nurse navigators are viewed by some as a "Band-Aid" for enormous failures in health systems, communications, and lapses in professional nursing leadership. Others envision navigation and navigators as potential solutions to the ever-expanding quagmire of disparate outcomes, fragmentation, and complexities associated with the delivery of cancer care in modern societies. It is apparent that navigation and navigators will be an ongoing presence in cancer care and even more broadly in the provision of care for people with other chronic conditions.

Conclusion

Throughout the United States and globally, nurse navigators facilitate care in all phases of the cancer prevention, detection, diagnosis, treatment, and transitional care continuum. Cancer care in the 21st century presents all professionals caring for patients with cancer and their families with new challenges and new rewards. Nurse navigators empower patients in decision making, advocate for and uphold the physical and psychosocial dimensions of care, and ensure that navigation services are accessible to all those affected by cancer.

References

Academy of Oncology Nurse and Patient Navigators. (n.d.). Helpful definitions. Navigation. Retrieved from http://www.aonnonline.org/about/definitions

American Cancer Society. (1989). *Cancer in the poor: A report to the nation.* Atlanta, GA: Author.

American College of Surgeons Commission on Cancer. (2012). *Cancer program standards 2012: Ensuring patient-centered care* [v.1.2.1, released January 2014]. Retrieved from http://www.facs.org/cancer/coc/programstandards2012.pdf

Annas, G.J., & Healey, J. (1974). The patient rights advocate. *Journal of Nursing Administration, 4*(3), 25–31.

Brown, C.G., Cantril, C., McMullen, L., Barkley, D.L., Dietz, M., Murphy, C.M., & Fabrey, L.J. (2012). Oncology Nurse Navigator Role Delineation Study: An Oncology Nursing Society report. *Clinical Journal of Oncology Nursing, 16,* 581–585. doi:10.1188/12.CJON.581-585

Buhler-Wilkerson, K. (1993). Bringing care to the people: Lillian Wald's legacy to public health nursing. *American Journal of Public Health, 83,* 1778–1786. Retrieved from http://www.ncbi.nlm.nih.gov/pmc/articles/PMC1694935/pdf/amjph00536-0124.pdf

Cantril, C., & Haylock, P.J. (2013). Patient navigation in the oncology care setting. *Seminars in Oncology Nursing, 29,* 72–90. doi:10.1016/j.soncn.2013.02.003

C-Change. (n.d.). Cancer patient navigation: Care for your community. Cancer patient navigation overview. Retrieved from http://www.cancerpatientnavigation.org

Central Area Health Education Center. (n.d.). The Affordable Care Act and patient navigation: Executive summary. Retrieved from http://www.centralctahec.org/downloads/Patient-Navigation-Exec-Summary.pdf

Christy, T.E. (1973). New privileges, new challenges, new responsibilities. *Nursing, 3*(11), 8–13.

Freeman, H.P. (2013). The history, principles, and future of patient navigation: Commentary. *Seminars in Oncology Nursing, 29,* 72–75. doi:10.1016/j.soncn.2013.02.002

Freeman, H.P., Muth, B.J., & Kerner, J.F. (1995). Expanding access to cancer screening and clinical follow-up among the medically underserved. *Cancer Practice, 3,* 19–30.

Freeman, H.P., & Reuben, S.H. (2001). *Voices of a broken system: Real people, real problems. President's Cancer Panel report of the chairman.* Bethesda, MD: National Institutes of Health, National Cancer Institute.

Freund, K.M., Battaglia, T.A., Calhoun, E., Dudley, D.J., Fiscella, K., Paskett, E., ... Roetzheim, R.G. (2008). National Cancer Institute Patient Navigation Research Program: Methods, protocol, and measures. *Cancer, 113,* 3391–3399. doi:10.1002/cncr.23960

Kennedy, J.F. (1962, March 15). Special message to the Congress on protecting the consumer interest. Retrieved from http://www.presidency.ucsb.edu/ws/?pid=9108

Kersbergen, A.L. (1996). Case management: A rich history of coordinating care to control costs. *Nursing Outlook, 44,* 169–172.

Little, D. (1967). The nurse specialist. *American Journal of Nursing, 67,* 552–556.

McMullen, L. (2013). Oncology nurse navigators and the continuum of cancer care. *Seminars in Oncology Nursing, 29,* 105–117. doi:10.1016/j.soncn.2013.02.005

Mitchell, P.H. (2008). Patient-centered care—A new focus on a time-honored concept. *Nursing Outlook, 56,* 197–198. doi:10.1016/j.outlook.2008.08.001

Montemuro, M.A. (1987). The evolution of the clinical nurse specialist: Response to the challenge of professional nursing practice. *Clinical Nurse Specialist, 1,* 106–110.

Oncology Nursing Society, Association of Oncology Social Work, & National Association of Social Workers. (2010). Oncology Nursing Society, the Association of Oncology Social Work, and the National Association of Social Workers joint position on the role of oncology nursing and oncology social work in patient navigation. *Oncology Nursing Forum, 37,* 251–252. Retrieved from http://ons.metapress.com/content/f2830241m137mg1m/fulltext.pdf

Patten, S., & Goudreau, K.A. (2012). The bright future for clinical nurse specialist practice. *Nursing Clinics of North America, 47,* 193–203, v. doi:10.1016/j.cnur.2012.02.009

Peplau, H. (2003). Specialization in professional nursing (1965). *Clinical Nurse Specialist, 17,* 3–9.

Planetree. (n.d.). About us. Retrieved from http://planetree.org/?page_id=510

Reverby, S.M. (1993). From Lillian Wald to Hillary Rodham Clinton: What will happen to public health nursing? *American Journal of Public Health, 83,* 1662–1663. Retrieved from http://www.ncbi.nlm.nih.gov/pmc/articles/PMC1694915/pdf/amjph00536-0008.pdf

Wald, L. (1900). Nurses' settlement. *American Journal of Nursing, 1,* 39. Retrieved from http://journals.lww.com/ajnonline/Citation/1900/10000/Nurses__Settlement.9.aspx

CHAPTER 2

Getting Started as a Nurse Navigator

Karyl D. Blaseg, RN, MSN, OCN®

Introduction

The origin of patient navigation is often credited to Harold P. Freeman, MD, who created a lay navigation program in Harlem, New York City, targeted toward improving the timeliness of breast cancer diagnosis and treatment for African American women (Freeman, 2004). Since then, as healthcare organizations have continued to develop innovative strategies for various initiatives focused on decreasing healthcare disparities, eliminating barriers to care, and improving the overall patient experience, the number of patient navigation programs has steadily increased. In addition, the scope of navigation has evolved and can now span the entire cancer continuum. With this growth and evolution, it is not surprising that great variability exists regarding the roles and responsibilities of navigators, as well as the minimum qualifications and training needed for optimal success.

Definitions

Although numerous definitions of patient navigation are found throughout the literature, most of these focus on interventions targeted toward reducing barriers to timely care. In general, navigators coordinate the overall care for patients with cancer and have often been referred to as the "glue that holds it all together" or the safety net that prevents patients from "falling through the cracks" (Gilbert et al., 2011, p. 233).

A qualitative synthesis of the patient navigation literature identified common elements of patient navigation definitions to include *individualized assistance*, with efforts targeted toward a *specific set of health services* and focused on *eliminating barriers to timely access to care*, provided for a *defined episode of care*, with a *specific endpoint* (Wells et al., 2008). Similarly, a joint position statement issued by the Oncology Nursing Society (ONS), the Association of Oncology Social Work (AOSW), and the National Association of Social Workers (NASW) defined patient navigation as "individualized assistance offered to patients, families, and caregivers to help overcome healthcare system barriers and facilitate timely access to quality health and psychosocial care from prediagnosis through all phases of the cancer experience" (ONS, AOSW, & NASW, 2010, p. 251).

Roles and Responsibilities

Navigation programs vary widely in focus and scope of services because of the unique needs of the population served and the particular objectives of the funding source or organization. However, despite this variability, fundamental navigation roles and responsibilities do exist. The literature is replete with content regarding the roles and responsibilities of navigators. Although these two terms can technically be differentiated into discrete concepts (that is, *role* referring to a customary function and *responsibility* relating to specific tasks one is accountable for), for the purposes of this chapter, the terms will be used interchangeably.

Identify and Resolve Barriers

Navigators reduce healthcare disparities through the identification and resolution of patient-level barriers and unmet needs (Freeman & Rodriguez, 2011; Stanley et al., 2013; Wells et al., 2008). Typical patient-oriented barriers relate to difficulty navigating healthcare bureaucracy; fear or mistrust; lack of resources (e.g., financial, insurance, transportation, lodging, child care); and communication, language, or cultural obstacles (Fiscella et al., 2011; Stanley et al., 2013; Vargas, Ryan, Jackson, Rodriguez, & Freeman, 2008; Wells et al., 2008). In addition, barriers within the healthcare system itself exist, including scheduling challenges, acceptance of uninsured patients, and quality-of-care concerns (Vargas et al., 2008). Wells et al. (2008) identified an important distinction with regard to resolution of barriers, stating that navigators tend to focus on eliminating barriers that affect individual access to care, whereas other healthcare personnel (such as patient advocates) may focus on resolution of more systemic issues.

Nurse navigators conduct comprehensive patient assessments to elicit information regarding physical, social, emotional, cultural, and spiritual needs; then, based on the individual needs and specific barriers identified, they collaborate with other healthcare professionals to develop a plan to address these (Freund et al., 2008; McDonald, 2011; Steinberg et al., 2006; Thygesen, Pedersen, Kragstrup, Wagner, & Mogensen, 2011). It is imperative for nurse navigators to establish a therapeutic relationship to ensure that even the most private of patients feel comfortable disclosing specific needs and concerns related to cancer care. Subsequent navigation interventions may include arranging for interpreter assistance or logistical support (such as transportation, lodging, or child care), providing referrals to financial assistance programs, advocating for appointments with oncology specialists, and connecting patients with available community support resources (Freund et al., 2008; McDonald, 2011; Nguyen & Kagawa-Singer, 2008; Stanley et al., 2013; Steinberg et al., 2006).

Coordinate Timely Access to Care and Seamless Transitions

Navigators coordinate timely access to care and ensure seamless transitions through an often-fragmented healthcare system (Freeman & Rodriguez, 2011; Stanley et al., 2013; Wells et al., 2008). Scheduling appointments with primary care, surgery, and oncology specialists, as well as connecting patients to social support services, is a large component of navigators' roles (Steinberg et al., 2006; Thygesen et al., 2011). In addition, nurse navigators must be knowledgeable of the typical pathways and protocols specific to their defined scope (whether this is the diagnostic, treatment, survivorship, or palliative care portions of the cancer continuum) to be able to appropriately respond when challenges arise requiring advocacy on behalf of patients. Familiarity not only with the healthcare systems but also with typical clinical challenges that individuals struggle with will enable nurse navigators to anticipate potential gaps or care issues and promptly intervene to ensure optimal patient experiences.

Facilitate Communication and Collaboration

Navigators facilitate communication between patients and healthcare providers (Horner et al., 2013; Stanley et al., 2013; Steinberg et al., 2006; Wells et al., 2008). Patients have reported difficulty in understanding the medical jargon that providers frequently use and have expressed a desire for navigators to be present during physician visits to translate information into simpler terms, thereby enhancing patient comprehension (Korber, Padula, Gray, & Powell, 2011).

Although patient education can be standardized according to cancer type and treatment options, a key function of navigators is the provision of tailored, culturally appropriate education and support (McDonald, 2011;

Stanley et al., 2013). Navigators orient individuals to the healthcare system and provide a wealth of information to both patients and families regarding available options (Fillion et al., 2012; Schwaderer & Itano, 2007; Wilcox & Bruce, 2010). Because patients commonly are overwhelmed with the cancer experience, nurse navigators reiterate, elucidate, and substantiate information previously presented by the multidisciplinary team (Korber et al., 2011) and provide anticipatory guidance throughout the cancer continuum (Francz & Simpson, 2013; Schwaderer & Itano, 2007). For example, when working with a 45-year-old patient undergoing multimodality treatment for breast cancer, a nurse navigator may provide a patient guidebook, links to online resources, and cancer-specific patient education materials, as well as attend all physician consultations during the treatment planning phase to help reinforce information and provide emotional support. The navigator may coach the patient on potential questions to ask the providers and suggest the use of a journal for note-taking during appointments so that the information is available for future reference. In addition, this patient may require referrals for rehabilitation or financial, psychosocial, or genetic counseling, as well as frequent telephone calls from the navigator for support during treatment. Although this approach may work well with this particular situation, nurse navigators must recognize that each patient is unique not only with regard to individual needs but also with the degree of support desired.

The importance of teamwork is well established in oncology and is especially true with nurse navigators, who often are viewed as the key to facilitating communication and collaboration among the multidisciplinary healthcare team. This starts with the development of collegial and trusting relationships among the various oncology team members (e.g., providers, nurses, ancillary personnel, clerical staff) based on shared goals of providing high-quality cancer care and exceptional patient experiences through coordination of care (Gilbert et al., 2011; Steinberg et al., 2006). Interacting with various members of the healthcare team to ensure the timely and appropriate scheduling and provision of healthcare services (Korber et al., 2011; Seek & Hogle, 2007) and referring cases for presentation at multidisciplinary conferences (McDonald, 2011) are two strategies used by navigators to facilitate multidisciplinary teamwork.

Provide Emotional Support

A cancer diagnosis frequently invokes fear, anxiety, and other emotional distress for both patients and families. Navigators provide basic emotional support ranging from mere presence and active listening to formal referrals for individual counseling services (Freund et al., 2008; Horner et al., 2013; Korber et al., 2011; McDonald, 2011; Steinberg et al., 2006; Thygesen et al., 2011). Specifically, nurse navigators assist patients in identifying issues they are struggling with, offer reassurances regarding coping abilities as appropriate, explore potential avenues for resolution, and encourage patient-centered decision making (Fillion et al., 2009; Schwaderer & Itano, 2007; Thygesen et al., 2011).

Nurse navigators must establish healthy boundaries when providing emotional support to patients and families. This begins with setting limits and clearly defining role expectations early in the navigator-patient relationship. The patient-navigator connection should be based on facilitating self-advocacy, self-management, and patient empowerment rather than allowing an overly dependent and enabling relationship to develop (Fillion et al., 2012; Thygesen et al., 2011). Nurse navigators should encourage patients to remain as autonomous and independent as possible. As needs are identified, it is important for navigators to educate patients on how to access available resources but not to take on that responsibility for patients. For example, if a patient has financial needs, the navigator should inform and connect the patient to available resources but should not assume the task of completing applications for charity care and financial assistance for the patient. Overnavigation can create unnecessary patient dependence upon the navigator, which can lead to difficulties in terminating the relationship once treatment is finished.

Other situations that might cause professional boundary issues between navigators and patients include disclosing of the navigator's personal information, spending time together outside of work, providing special treatment or care, and giving or receiving gifts. When a boundary issue is identified, it is important for the navigator to honestly acknowledge the situation and immediately attempt to restore the therapeutic relationship.

Additional Key Responsibilities

The preceding roles and responsibilities are by no means intended to be all-encompassing. Rather, these are some of the customary functions and tasks that nurse navigators are frequently accountable for. A role delineation study conducted by Brown, Cantril, et al. (2012) identified direct care and collaboration with healthcare providers to coordinate care as the two largest aspects of nurse navigators' roles, comprising approximately 40% and 27%, respectively, of the navigators' time. Specific tasks identified in the study are depicted in Figure 1-3 in Chapter 1. Other duties identified in the delineation study included marketing and public relations (20%), community outreach and education (9%), and program development and administration (5%) (Brown, Cantril, et al., 2012). In this rapidly evolving field, one must acknowledge that roles and responsibilities are as unique as individual programs and will likely continue to evolve as programs strive to meet the distinct needs of the patients and communities served.

Desired Qualities

Cultural Competence

Cultural competence and sensitivity is an important quality for a navigator (Freeman, 2004; Petereit et al., 2008). Cultural competence in health care involves

> understanding the importance of social and cultural influences on patients' health beliefs and behaviors; considering how these factors interact at multiple levels of the healthcare delivery system (e.g., at the level of structural processes of care or clinical decision making); and, finally, devising interventions that take these issues into account to assure quality healthcare delivery to diverse patient populations. (Betancourt, Green, Carrillo, & Ananeh-Firempong, 2003, p. 297)

Considering that most navigation programs strive to reduce healthcare disparities, one can appreciate the importance for navigators to understand the diverse communities and populations served (Nguyen & Kagawa-Singer, 2008). This goes beyond mere language barriers and includes recognizing the unique needs and challenges faced, as well as establishing trust with the communities served to create effective health partnerships (Petereit et al., 2008). For optimal cultural competence and sensitivity, some literature sources have asserted that navigators should be members of the community or culture served (Freeman & Chu, 2005; Vargas et al., 2008).

Communication Skills

Superb and adaptable communication skills are essential for navigators when conversing with other healthcare professionals. Navigators often serve as a communication bridge among various members of the multidisciplinary team. Healthcare teams rely on nurse navigators to synthesize key information and share it with others in an efficient and effective manner. Thus, active listening, confidence, a willingness to clarify understanding, and the ability to articulate clearly are all crucial skills to possess. In addition, as patient advocates, navigators must feel comfortable speaking up and bringing forward concerns that others may not want to hear.

Communication skills are equally as important for navigators in working with patients and families. Not only must navigators display approachability, sincerity, and patience when communicating, as mentioned previously, but they also often serve as medical terminology and technology interpreters for patients. Nurse navigators must be able to condense and summarize complex medical information as delivered by physicians and present it in more simplistic layman's terms for optimal patient and family understanding (Horner et al., 2013; Vargas et al., 2008). In a study of 56 navigation programs funded by the Avon Foundation for Women, 90% of program directors identified communication as a vital skill. Other essential traits related to communication included interpersonal and listening skills (93%) and maintaining confidentiality (86%) (Stanley et al., 2013).

Familiarity With Disease Processes

Nurse navigators must be knowledgeable in aspects of the oncology continuum specific to their focus and scope of services. For some, this may be limited to the screening or diagnostic phases, whereas for others it may include a broader portion of the spectrum (e.g., from diagnosis through completion of treatment and/or survivorship). A sound oncology background proves invaluable to nurse navigators when working to coordinate the complexities of care associated with diagnostic and treatment modalities (Seek & Hogle, 2007).

Being well versed in specific oncology interventions (i.e., surgical oncology, medical oncology, and radiation oncology) enables navigators to provide more informative anticipatory guidance, as well as comprehensive education regarding treatment risks and early detection of toxicities (Wilcox & Bruce, 2010). Often patients turn first to navigators when questions, issues, or concerns arise; therefore, nurse navigators must possess keen assessment and triage skills related to toxicities and symptom management, along with a broad understanding of best supportive care practices (Horner et al., 2013). Brown, Cantril, et al. (2012) identified key knowledge areas as part of the nurse navigation role delineation study (see Figure 1-3 in Chapter 1).

Knowledge of Resources

In today's ever-changing healthcare environment, navigators must recognize that a working knowledge of case management principles may be useful, if not essential, in advocating for necessary care (Seek & Hogle, 2007). It is vital for navigators to be thoroughly familiar with the healthcare system or systems used by the community and populations served, as well as internal and external resources. To remove barriers to care, navigators must maintain a current working knowledge of eligibility criteria for community resources and then appropriately connect patients to these. External resources often have limited funding, so it is essential for navigators to maintain close relationships with community agencies and keep abreast of any changes in eligibility criteria or program closures. In addition, these community connections facilitate the navigator's awareness as new resources emerge. See Figure 2-1 for examples of resources as identified by Brown, Bornstein, and Wilcox (2012).

Figure 2-1. Examples of Commonly Used Internal and External Resources

Internal Resources
- Patient financial services
- Pharmacy
- Spiritual services
- Nutrition
- Community medical clinic
- Behavioral health

External Resources
- Primary care
  - Private offices and clinics
- Cancer care coalition support services (local)
  - American Cancer Society
  - Cancer Support Community
  - Leukemia and Lymphoma Society
  - TideWell Hospice
- General community resources
  - Senior
  - Mental health
  - Patient advocacy
  - Disability
  - Nutrition
  - Legal
- Prescription options
- Transportation services
- Financial services
  - Social Security
  - Department of children and families
  - Co-pay assistance programs
  - Financial assistance programs
- National resources
  - Cancer site-specific
  - Fertility
  - Patient advocacy
  - Cancer survivorship

Note. From "Partnership and Empowerment Program: A Model for Patient-Centered, Comprehensive, and Cost-Effective Care," by C. Brown, E. Bornstein, and C. Wilcox, 2012, *Clinical Journal of Oncology Nursing, 16,* p. 16. doi:10.1188/12.CJON.15-17. Copyright 2012 by the Oncology Nursing Society. Reprinted with permission.

Leadership Skills

Efficient organizational and time management skills are essential when coordinating the optimal patient experience through the complex healthcare system (Seek & Hogle, 2007). Navigators must be self-directed and able to work autonomously with minimal supervision in order to effectively advance program initiatives. This is especially true considering that navigation programs may consist of only one or two individuals who are responsible for program development and implementation. Navigators must demonstrate personal and professional accountability with a commitment to the profession and lifelong learning. The job of navigators is that of problem solver and change agent; thus, navigators must enjoy challenges, be able to think critically, and remain flexible to possibilities (Vargas et al., 2008). Skills of nurse navigators as defined in the role delineation study by Brown, Cantril, et al. (2012) are depicted in Figure 1-3 in Chapter 1.

Prerequisites

Education

Historically, navigator positions were assumed by lay community members who were often either cancer survivors or members of the communities served (Steinberg et al., 2006). Advantages to this model included lower program costs and increased cultural sensitivity and awareness of specific barriers experienced by the target population.

Over time, patient navigation models evolved, and positions are now held by a variety of healthcare professionals, including nurses, social workers, health educators, and advanced practice nurses (Gilbert et al., 2011; Wilcox & Bruce, 2010). Although these models obviously incur higher salary expenditures, the benefits of using healthcare professionals (specifically nurses) as navigators include the ability to provide in-depth education regarding disease processes, treatment modalities, and self-care strategies, as well as emotional support throughout the cancer journey. In addition, nurses are able to assess challenging clinical situations or conditions and subsequently implement nursing interventions to increase the overall quality of care and patient experience (Pedersen & Hack, 2011; Seek & Hogle, 2007).

The literature abounds with studies examining the positive impact that navigators have in various settings. While some studies have demonstrated benefits through the use of lay navigators in reducing healthcare disparities and achieving program goals (Burhansstipanov et al., 1998; Ell et al., 2002), others have chosen to use healthcare professionals for a more extensive navigation scope and have reported significant positive outcomes as well (Fillion et al., 2006; Seek & Hogle, 2007). Blended navigation programs also exist, which successfully combine the best aspects of the two models and use lay and professional navigators (Gabram et al., 2008; Hiatt et al., 2001; Petereit et al., 2008; Weinrich et al., 1998). In fact, in their joint position statement, ONS, AOSW, and NASW asserted that "patient outcomes are optimal when a social worker, nurse, and lay navigator (defined as a trained nonprofessional or volunteer) function as a multidisciplinary team" (ONS et al., 2010, p. 251).

Although no consensus has been reached as to the best educational preparation for navigators, one could assert that the nurse navigator role is optimally filled by a bachelor's-prepared RN. In one integrated review of 15 navigation research studies, 11 navigation roles were filled by bachelor's-prepared RNs (Case, 2011). Membership data from the National Coalition of Oncology Nurse Navigators (NCONN) indicate that 47% of more than 1,000 members hold a bachelor's degree (Francz & Simpson, 2013). Furthermore, a review of *The Essentials of Baccalaureate Education for Professional Nursing Practice* developed by the American Association of Colleges of Nursing (2008) revealed that most, if not all, of the nine essentials (outlined in Figure 2-2) have direct correlation to core patient navigation concepts.

Experience

No standard has been established regarding the prerequisite experience needed for optimal success as a navigator. When a program is using lay navigators, consideration is often given to individuals who are familiar with the community and population served (that is, either having experienced cancer themselves or being a member of the identified community) (Steinberg et al., 2006).

When a program is using healthcare professionals as navigators, previous experience in the field of oncology is beneficial. Familiarity with cancer biology and disease progression, treatments and typical toxicities, and symptom management proves invaluable in proactively anticipating and guiding individuals through the cancer journey (Wilcox & Bruce, 2010). Oncology nurses are skilled in holistic patient assessment, cognizant of available resources, proficient in patient education, and accustomed to the principles of teamwork and multidisciplinary collaboration in cancer care (Fillion et al., 2006; Gilbert et al., 2011).

Ultimately, certification in oncology nursing is ideal for nurse navigators. A license indicates that a nurse has demonstrated the minimum knowledge required for general practice, whereas certification validates that the nurse has obtained specialized knowledge and experience in a particular field and further demonstrates one's commitment to the specialty (Oncology Nursing Certification Corporation, n.d.).

Figure 2-2. The Essentials of Baccalaureate Education for Professional Nursing Practice

Essential I: Liberal Education for Baccalaureate Generalist Nursing Practice
A solid base in liberal education provides the cornerstone for the practice and education of nurses.

Essential II: Basic Organizational and Systems Leadership for Quality Care and Patient Safety
Knowledge and skills in leadership, quality improvement, and patient safety are necessary to provide high-quality health care.

Essential III: Scholarship for Evidence-Based Practice
Professional nursing practice is grounded in the translation of current evidence into one's practice.

Essential IV: Information Management and Application of Patient Care Technology
Knowledge and skills in information management and patient care technology are critical in the delivery of quality patient care.

Essential V: Health Care Policy, Finance, and Regulatory Environments
Healthcare policies, including financial and regulatory, directly and indirectly influence the nature and functioning of the healthcare system and thereby are important considerations in professional nursing practice.

Essential VI: Interprofessional Communication and Collaboration for Improving Patient Health Outcomes
Communication and collaboration among healthcare professionals are critical to delivering high-quality and safe patient care.

Essential VII: Clinical Prevention and Population Health
Health promotion and disease prevention at the individual and population level are necessary to improve population health and are important components of baccalaureate generalist nursing practice.

Essential VIII: Professionalism and Professional Values
Professionalism and the inherent values of altruism, autonomy, human dignity, integrity, and social justice are fundamental to the discipline of nursing.

Essential IX: Baccalaureate Generalist Nursing Practice
The baccalaureate-graduate nurse is prepared to practice with patients, including individuals, families, groups, communities, and populations across the life span and across the continuum of healthcare environments.
The baccalaureate graduate understands and respects the variations of care, the increased complexity, and the increased use of healthcare resources inherent in caring for patients.

Note. From *The Essentials of Baccalaureate Education for Professional Nursing Practice* (pp. 3–4), by the American Association of Colleges of Nursing, October 2008, Washington, DC: Author. Copyright 2008 by the American Association of Colleges of Nursing. Reprinted with permission.

Training

Orientation

Successful onboarding (introduction, training, and cultural integration) is critical for navigators. First, navigators must become familiar with the organization's mission, vision, values, culture, and core business objectives and strategies. Although this may seem somewhat superfluous for navigators who are anxious to get their "boots on the ground," this information is essential to understand how the navigator role interfaces with others and contributes to the organization's strategic mission.

Oftentimes, a preceptor is assigned to orient the navigator to the department. In the event this does not occur, the navigator should proactively seek out potential mentors who can assist in gaining a better understanding of the department's values, norms, and standards. An orientation checklist should be provided to familiarize the navigator with basic aspects of the position, department, and organization. Specific components of an orientation checklist might include

- Key organizational information (e.g., mission, vision, leadership structures, key policies)
- Facility tours of all pertinent clinical and nonclinical areas
- Introduction to members of the multidisciplinary team
- Communication mechanisms
- Risk and safety considerations
- Documentation/electronic medical record systems
- Strategies for coordinating care
- Patient education materials and community resources
- Professional development opportunities.

When completing an orientation checklist, the preceptor should indicate the method for validating initial competence (i.e., how the content was covered) and then date and initial each item. Figure 2-3 provides a simplified example of an orientation checklist.

Although extensive hands-on training is necessary to successfully orient an individual to the navigation role (Vargas et al., 2008), formalized education with content related to cancer, communication, roles and responsibilities, and available resources also is essential. Specifically, ONS, AOSW, and NASW asserted that

> nurses and social workers in oncology who perform navigation services should have education and knowledge in community assessment, cancer program assessment, resolution of system barriers, the cancer continuum, cancer health disparities, cultural competence, and the individualized provision of assistance to patients with cancer, their families, caregivers, and survivors at risk. (ONS et al., 2010, p. 251)

Figure 2-3. Billings Clinic Orientation Checklist and Initial Assessment of Competence for Patient Navigators

ORIENTATION AND INITIAL COMPETENCE ASSESSMENT CHECKLIST FOR BILLINGS CLINIC PATIENT NAVIGATORS

Topic	Method of Validation	Date	Validator's Initials
Organizational Information			
• Mission	☐D ☐S ☐R ☐ED ☐W ☐T ☐I		
• Vision	☐D ☐S ☐R ☐ED ☐W ☐T ☐I		
• Senior leadership	☐D ☐S ☐R ☐ED ☐W ☐T ☐I		
• Organizational chart	☐D ☐S ☐R ☐ED ☐W ☐T ☐I		
• Department plan of care	☐D ☐S ☐R ☐ED ☐W ☐T ☐I		
• Job description	☐D ☐S ☐R ☐ED ☐W ☐T ☐I		
• Professional appearance	☐D ☐S ☐R ☐ED ☐W ☐T ☐I		
• Time and attendance	☐D ☐S ☐R ☐ED ☐W ☐T ☐I		
Facility			
• [List each area to be in-troduced to]	☐D ☐S ☐R ☐ED ☐W ☐T ☐I		
• Parking	☐D ☐S ☐R ☐ED ☐W ☐T ☐I		
Team Members			
• [List pertinent clinical pro-viders and staff, as well as non-clinical staff/vol-unteers/leaders]	☐D ☐S ☐R ☐ED ☐W ☐T ☐I		
Communication			
• Meetings, huddles	☐D ☐S ☐R ☐ED ☐W ☐T ☐I		
• Phone/email etiquette	☐D ☐S ☐R ☐ED ☐W ☐T ☐I		
• Paging system	☐D ☐S ☐R ☐ED ☐W ☐T ☐I		
• SBAR for patient hand-offs	☐D ☐S ☐R ☐ED ☐W ☐T ☐I		
Safety and Risk			
• Disaster/emergency pre-paredness plans	☐D ☐S ☐R ☐ED ☐W ☐T ☐I		
• Patient safety goals and initiatives	☐D ☐S ☐R ☐ED ☐W ☐T ☐I		

(Continued on next page)

Figure 2-3. Billings Clinic Orientation Checklist and Initial Assessment of Competence for Patient Navigators *(Continued)*			
Topic	**Method of Validation**	**Date**	**Validator's Initials**
• Infection control policies and resources	☐D ☐S ☐R ☐ED ☐W ☐T ☐I		
• MSDS web site	☐D ☐S ☐R ☐ED ☐W ☐T ☐I		
• Occurrence and injury reporting systems	☐D ☐S ☐R ☐ED ☐W ☐T ☐I		
• HIPAA/confidentiality	☐D ☐S ☐R ☐ED ☐W ☐T ☐I		
Patient Satisfaction			
• Surveys and feedback mechanisms	☐D ☐S ☐R ☐ED ☐W ☐T ☐I		
• Service recovery	☐D ☐S ☐R ☐ED ☐W ☐T ☐I		
Care Coordination			
• Scheduling software/protocols	☐D ☐S ☐R ☐ED ☐W ☐T ☐I		
• Multidisciplinary clinic coordination	☐D ☐S ☐R ☐ED ☐W ☐T ☐I		
• Navigation standard operating practices	☐D ☐S ☐R ☐ED ☐W ☐T ☐I		
Office Essentials			
• Office/space for personal belongings	☐D ☐S ☐R ☐ED ☐W ☐T ☐I		
• Computer and software programs	☐D ☐S ☐R ☐ED ☐W ☐T ☐I		
• [List various office equipment]	☐D ☐S ☐R ☐ED ☐W ☐T ☐I		
• Office supplies	☐D ☐S ☐R ☐ED ☐W ☐T ☐I		
• Business cards	D S R ED W T I		
Patient Education and Community Resources			
• [List patient education materials and resources]	☐D ☐S ☐R ☐ED ☐W ☐T ☐I		
• [List local resources and support groups]	☐D ☐S ☐R ☐ED ☐W ☐T ☐I		

(Continued on next page)

Figure 2-3. Billings Clinic Orientation Checklist and Initial Assessment of Competence for Patient Navigators *(Continued)*			
Topic	Method of Validation	Date	Validator's Initials
EMR Functions			
• [List key functions the navigator will perform within the EMR]	□D □S □R □ED □W □T □I		
Professional Development			
• ONS – national membership and local chapter activities	□D □S □R □ED □W □T □I		
• [List other continuing education offerings]	□D □S □R □ED □W □T □I		
• Tumor conference schedule	□D □S □R □ED □W □T □I		
• Public relations and marketing opportunities	□D □S □R □ED □W □T □I		
Additional Items (please list)			
	□D □S □R □ED □W □T □I		
	□D □S □R □ED □W □T □I		

D = demonstrates, S = discusses, R = reviews audio/visual or written material, ED = evidence of daily work, W = written testing, T = tour, I = personal introduction; EMR—electronic medical record; HIPAA—Health Insurance Portability and Accountability Act; MSDS—Material Safety Data Sheets; ONS—Oncology Nursing Society; SBAR—situation, background, assessment, and recommendation

Note. Figure courtesy of the Billings Clinic. Used with permission.

Wells et al. (2008) identified components of standardized training provided as part of the Patient Navigation Research Program (PNRP). The PNRP was founded in 2005 by the National Cancer Institute's Center to Reduce Cancer Health Disparities to study the efficacy and cost-effectiveness of community-based navigation programs. Content for the PNRP training program included the basic biology of cancer development (including principles of screening, diagnosis, and treatment), typical barriers to care, available resources, principles of communication, and the importance of cultural sensitivity (Wells et al., 2008). Calhoun et al. (2010) further detailed a collaborative training program for three large multisite navigation programs: the PNRP, the American Cancer Society Patient Navigator Program, and the Centers for Medicare and Medicaid Services' Cancer Prevention and Treatment Demonstration Project. Content outlined for this collaborative training program was similar to that identified by Wells et al. (2008) but included information regarding the importance of clinical trials in oncology care and the ethical conduct of research (Calhoun et al., 2010).

A growing number of nationally recognized patient navigation training programs have been developed. The Harold P. Freeman Patient Navigation Institute offers formal training both as a two-day course and through online learning modules (Harold P. Freeman Patient Navigation Institute, 2013). Similarly, the Colorado Patient Navigator Training Program offers both face-to-face and web-based learning opportunities (Patient Navigator Training Collaborative, n.d.). The Smith Center for Healing and the Arts (n.d.) provides an extensive in-person training course, as does EduCare (n.d.), albeit this program is specific to breast cancer navigation only. Although each program is unique in its specific curriculum, the topics covered are comparable to those previously mentioned, including the navigator role, an overview of cancer biology and treatments, barriers to care, community resources, cancer research, communication, and cultural sensitivity. Prior to enrolling in any of the aforementioned patient navigation training programs, due diligence is needed to ensure the curriculum and training focus are appropriate to the needs of one's own program.

After initial orientation and training, navigators must commit to lifelong learning and the pursuit of ongoing continuing education. This is essential in order for navigators to remain knowledgeable about practice changes and current advances in treatments and symptom management. Today, it is relatively easy for navigators to engage in continuing education, including face-to-face educational offerings, online opportunities (which can be synchronous or asynchronous), and journal articles offering continuing education credit. Locally, nurse navigators may seek continuing education from multidisciplinary case conferences, local nursing associations, and other healthcare organizations. Regionally and nationally, nurse navigators have an increasing array of navigation-specific education available. Currently, both the Academy of Oncology Nurse and Patient Navigators (AONN+) and NCONN offer conferences with topics tailored to the needs of nurse navigators. ONS supports a special interest group for nurse navigators and often has multiple sessions at its annual conference pertinent to navigation. Furthermore, Breast Patient Navigation Certification has been developed by the National Consortium of Breast Centers (NCBC) as a means to demonstrate specific knowledge and skills pertaining to breast navigation.

Core Competencies

Competence is the validation of knowledge, skills, and attitudes needed to accomplish the defined responsibilities of a position. A comprehensive competency framework, inclusive of initial assessment of competence as well as ongoing assessment, is essential to ensure that navigators are qualified and safe in performing assigned duties.

Specific to nurse navigation, NCONN (2013) was the first national organization to develop a set of core navigation competencies. Originally published in 2009, the competencies were intended to serve as a framework for the role of the navigator and focused on five general categories: professional, legal, and ethical nursing practice; health promotion and health education; management and leadership; advocacy; and personal effectiveness and professional development (Francz & Simpson, 2013). Figure 2-4 lists the five specific competency statements as defined by NCONN.

ONS formed a project team in 2012 to define oncology nurse navigator competencies. Competencies were drafted based on a review of the literature and underwent extensive field review yielding recommendations related to the scope of content and wording changes before being released to the oncology nursing community (ONS, 2013). Figure 2-5 outlines the oncology nurse navigator core competencies as defined by ONS.

Figure 2-4. Oncology Nurse Navigator Core Competencies 2013, as Defined by the National Coalition of Oncology Nurse Navigators

Competence Area 1: Professional, Legal, and Ethical Nursing Practice
The Oncology Nurse Navigator will integrate the philosophy of nursing care and evidence-based practice into care of the oncology patient.

Competence Area 2: Health Promotion and Health Education
The Oncology Nurse Navigator will perform an assessment of the patient's current health status to address health promotion needs, functional status, developmental and lifestyle issues to maximize health outcomes. The ONN will implement specific therapeutic modalities to facilitate individualized care to the oncology patient in collaboration with the multidisciplinary team.

Competence Area 3: Management and Leadership
The Oncology Nurse Navigator will promote the role of patient navigation to the public market and health care industry to ensure preservation of the role and advancement of the profession.

Competence Area 4: Advocacy
The Oncology Nurse Navigator will guide and direct the patient through a collaborative environment of health care disciplines to maintain dignity and autonomy of the individual patient.

Competence Area 5: Personal Effectiveness and Professional Development
The Oncology Nurse Navigator will strive for optimal quality of nursing care through continued self-evaluation and program analysis that is adaptable to patient and community needs.

Note. From *Oncology Nurse Navigator Core Competencies 2013* (pp. 12–17), by National Coalition of Oncology Nurse Navigators, 2013, Rockville, MD: Author. Copyright 2013 by the National Coalition of Oncology Nurse Navigators. Reprinted with permission.

Figure 2-5. Oncology Nurse Navigator Core Competencies, as Defined by the Oncology Nursing Society

Introduction
The oncology nurse navigator (ONN) demonstrates critical thinking and uses the nursing process to assess and meet the needs of patients by providing care coordination throughout the cancer continuum. He or she works within the domains of the patient and family unit and the healthcare delivery system to improve health, treatment, and end-of-life outcomes. This is accomplished through competent practice in the following functional areas.

Competency Category 1: Professional Role
The ONN demonstrates professionalism within both the workplace and the community through respectful interactions and effective teamwork. The nurse works to promote and advance the role of the ONN and takes responsibility to pursue personal professional growth and development. The ONN
1. Promotes lifelong learning and evidence-based practice, by self and others, to improve the care of patients with a past, current, or potential diagnosis of cancer
2. Demonstrates effective communication with peers, members of the multidisciplinary healthcare team, and community organizations and resources
3. Contributes to the knowledge base of the healthcare community and in support of the ONN role through activities such as involvement in professional organizations, presentations, publications, and research
4. Contributes to ONN program development, implementation, and evaluation within the healthcare system and community
5. Disseminates knowledge of the ONN role to other healthcare team members through peer education, mentorship, and preceptor experiences
6. Obtains or develops oncology-related educational materials for patients, staff, and community members as appropriate
7. Participates in the tracking of metrics and patient outcomes, in collaboration with administration, to document and evaluate outcomes of the navigation program and report findings to the cancer committee
8. Collaborates with the cancer committee and administration to perform and evaluate data from the community needs assessment to identify areas of improvement that will affect the patient navigation process and program and participate in quality improvement based on identified service gaps
9. Promotes a patient- and family-centered care environment for ethical decision making and advocacy for patients with cancer
10. Establishes and maintains professional role boundaries with patients, caregivers, and the multidisciplinary care team in collaboration with the manager as defined by the job description
11. In collaboration with other members of the healthcare team, builds partnerships with local agencies and groups that may assist with cancer patient care, support, or educational needs.

Competency Category 2: Education
The ONN provides appropriate and timely education to patients, families, and caregivers to facilitate understanding and support informed decision making. The ONN
1. Assesses educational needs of patients, families, and caregivers, taking into consideration barriers to care (e.g., literacy, language, cultural influences, comorbidities)

(Continued on next page)

Figure 2-5. Oncology Nurse Navigator Core Competencies, as Defined by the Oncology Nursing Society *(Continued)*

2. Provides and reinforces education to patients, families, and caregivers about diagnosis, treatment options, side effect management, and post-treatment care and survivorship
3. Educates patients, families, and caregivers on the role of the ONN
4. Orients and educates patients, families, and caregivers to the cancer healthcare system, multidisciplinary team member roles, and available resources
5. Promotes autonomous decision making by patients through the provision of personalized education and support
6. As part of the multidisciplinary team, provides education and reinforces to patients, families, and caregivers the significance of adherence to treatment schedules, protocols, and follow-up
7. Assesses and promotes healthy lifestyle choices and self-care strategies for patients through education and appropriate referrals to ancillary services
8. Provides anticipatory guidance, education, and appropriate referrals to assist patients in coping with the diagnosis of cancer and its potential or expected outcomes
9. Promotes awareness of clinical trials to patients, families, and caregivers.

Competency Category 3: Coordination of Care
The ONN facilitates the appropriate and efficient delivery of healthcare services, both within and across systems, to promote optimal outcomes while delivering patient-centered care. The ONN

1. Assesses patient needs upon initial encounter and periodically throughout navigation, matching unmet needs with appropriate services and referrals and support services, such as dietitians, providers, social work, and financial services
2. Identifies potential and realized barriers to care (e.g., transportation, child care, elder care, housing, language, culture, literacy, role disparity, psychosocial, employment, financial, insurance) and facilitates referrals as appropriate to mitigate barriers
3. Develops and/or uses appropriate assessment tools (e.g., Distress Thermometer, pain scale, fatigue scale, performance status) to promote a consistent, holistic plan of care
4. Facilitates timely scheduling of appointments, diagnostic testing, and procedures to expedite the plan of care and to promote continuity of care
5. Participates in coordination of the care plan with the multidisciplinary team, promoting timely follow-up on treatment and supportive care recommendations
6. Facilitates individualized care within the context of functional status, cultural considerations, health literacy, psychosocial and spiritual needs for patients, families, and caregivers
7. Demonstrates knowledge of clinical guidelines (e.g., National Comprehensive Cancer Network, American Joint Committee on Cancer) and specialty resources (e.g., ONS Putting Evidence Into Practice resources) throughout the disease process
8. Assists in the identification of candidates for genetic counseling and facilitates appropriate referrals
9. Supports a smooth transition of patients from active treatment into survivorship or end-of-life care
10. Uses an ethical framework regarding patient care to assist patients with cancer with issues related to treatment goals, advance directives, palliative care, and end-of-life concerns

(Continued on next page)

Figure 2-5. Oncology Nurse Navigator Core Competencies, as Defined by the Oncology Nursing Society *(Continued)*

11. Ensures documentation of patient encounters and provided services
12. Applies basic knowledge of insurance processes (e.g., Medicare, Medicaid, third-party payers) and their impact on staging, referrals, and patient care decisions toward establishing appropriate referrals, as needed.

Competency Category 4: Communication
The ONN demonstrates interpersonal communication skills that enable exchange of ideas and information effectively with patients, families, and colleagues at all levels. This includes writing, speaking, and listening skills. The ONN
1. Builds therapeutic and trusting relationships with patients, families, and caregivers through effective communication and listening skills
2. Acts as a liaison between the patients, families, and caregivers and the providers to optimize patient outcomes
3. Advocates for patients to promote optimal care and outcomes
4. Provides psychosocial support to and facilitates appropriate referrals for patients, families, and caregivers, especially during periods of high emotional stress and anxiety
5. Empowers patients and families through education and encouragement to self-advocate and communicate their needs
6. Adheres to established regulations concerning patient information and privacy
7. Ensures that communication is culturally sensitive
8. Facilitates communication among members of the multidisciplinary cancer care team to prevent fragmented or delayed care that could adversely affect patient outcomes.

Note. From *Oncology Nurse Navigator Core Competencies,* by the Oncology Nursing Society, 2013, Pittsburgh, PA: Author. Copyright 2013 by the Oncology Nursing Society. Reprinted with permission.

Succeeding in the Role

Getting started as a navigator is an exciting endeavor. Indeed, the opportunity to work with patients to remove barriers to care and facilitate timely coordinated services, with the ultimate goal of improving healthcare outcomes, can be very rewarding. However, there are some important program matters to discuss and confirm up front with program administrators and key stakeholders to ensure overall success in the role.

First, it is important to develop a job description that defines a clear scope of practice for patient navigation; that is, when does navigation start, and when does it end for the specific position created? Tasks and aspects of care for which the navigator is accountable for should be specified and should not significantly overlap with others' roles and responsibilities (Freeman & Rodriguez, 2011). All too often, in the haste to initiate a navigation program, thorough consideration is not given to these basic fundamentals. Instead, assorted tasks are assigned to navigators as a mechanism to ensure a sense of productivity and value associated with the role. This unfortunately can result in navigators assuming responsibility for aspects of others' roles without careful consideration to clearly delineate roles based on scope of services, community and organizational needs, and the qualifications and past experiences the navigator brings to the position. This lack of clarity can be further perpetuated when others look to defer any difficulties associated with an individual's circumstances to navigators for resolution. Figure 2-6 depicts an example of one program's nurse navigator job description.

Figure 2-6. Billings Clinic Job Description for Patient Care Navigator

BILLINGS CLINIC JOB DESCRIPTION

JOB TITLE

Patient Care Navigator

REPORTS TO	EVALUATES
Manager	None
INTERNAL RELATIONSHIPS	EXTERNAL RELATIONSHIPS
Billings Clinic staff and customers	Public, vendors, regulatory agencies, and other healthcare providers

PURPOSE/DISTINGUISHING CHARACTERISTICS
The incumbent in this position acts as an advocate for patients serving as the primary point of contact and is responsible for coordinating the care and services of the identified patient populations for an extended period of time across the continuum of care for both inpatient and outpatient services; promoting effective resource utilization; assuming a leadership role with the multidisciplinary team to achieve an optimal clinical outcome.

Essential Job Functions

DESCRIPTION
1. Supports and models behaviors consistent with the mission and philosophy of Billings Clinic and department/service.
2. Demonstrates Patient Service Excellence.
    a) Demonstrates excellence in communication skills and patient interactions.
    b) Demonstrates ability to work as a team member intra- and interdepartmentally.
    c) Adheres to Personal Service Excellence skills.
3. Facilitates the coordination of patient care services to assure excellence in patient care and patient flow; includes coordinating care, treatment and communication among the medical team.
    a) Follows patient through the care continuum/experience, eliminating operational (such as scheduling, test results, etc.) barriers to services.
    b) Works closely with other healthcare disciplines to ensure timely appointments, results reporting, financial need referrals, communication, patient care, and follow-up.

(Continued on next page)

Figure 2-6. Billings Clinic Job Description for Patient Care Navigator
(Continued)

4. Facilitates the development, implementation, and adherence to clinical and evidence-based guidelines, as appropriate, to ensure optimal clinical outcomes.
   a) Ensures follow-up has occurred regarding patient clinical and non-clinical care to include adherence to plans of care, resource utilization, and general progress utilizing care conferences as necessary.
   b) Works in collaboration with the medical team to develop and implement clinical guidelines. Facilitates the adherence of the guidelines through regular evaluation and auditing of clinical practice.
   c) Works with care team to assure direct care needs are met, assisting as needed or assigned.
5. Demonstrates expertise in educational and resourcing services.
   a) Participates in educational activities related to patient/community, clinical operation, and process issues on an ongoing basis.
   b) Collaborates with other healthcare providers in developing, implementing, and evaluating educational materials for patients and families.
   c) Facilitates intra-departmental relationships in an effort to provide necessary resources to and for the patient.
   d) Interfaces with other members/disciplines within the healthcare teams for appropriate referrals/services.
   e) Aware of and assists with financial needs of the patients.
   f) Identifies and accesses appropriate social services, including resources to assist caregivers to support treatment.
   g) Develops options for complementary and integrative care.
6. Contributes to an environment of quality and process improvement.
   a) Ensures accurate and timely data collection and entry into patient database as indicated by department guidelines.
   b) Directs and coordinates identified quality assessment and improvement activities to assure quality patient services are provided through audits and reviews of other identified evaluation tools.
   c) Ensures patient care activities for the department services are monitored monthly through audits and reviews.
   d) Ensures and enhances facility, safety, and regulatory outcomes.
      i) Complies with all applicable laws, regulations, and accrediting agencies.
      ii) Complies with all Billings Clinic policies.
7. Works in collaboration with Leadership team to ensure hospital and clinic departmental goals and objectives are met.
   a) Supports the hospital and clinic departmental goals.
   b) Contributes to community activities sponsored by the department.
   c) Develops patient referral services by relationship-building strategies with physicians not related to the department.
   d) Performs other duties as assigned or needed to meet the needs of the department/organization.
8. Works as an active team member and effective communicator.
   a) Demonstrates effective internal and external communication strategies, written and verbal, to assure a collaborative environment.
   b) Ensures appropriate and timely documentation.
   c) Demonstrates a productive work ethic while on duty.
   d) Works consistently as an active team player, inter- and intra-departmentally.

(Continued on next page)

Figure 2-6. Billings Clinic Job Description for Patient Care Navigator
(Continued)

9. Identifies needs and sets goals for own growth and development; meets all mandatory organizational and departmental requirements.
10. Maintains competency in all organizational, departmental, and outside agency environmental, employee or patient safety standards relevant to job performance.

Additional Duties for Breast Diagnostic Navigator

11. Facilitates the coordination of patient care services to assure excellence in patient care and patient flow.
    a) Follows patient from abnormal mammogram through diagnosis.
    b) Provides seamless patient flow from abnormal mammogram to diagnosis and referral to breast cancer Patient Care Navigator.
       i) Facilitates breast biopsy scheduling.
       ii) Facilitates breast biopsy education.
12. Facilitates the development, implementation, and adherence to clinical and research guidelines, as appropriate, to ensure optimal clinical outcomes.
    a) Ensures each patient scheduled for a screening mammogram has had a clinical breast exam within acceptable time frame.
13. Demonstrates expertise in educational and resourcing services.
    a) Facilitates relationship between physicians, vendors, departments, and the breast multidisciplinary program.
    b) Interfaces with finance and breast imaging services to meet the financial needs of the patients.

Additional Duties for Outreach Regional Navigator

14. Collaborates with local individuals, agencies, and organizations to facilitate the increased availability of community-based care services.
    a) Facilitates research participation opportunities through outreach clinics.
    b) Facilitates increased utilization of telemedicine in connecting rural patients and providers to Billings Clinic resources.
    c) Coordinates opportunities to increase prevention awareness and offer early-detection screening programs in outreach areas.
15. Develops and implements regional care protocols, resulting in reduced time to problem resolution and improved quality of care.
    a) Interfaces with local and outreach providers in addressing care navigation concerns.
    b) Identifies community support services in underserved and frontier areas and facilitates utilization of these services.
16. Advocates for the individual and collective needs of patients in rural and frontier areas.
    a) Facilitates relationship-building between physicians, agencies, and organizations.
    b) Interfaces with physicians, agencies, and organizations to meet the medical, social, and financial needs of patients.

(Continued on next page)

Figure 2-6. Billings Clinic Job Description for Patient Care Navigator *(Continued)*

KNOWLEDGE, SKILLS AND ABILITIES
KNOWLEDGE OF:
- Billings Clinic policy and procedures, both organizational and departmental
- Personal computers, hardware and software
- Microsoft Office Programs (i.e., Windows, Outlook, Word, Excel, etc.)
- Billings Clinic Code of Business Conduct
- Billings Clinic Corporate Compliance Program
- HIPAA and confidentiality requirements
- Patient's/resident's rights
- Patient safety standards
- Customer service techniques and Personal Service Excellence skills
- Community resources
- Infection control and safety practices and procedures
- Nursing theory and practice to assess, provide, and evaluate quality patient care
- Advanced nursing assessments and procedures assessment, patient education, provider education, planning, evaluation

SKILL IN:
- Professional communication skills, both verbal and written
- Strong organizational skills
- Skill in utilizing personal computers with basic computer skills in word processing and data management using Microsoft Office programs
- Conflict resolution

ABILITY TO:
- Incorporate population-specific needs into all aspects of communication and patient care; scope of services provided will encompass age groups from infant through geriatric
- Communicate clearly and effectively, both verbal and written
- Establish and maintain collaborative relationships
- Work independently

COMPLEXITY AND DIFFICULTY
- Ability to define and implement an evolving role of patient-centered care delivered in a complex integrated healthcare system which includes setting common goals, merging resources, providing education, and cross training of roles.
- Must be able to work with a variety of diverse and complex patients, families, and both internal and external healthcare providers.
- Accountable to provide clinically sound information

MINIMUM QUALIFICATIONS
- Graduate of an accredited school of nursing, bachelor's degree in nursing preferred.
- Current Montana/Wyoming RN license.
- Two (2) years clinical practice experience, 5 years of service line experience preferred.
- Healthcare Provider CPR certification.
- One (1) year demonstrated computer experience dealing with word processing and data management.
- Or an equivalent combination of education and experience relating to the above tasks, knowledge, skills and abilities will be considered.

(Continued on next page)

Figure 2-6. Billings Clinic Job Description for Patient Care Navigator *(Continued)*
Additional Qualifications for Breast Diagnostics • Demonstrated clinical breast exam proficiency, certification preferred or to be obtained within six (6) months of hire **Additional Qualifications for Outreach Regional Navigator** • Valid Montana driver's license and the ability to be insured to operate Billings Clinic vehicles.
WORKING CONDITIONS • Normal patient care and office work environments • Regional Navigator will be required to travel to outreach facilities **Blood Borne Pathogen Category:** Category I: Tasks that involve exposure to blood, body fluids or tissues. **Airborne Contaminant Category:** Category I: Tasks that routinely require activities that may involve exposure to airborne contaminants.
The above is intended to describe the general content of and requirements of the performance of this job. It is not to be construed as an exhaustive statement of duties, responsibilities or requirements.
CPR—cardiopulmonary resuscitation; HIPAA—Health Insurance Portability and Accountability Act *Note.* Figure courtesy of the Billings Clinic. Used with permission.

Steinberg et al. (2006) identified the importance of establishing standard operating procedures (SOPs) within navigation programs to clearly delineate roles, responsibilities, and expectations placed upon navigators. Content to consider addressing in SOPs might include incoming referral processes, coordination of multidisciplinary clinic evaluations, points of patient contact, attendance at patient appointments, assessment and documentation standards, patient education, referral initiation for ancillary services, and alternate coverage during navigator absences. Examples of SOPs are depicted in Figure 3-5 in Chapter 3.

Identifying key program metrics is also an important consideration when getting started as a navigator. Program administrators and key stakeholders are always very interested in proving the value of the navigation program. In addition to patient volumes, meaningful measures should be identified based on the goals and objectives of the navigation program and then clearly defined to ensure consistency and integrity of the data collected. Chapter 9 provides further detail regarding possible program metrics, data sources, and tracking mechanisms.

Conclusion

The definitions, roles, and responsibilities of navigators have rapidly developed over the past 20 years and will likely undergo additional evolution as programs continue to mature and advance. Patient navigation has been notably summarized by Wells et al. (2008) as individualized assistance, with efforts targeted toward a specific set of health services and focused on eliminating barriers to timely access to care, provided for a defined episode of care, with a specific endpoint.

Roles and responsibilities common to most navigators include facilitating communication and collaboration, coordinating timely access to care and seamless transitions, identifying and resolving barriers, and providing emotional support. When starting as a navigator, it is important to understand the scope of one's job description and work collaboratively with program administrators and stakeholders to ensure consensus regarding fundamental duties.

Qualities frequently associated with successful navigators include cultural competence, superb communication skills, familiarity with cancer biology and the care continuum, knowledge of community resources, and generalized leadership skills. However, even if navigators come with the qualities and experiences discussed herein, it is nonetheless imperative to invest time in a thorough orientation, as well as ongoing professional and program development. Overall, opportunities abound for navigators in healthcare settings, and working as a navigator can be extremely rewarding for those who enjoy patient advocacy, support, and empowerment.

References

American Association of Colleges of Nursing. (2008, October). *The essentials of baccalaureate education for professional nursing practice.* Retrieved from http://www.aacn.nche.edu/education-resources/baccessentials08.pdf

Betancourt, J.R., Green, A.R., Carrillo, J.E., & Ananeh-Firempong, O., II. (2003). Defining cultural competence: A practical framework for addressing racial/ethnic disparities in health and health care. *Public Health Reports, 118,* 293–302. Retrieved from http://www.ncbi.nlm.nih.gov/pmc/articles/PMC1497553/pdf/12815076.pdf

Brown, C., Bornstein, E., & Wilcox, C. (2012). Partnership and empowerment program: A model for patient-centered, comprehensive, and cost-effective care. *Clinical Journal of Oncology Nursing, 16,* 15–17. doi:10.1188/12.CJON.15-17

Brown, C.G., Cantril, C., McMullen, L., Barkley, D.L., Dietz, M., Murphy, C.M., & Fabrey, L.J. (2012). Oncology Nurse Navigator Role Delineation Study: An Oncology Nursing Society report. *Clinical Journal of Oncology Nursing, 16,* 581–585. doi:10.1188/12.CJON.581-585

Burhansstipanov, L., Wound, D.B., Capelouto, N., Goldfarb, F., Harjo, L., Hatathlie, L., ... White, M. (1998). Culturally relevant "navigator" patient support. The Native sisters. *Cancer Practice, 6,* 191–194. doi:10.1046/j.1523-5394.1998.006003191.x

Calhoun, E.A., Whitley, E.M., Esparza, A., Ness, E., Greene, A., Garcia, R., & Valverde, P.A. (2010). A national patient navigator training program. *Health Promotion Practice, 11,* 205–215. doi:10.1177/1524839908323521

Case, M.A.B. (2011). Oncology nurse navigator: Ensuring safe passage. *Clinical Journal of Oncology Nursing, 15,* 33–40. doi:10.1188/11.CJON.33-40

EduCare. (n.d.). Breast health navigator training. Retrieved from http://www.educareinc.com/training_nav.php

Ell, K., Vourlekis, B., Muderspach, L., Nissly, J., Padgett, D., Pineda, D., … Lee, P.J. (2002). Abnormal cervical screen follow-up among low-income Latinas: Project SAFe. *Journal of Women's Health and Gender-Based Medicine, 11,* 639–651. doi:10.1089/152460902760360586

Fillion, L., Cook, S., Veillette, A.M., de Serres, M., Aubin, M., Rainville, F., … Doll, R. (2012). Professional navigation: A comparative study of two Canadian models. *Canadian Oncology Nursing Journal, 22,* 257–277.

Fillion, L., de Serres, M., Cook, S., Goupil, R.L., Bairati, I., & Doll, R. (2009). Professional patient navigation in head and neck cancer. *Seminars in Oncology Nursing, 25,* 212–221. doi:10.1016/j.soncn.2009.05.004

Fillion, L., de Serres, M., Lapointe-Goupil, R., Bairati, I., Gagnon, P., Deschamps, M., … Demers, G. (2006). Implementing the role of patient-navigator nurse at a university hospital centre. *Canadian Oncology Nursing Journal, 16,* 11–17, 5–10.

Fiscella, K., Ransom, S., Jean-Pierre, P., Cella, D., Stein, K., Bauer, J.E., … Walsh, K. (2011). Patient-reported outcome measures suitable to assessment of patient navigation. *Cancer, 117*(Suppl. 15), 3603–3617. doi:10.1002/cncr.26260

Francz, S.L., & Simpson, K.D. (2013). Oncology nurse navigators: A snapshot of their educational background, compensation, and day-to-day roles and responsibilities. *Oncology Issues, 28*(1), 36–43.

Freeman, H.P. (2004). A model patient navigation program: Breaking down barriers to ensure that all individuals with cancer receive timely diagnosis and treatment. *Oncology Issues, 19*(5), 44–46.

Freeman, H.P., & Chu, K.C. (2005). Determinants of cancer disparities: Barriers to cancer screening, diagnosis, and treatment. *Surgical Oncology Clinics of North America, 14,* 655–669, v. doi:10.1016/j.soc.2005.06.002

Freeman, H.P., & Rodriguez, R.L. (2011). History and principles of patient navigation. *Cancer, 117*(Suppl. 15), 3539–3542. doi:10.1002/cncr.26262

Freund, K.M., Battaglia, T.A., Calhoun, E., Dudley, D.J., Fiscella, K., Paskett, E., … Roetzheim, R.G. (2008). National Cancer Institute Patient Navigation Research Program: Methods, protocol, and measures. *Cancer, 113,* 3391–3399. doi:10.1002/cncr.23960

Gabram, S.G.A., Lund, M.J.B., Gardner, J., Hatchett, N., Bumpers, H.L., Okoli, J., … Brawley, O.W. (2008). Effects of an outreach and internal navigation program on breast cancer diagnosis in an urban cancer center with a large African-American population. *Cancer, 113,* 602–607. doi:10.1002/cncr.23568

Gilbert, J.E., Green, E., Lankshear, S., Hughes, E., Burkoski, V., & Sawka, C. (2011). Nurses as patient navigators in cancer diagnosis: Review, consultation and model design. *European Journal of Cancer Care, 20,* 228–236. doi:10.1111/j.1365-2354.2010.01231.x

Harold P. Freeman Patient Navigation Institute. (n.d.). The program. Retrieved from http://www.hpfreemanpni.org/the-program

Hiatt, R.A., Pasick, R.J., Stewart, S., Bloom, J., Davis, P., Gardiner, P., … Stroud, F. (2001). Community-based cancer screening for underserved women: Design and baseline findings from the Breast and Cervical Cancer Intervention Study. *Preventive Medicine, 33,* 190–203. doi:10.1006/pmed.2001.0871

Horner, K., Ludman, E.J., McCorkle, R., Canfield, E., Flaherty, L., Min, J., … Wagner, E.H. (2013). An oncology nurse navigator program designed to eliminate gaps in early cancer care. *Clinical Journal of Oncology Nursing, 17,* 43–48. doi:10.1188/13.CJON.43-48

Korber, S.F., Padula, C., Gray, J., & Powell, M. (2011). A breast navigator program: Barriers, enhancers, and nursing interventions. *Oncology Nursing Forum, 38,* 44–50. doi:10.1188/11.ONF.44-50

McDonald, C. (2011). A first-hand look at the role of the breast cancer nurse navigator. *Care Management, 17*(5), 11–13, 27–28. Retrieved from http://www.jcaremanagement.com/pdf_nonmember/6CM_dec2011_jan2012.pdf

National Coalition of Oncology Nurse Navigators. (2013). *Oncology nurse navigator core competencies 2013.* Rockville, MD: Author.

Nguyen, T.-U.N., & Kagawa-Singer, M. (2008). Overcoming barriers to cancer care through health navigation programs. *Seminars in Oncology Nursing, 24,* 270–278. doi:10.1016/j. soncn.2008.08.007

Oncology Nursing Certification Corporation. (n.d.). Why should you get certified? Retrieved from http://www.oncc.org/TakeTest/WhyGetCertified

Oncology Nursing Society. (2013). *Oncology nurse navigator core competencies.* Retrieved from http://beta.ons.org/sites/default/files/ONNCompetencies.pdf

Oncology Nursing Society, Association of Oncology Social Work, & National Association of Social Workers. (2010). Oncology Nursing Society, the Association of Oncology Social Work, and the National Association of Social Workers joint position on the role of oncology nursing and oncology social work in patient navigation. *Oncology Nursing Forum, 37,* 251–252. Retrieved from http://ons.metapress.com/content/f2830241m137mg1m/fulltext.pdf

Patient Navigator Training Collaborative. (n.d.). Colorado Patient Navigator Training Program. Retrieved from http://www.patientnavigatortraining.org

Pedersen, A.E., & Hack, T.F. (2011). The British Columbia Patient Navigation Model: A critical analysis. *Oncology Nursing Forum, 38,* 200–206. doi:10.1188/11.ONF.200-206

Petereit, D.G., Molloy, K., Reiner, M.L., Helbig, P., Cina, K., Miner, R., ... Roberts, C.R. (2008). Establishing a patient navigator program to reduce cancer disparities in the American Indian communities of Western South Dakota: Initial observations and results. *Cancer Control, 15,* 254–259. Retrieved from http://www.moffitt.org/File%20Library/Main%20Nav/ Research%20and%20Clinical%20Trials/Cancer%20Control%20Journal/v15n3/254.pdf

Schwaderer, K.A., & Itano, J.K. (2007). Bridging the healthcare divide with patient navigation: Development of a research program to address disparities. *Clinical Journal of Oncology Nursing, 11,* 633–639. doi:10.1188/07.CJON.633-639

Seek, A.J., & Hogle, W.P. (2007). Modeling a better way: Navigating the healthcare system for patients with lung cancer. *Clinical Journal of Oncology Nursing, 11,* 81–85. doi:10.1188/07. CJON.81-85

Smith Center for Healing and the Arts. (n.d.). Patient navigation training in integrative cancer care. Retrieved from http://www.smithcenter.org/integrative-patient-navigation/patient -navigation-training-integrative-cancer-care.html

Stanley, S., Arriola, K.J., Smith, S., Hurlbert, M., Ricci, C., & Escoffery, C. (2013). Reducing barriers to breast cancer care through Avon Patient Navigation Programs. *Journal of Public Health Management and Practice, 19,* 461–467. doi:10.1097/PHH.0b013e318276e272

Steinberg, M.L., Fremont, A., Khan, D.C., Huang, D., Knapp, H., Karaman, D., ... Streeter, O.E., Jr. (2006). Lay patient navigator program implementation for equal access to cancer care and clinical trials: Essential steps and initial challenges. *Cancer, 107,* 2669–2677. doi:10.1002/cncr.22319

Thygesen, M.K., Pedersen, B.D., Kragstrup, J., Wagner, L., & Mogensen, O. (2011). Benefits and challenges perceived by patients with cancer when offered a nurse navigator. *International Journal of Integrated Care, 11,* e130. Retrieved from http://www.ncbi.nlm.nih.gov/ pmc/articles/PMC3225241

Vargas, R.B., Ryan, G.W., Jackson, C.A., Rodriguez, R., & Freeman, H.P. (2008). Characteristics of the original patient navigation programs to reduce disparities in the diagnosis and treatment of breast cancer. *Cancer, 113,* 426–433. doi:10.1002/cncr.23547

Weinrich, S.P., Boyd, M.D., Weinrich, M., Greene, F., Reynolds, W.A., Jr., & Metlin, C. (1998). Increasing prostate cancer screening in African American men with peer-educator and client-navigator interventions. *Journal of Cancer Education, 13,* 213–219. doi:10.1080/08858199809528549

Wells, K.J., Battaglia, T.A., Dudley, D.J., Garcia, R., Greene, A., Calhoun, E., ... Raich, P.C. (2008). Patient navigation: State of the art or is it science? *Cancer, 113,* 1999–2010. doi:10.1002/cncr.23815

Wilcox, B., & Bruce, S.D. (2010). Patient navigation: A "win-win" for all involved. *Oncology Nursing Forum, 37,* 21–25. doi:10.1188/10.ONF.21-25

CHAPTER 3

How to Start and Expand a Nurse Navigation Program

Nadesda A. Mack, RN, BSN, MBA, OCN®,
and Lisa Shalkowski, RN, BSN, MSHA

Introduction

Patient navigation is not a new paradigm in oncology care. Patients have been informally navigated in physician offices, hospitals, and outpatient departments for many years. Nurses, social workers, and lay colleagues perform navigation functions in a multitude of settings and circumstances and under many different names, including care management, care coordination, and patient-centered care. This informal model, however, is often inconsistent, unorganized, and inadequate in meeting the multifaceted needs of patients with cancer.

Oncology care has become increasingly more complex, requiring multiple subspecialty evaluations and testing. Patients and families can experience extreme anxiety and difficulty coping because of abundant but conflicting and confusing information from the Internet, lack of knowledge about and availability of clinical trials, financial and psychosocial burdens, and the stigma of the disease itself. All this is occurring at a time when patients are faced with complicated and often life-altering decisions. Given these factors, a formal, consistent, and comprehensive approach to the support of patients with cancer is necessary.

Creating a Navigation Program

As the need and value of navigation become more evident, accrediting bodies such as the American College of Surgeons (ACoS) Commission on Cancer (CoC) are requiring that a formalized process be in place to support patients with cancer. Standard 3.1 of the ACoS CoC cancer program standards will be an accreditation requirement as of 2015. The standard reads:

Patient navigation in cancer care refers to individualized assistance offered to patients, families, and caregivers to help overcome healthcare system barriers and facilitate timely access to quality medical and psychosocial care and can occur from prior to a cancer diagnosis through all phases of the cancer experience. (ACoS CoC, 2012, p. 75)

Compliance requires a community needs assessment every three years, establishment of a patient navigation process and identification of resources, yearly assessment of the process and barriers to care, and yearly modification or enhancement of the process as indicated by the community needs assessment (ACoS CoC, 2012).

Assessing Need

The first step in the design and establishment of a navigation program needs to be a program-wide gap analysis. Understanding the current state of patient navigation in the organization is essential to the success of building a formalized navigation program. System issues and gaps need to be identified and corrected to ensure support of the initiative. A multipronged approach assessing current practice, patient and community needs, and stakeholder perspectives and concerns needs to be performed.

All areas within the oncology continuum need to be evaluated. For example, Lehigh Valley Health Network in Allentown, Pennsylvania, conducted an extensive needs assessment and analysis as part of its navigation program planning. From diagnostic evaluation to survivorship, each department within the cancer program was required to participate in the effort. Leadership carved out four hours to create an initial draft of the current oncology patient experience. A manager and a staff member from every oncology department were invited to a 30-minute session to identify and map the journey of the patient with cancer. Sticky notes were used to represent each touchpoint in the continuum, and a conference room wall was used to display each map. Problem areas were flagged as leaders asked probing questions about decision making and patient flow. Over subsequent weeks, all cancer center staff members were invited to review the maps, make appropriate changes, and provide insightful notes. Leadership then created a map of the ideal patient flow and compared it to the current state. Frontline staff again participated in the evaluation of the model and offered comments and suggestions to improve the design. Staff involvement led to robust discussions across departmental silos and resulted in a better appreciation and understanding of the total oncology patient experience.

Next steps included a survey of current patients with cancer and their families regarding the patient experience. Project leaders in multiple departments throughout the cancer program conducted face-to-face interviews using a standard tool (see Figure 3-1). Patients with a variety of diagnoses and treatments and their caregivers were interviewed. The initial responses were positive, and it was not until patients were asked open-ended questions targeting improvements in the cancer experience that real prob-

---

Figure 3-1. Lehigh Valley Health Network's Gap Analysis Interview Tool

1. Have you had any difficulty with the following:

   - Getting appointments   ☐ Yes   ☐ No
   - Getting results   ☐ Yes   ☐ No
   - Knowing what to do should symptoms occur?   ☐ Yes   ☐ No

   If yes, what was the problem?_____

   _____

   _____

2. Did anyone discuss resources available to you outside   ☐ Yes   ☐ No
   of this department, such as nutrition, financial or support
   counseling?

3. How would you rate the coordination between your many physicians?

   ☐ Outstanding
   ☐ Very Good
   ☐ Fair
   ☐ Poor
   ☐ Nonexistent

4. Did someone review your treatment plan with you?   ☐ Yes   ☐ No

5. Did you receive a written plan of care?   ☐ Yes   ☐ No

6a. Has anyone checked in on you without you calling?   ☐ Yes   ☐ No

6b. Would this be something you would like?   ☐ Yes   ☐ No

7. Do you have any unanswered questions?   ☐ Yes   ☐ No

   _____

   _____

   _____

8. Do you feel you have received enough information and enough time to discuss it with
   those providing it?

   Enough information   ☐ Yes   ☐ No
   Enough time   ☐ Yes   ☐ No

9. Do you have any unmet needs?   ☐ Yes   ☐ No

(Continued on next page)

Figure 3-1. Lehigh Valley Health Network's Gap Analysis Interview Tool
(Continued)

If yes, what are they? _____
_____
_____
_____

10. Where could you have used more help during your cancer journey?

☐ At diagnosis

☐ During treatment planning

☐ During treatment

☐ With financial needs

☐ Support for family

☐ Coordinating with physicians

☐ Other _____
_____
_____
_____

Type of treatment

☐ Surgery

☐ Radiation

☐ Chemotherapy

Type of cancer

_____
_____
_____

Treatment facility

_____
_____
_____

Note. Figure courtesy of Lehigh Valley Health Network. Used with permission.

lem areas were uncovered. Lack of coordination between specialists, insurance issues, financial concerns, and psychosocial problems were specifically identified as areas of disconnect. Although the cancer program had an extensive support services department, patients were unaware of the services available. Communication gaps were revealed; specifically, no process was in place for ensuring that patients received comprehensive information regarding specialty services. Each provider assumed that another was discussing the needed information.

The third step in the complete gap analysis involved conducting a community needs assessment. In 2015, this will be necessary to meet the CoC's navigation standard. According to CoC Standard 3.1, a needs assessment should identify the needs of the population served, the potential to improve cancer health disparities, and gaps in resources (ACoS CoC, 2012). The comprehensive community needs assessment conducted by this organization revealed that disparate populations of the community had significant unmet needs. Language, cultural, and psychosocial barriers existed that prevented informed decision making and resulted in poorer outcomes. The information did not come as a surprise to administration.

As far back as 1989, the American Cancer Society's *Cancer in the Poor: A Report to the Nation* described significant obstacles that poorer populations face in accessing cancer care services that prevent these individuals from obtaining needed care. Such obstacles include widespread financial barriers, logistical barriers, and sociocultural barriers (Wells et al., 2008). The report led to the American Cancer Society's partnership with Harold P. Freeman, MD, in Harlem in 1990 and the development of the first structured patient navigation programs.

Once a gap analysis has been performed, one important final step must be completed when developing and implementing a navigation program: open dialogue with key stakeholders. These individuals' perspectives and concerns are paramount in the success of any navigation program. Primary care and specialty physicians, social workers, financial counselors, and frontline staff in offices and departments provide insight about the unmet needs and challenges that patients face. When key stakeholders misunderstand patient navigation, it can be viewed as suspect. Interference with the patient-physician relationship is often the primary concern. However, once value is demonstrated and stakeholders observe the enhancement of integrated care and comprehensive support provided to patients and families, navigation is embraced. The process is often slow because trust must be earned and value to the entire team demonstrated. However, it is well worth the effort.

Moving forward, assessment tools such as the National Cancer Institute Community Cancer Centers Program's (NCCCP) Navigation Assessment Tool (NAT), as discussed further in Chapter 9, can be used as a framework for goal setting and benchmarking. The 16 categories of NAT, as outlined in Figure 3-2, provide the building blocks of essential navigation program infrastructure (Swanson, Strusowski, Mack, & Degroot, 2012). From basic program development to the demonstrated metrics of a sophisticated navigation program, the NAT can assist with moving a program forward in an organized and systematic fashion.

Structure

When an organization is beginning the development of a navigation program, it is essential to consider the overall objectives it would like to accom-

---

Figure 3-2. Categories of the National Cancer Institute Community Cancer Centers Program Navigation Assessment Tool

- Key stakeholders
- Community partnerships
- Acuity system and risk-factor identification
- Quality improvement
- Marketing
- Percentage of patients offered navigation
- Continuum of care
- Support services
- Reporting tools
- Financial assessment
- Focus on disparate populations
- Navigator responsibilities
- Patient identification
- Navigator training
- Engagement with clinical trials
- Multidisciplinary conference involvement

Note. Based on information from Swanson et al., 2012.

---

plish by providing this service. In addition to industry standards set forth by ACoS CoC to address patients' concerns and improve the care of patients with cancer by ensuring patient-centered care, an organization should identify issues unique to the program that can be addressed for improvement (ACoS CoC, 2011). Examples of areas for consideration and examination are customer service experiences, business objectives, and patient satisfaction scores.

When first confronted with the possibility of having cancer, individuals are forced into a new, unknown, and challenging world that requires them to deal with

- Decision-making tasks involving difficult and confusing choices, which must be performed in a condensed period of time leading to additional decisions and challenges
- Practical tasks, such as scheduling and following through with multiple appointments, often over an extended period of seven to nine months of active treatment
- Psychological tasks, such as the processing of new information, working the cancer diagnosis into family and home life, and integrating the clinical tasks with the emotional features of cancer.

Based on Freeman's (2006) innovative research, the patient navigation model was originally developed to reduce disparities in breast cancer care treatment and mortality rates for minority women. Ongoing research has demonstrated that the navigation model can support all patients with cancer and their families by providing seamless, coordinated, and timely care (Vargas, Ryan, Jackson, Rodriguez, & Freeman, 2008).

One strategy when starting a navigation program might be to build a personalized navigation model targeted to differentiate oncology services within the community, while offering patients with cancer a superior customer experience. Designing a unique program and providing services not otherwise widely available creates a market differentiator from local competitors. To better understand which services would be of value, program planners should include physicians, patients, caregivers, and other community members to gain stakeholders' perspectives. Recognizing that what works for one organization may not work for another because of staffing, volumes, or logistics also is essential. Assessment and analysis of an organization's current state, knowledge of patients' and caregivers' experiences and wants, and physician buy-in and support are all essential elements to investigate and gather before designing and launching a navigation program.

Another consideration may be to start a navigation program by first piloting it with one tumor type. Depending on the current state evaluation, an organization may decide to start small, allowing for greater ease in evaluating and monitoring navigation program outcomes. Analyzing cancer registry volumes according to tumor type can be a first step in determining a pilot's focus. Considerations when analyzing registry data might include identifying tumor sites treated at an organization that is experiencing patient retention problems or in which case volumes may be low or declining. Another consideration is identifying specific opportunities for improvement in a tumor site with established stakeholder engagement and enthusiasm for navigation services. Once the focus for the pilot is identified and the program is implemented, it is then critical to carefully monitor as the pilot proceeds and allow for program deviations when necessary. To properly gauge the pilot's success, consideration should be given to conducting the pilot for a minimum of 6–12 months.

The Design for Six Sigma methodology is another approach one might consider when developing a navigation program (Chowdhury, 2002). Although this methodology originated in the manufacturing industry, it is widely applied to other industries and has shown great success in healthcare. The overall premise is focused on eliminating variation and wasteful processes in order to design an end product of near perfection. The tools used with the Six Sigma methodology precisely define processes that allow for the identification of opportunities for workflow improvement and simplification of practices whenever possible. The use of this approach requires more work upfront, but reduces the likelihood of redesign in the future; therefore, increasing the chances of successfully meeting desired objectives and goals (Chowdhury, 2002). Primary goals one might consider in building a navigation program could include meeting customer expectations, improving the patient and caregiver experience, and ensuring patients receive quality care within suitable time frames.

The development of systems, structures, and processes will allow for timely access to navigators and to services that better prepare patients with cancer and their families for the cancer journey by providing information and education along the way. The intent of program innovation, or creating a new program from thorough research and preparation, is to provide coordinated access to timely care, as well as, to increase access to supportive, rehabilitative, palliative care, and survivorship services. In addition, other objectives include strengthening and supporting the role of primary care providers (PCPs) and community-based specialists in cancer care and improving relationships among cancer team members.

When forming the framework for a navigation program, an initial step is to conduct research to collect pertinent information to aid in decision making. General actions for successful program planning also include

- Identifying successful programs
- Performing a literature search
- Understanding a successful initiative requires an assessment of needs, commitment, and resources
- Creating a shared vision
- Engaging qualified staff with the appropriate skills, experience, and credentials
- Securing the support, motivation, and buy-in of all stakeholders involved.

Many factors should be evaluated before a successful, effective program can be implemented. The importance of a systematic design, using qualitative and quantitative information to gain insight for program development, cannot be overemphasized. This includes researching other organizations that have developed best practice navigation programs; many are open to site visits and telephone interviews with the personnel responsible for starting the program and staff working within the program such as navigators and social workers. The primary objective of such activities is to understand how each model or method works and identify components crucial for success. Figure 3-3 provides a guide of potential questions to consider when conducting informal research of best practice navigation programs.

Another step when designing the navigation program structure is to obtain input from customers, through focus groups with patients and caregivers, including those treated at the facility, as well as, elsewhere in the community. Focus group interviews should be carried out with more than one group and specific customer needs. Questions should center on actual navigator interactions with patients and physicians, as well as resources used. This practice allows an organization to pinpoint the "whats" that customers are looking for and to identify services considered important to incorporate into a navigation program (see Figure 3-4).

Feedback should be obtained from PCPs, specialists, and office personnel within the community to determine critical components of quality care and service delivery as experienced by these groups. This data can be gath-

Figure 3-3. Information to Gather From Established Navigation Programs

Process and Services Provided
- What prompted the development of this program? Was customer feedback obtained, and if so, how was this done?
- Describe the program's evolution.
  - What is the scope of services?
  - Are there common touchpoints during a care path between the navigators and patients?
  - Is a patient transportation service integrated with the patient navigator program?
  - How does the navigator service integrate with the preregistration process?
  - Describe how insurance referrals are obtained.
- Please share high-level process steps.
- How are patients identified and connected to the service?
- Does the organization's call center support the navigation program through its scheduling function?
- How do patient navigators and schedulers interface?
- What scheduling software is used?
- Does the patient navigator facilitate referrals to services outside the organization? If so, how?
- How is information sent from the navigator to the patient? Is it standardized or personalized?
- What are the backgrounds of the patient navigators (clinical/nonclinical)?
- What are the core responsibilities outlined within the navigator job description?
- What is the reporting structure for the patient navigators?
  - What is the staffing complement of the patient navigators, and how was this initially determined?
- Please describe how the organization addresses relevant Health Insurance Portability and Accountability Act (HIPAA) regulations with regard to navigation.

Interactions
- Describe how the patient navigators interact with physician offices.
- Describe how the patient navigators interact with a patient's family and/or caregivers.
- To what extent, if any, is there collaboration with third-party payers?
  - What is the level of buy-in for the program from the physician community (private and owned practices if applicable)?
- How has timeliness of care been improved with the integration of navigators in the organization?

Resources/Utilization of Service
- What start-up resources (e.g., time, dollars) were required?
- What are the funding sources for the program?
- What is the utilization of the service? (current, growth trend?)
  - What functions of the program are assessed to measure success? What metrics are used to measure performance?
- Are there productivity measures for the navigators? What is optimal productivity?
  - To what extent is the patient navigator service marketed to key customer group(s) as well as, to the community in general? What strategies are used?

Lessons Learned
- What were the greatest challenges to successfully implementing the program?
- What could be done differently with benefit of hindsight?

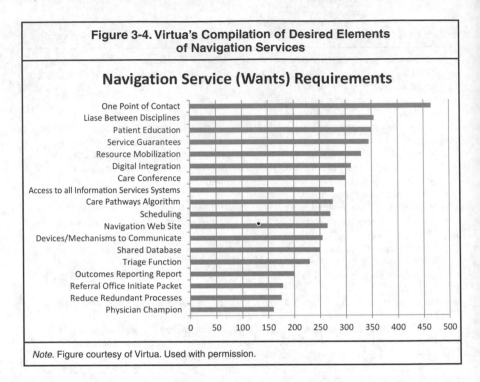

Figure 3-4. Virtua's Compilation of Desired Elements of Navigation Services

Note. Figure courtesy of Virtua. Used with permission.

ered by distributing a survey inclusive of questions to solicit opinions on current services and the projected value of the proposed navigation program. The survey should be comprised of a demographic section, a question section, and an open response section.

Implementation

Once the needs assessment has been conducted and preliminary research collected, it is time to translate customer needs and expectations into measurable outcomes, which can be built into the navigation program design. Development of short-term and long-term goals should be mapped out along with an evaluation plan, which includes specifics of "who, what, and when." Strategy should be addressed, as well as processes, education, and timelines as key objectives for implementation. It is important to include identification of the "whats" for program development; in other words, what components or important features do customers, internal and external, find as a valuable service.

Program implementation also involves developing the navigator's job description, outlining the orientation and training plan, securing necessary equipment, and defining standard operating procedures, policies, and process flow maps. Figures 3-5, 3-6, and 3-7 depict examples of standard operating procedures, policies, and process flow maps respectively; each of these tools provides step-by-step guides of operational functions for a navigation program.

Figure 3-5. Virtua's Navigation Program Standard Operating Procedures

PROCEDURE: Review Referrals
- Director or other designee as assigned will review patient referrals, both faxed referrals and via navigation database, and assign to navigator within 24 hours of referral.
- Navigator will check fax machine and log onto Navigation database **daily** to check for new referrals.
- Patient is now in "active status."
- At end of each week navigator contacts offices to establish check and balance for referrals.

PROCEDURE: Patient Contact
- Within 24 hours of assignment, navigator will contact patient either by phone or face-to-face meeting. Navigator may provide information over the phone or schedule a meeting with the patient.
- When contacting the patient by phone, document in database if a message was left if not able to speak with the patient. Always check physician intake form for permission to leave messages on voicemail.
- When contact is made with patient:
  - Introduce yourself and use the Introduction phone script.
  - Follow standard operating procedure of phone script.
  - Explain your role.
- Review binder sections needed at this time:
  - Address illness, understanding, and provide clarification.
  - Assist patients in understanding treatment options and resources available, including educating eligible patients about appropriate clinical research studies and technologies.
  - Offer psychosocial support and access to resources.
- Review physician orders and assist patient as needed:
  - Fill in navigator intake form during initial contact and input information into database. Or enter information directly into database.
  - Send Introduction letter to referring physician within 10 days of referral.
  - Once a patient is in the navigation program, it is the navigator's responsibility to monitor and follow that patient through the care continuum.

PROCEDURE: Treatment Planning Conference
- Coordinate meeting.
- Prepare patient summary.
- Assess opportunity for clinical trials.
- Review treatment plan against standard of care National Comprehensive Cancer Network guidelines.
- Document appropriately in database and follow recommendations.
- Introduction letter sent to referring physician/primary care physician (PCP) within 5 business days.

(Continued on next page)

Figure 3-5. Virtua's Navigation Program Standard Operating Procedures *(Continued)*

PROCEDURE: Develop Action Plan
- Review physician orders and assist patient as needed.
- Include referrals needed, explain referral process and facilitate scheduling appointments if necessary with surgeon, medical oncologist, radiation oncologist, genetic counseling, and other necessary services.
- Education needed: understanding of illness, emotional impact, treatment options, approximate timetable, pre- and post-surgery.
- Provide appropriate resources in a timely manner to meet patient's specific needs, such as local and national resource list in a binder.
- Provide post-procedure/treatment follow-up assessment and education.
- Put plan in database, including all treatment referrals, appointments, referrals to support services, and barriers to care.
- Send itinerary to patient (email or hardcopy).

PROCEDURE: Ongoing Documentation
- Check daily Task List and document as necessary to keep patient record up to date.
- Contact patient at diagnosis, high stress points, pre- and post-surgery, time of initiation of therapy and any other flag touchpoints as per navigator task list.
- Document noncompliance.
- Document side effects.
- Document handoffs between disciplines and use handoff script if applicable.
- Monitor treatment plan of care and document treatment.

PROCEDURE: Breast Conference
- Plan agenda.
- Attend conferences.

PROCEDURE: Handoffs Between Disciplines
- Call appropriate office and use handoff script.
- Document handoffs between disciplines in database.

PROCEDURE: Surveillance Plan
- Contact disciplines and develop surveillance plan for next 6 months post treatment.
- Discuss with patient further education and connection to resources.
- Identify barriers.
- Email social worker with patient contact information.
- Within 5 business days of treatment conclusion, send letter and surveillance plan to the referring physician/PCP and patient.
- Send patient satisfaction survey to patient with surveillance letter.
- Contact patient to confirm receipt of letter at end of treatment.
- At end of treatment phase, have conversation with patient regarding change of contact information.
- At end of treatment phase, change patient status to "surveillance" in database.

PROCEDURE: End Service/End of Surveillance (6 months post treatment conclusion)
- Last contact phone call, change patient status to "inactive" in database.

Note. Figure courtesy of Virtua. Used with permission.

Figure 3-6. Virtua's Policy Regarding Breast Health Navigation Services

POLICY:
It is the policy of _____ to actively provide care continuity throughout the patient experience in the cancer care system. The breast health navigator ensures breast health patients receive appropriate referrals in a timely manner.

PROCEDURES:
The breast health navigator:
1. Provides patient information about available services, resources, and/or support groups (internal and external) and discusses available community resources.
2. Provides appropriate resources in a timely manner to meet specific patients' needs.
3. Provides patient education and develops patient education tools.
4. Considers language, culture, and age in choosing referral options.
5. Serves as a liaison between the patient and medical staff and services.
6. Explains the referral process with patients and facilitates appointments as needed.
7. Forms relationships with key customers and provides contact information (business cards, etc.) to staff.
8. Attends care conferences, documents appropriately, and carries out physician recommendations.
9. Documents interventions.
10. Serves as a patient advocate by guiding patients through and around barriers in the healthcare system.
11. Monitors patient during the course of care.

Note. Figure courtesy of Virtua. Used with permission.

The development of a comprehensive job description for the navigator position is critical. Ensuring the right person is hired and defining the scope of responsibilities are essential to the success of the navigation program. Nursing and oncology experience are necessary, and case management experience can be of benefit. Each organization, however, must design the job description according to the specific environment and available nursing resources. For example, those with a large cadre of nurses may require three to five years of nursing experience with oncology certified nurse (OCN®) certification. In other areas, limited nursing resources may necessitate decreasing requirements to one to two years of nursing experience with OCN® certification obtained within two years of hire.

Launching the program, spreading the word, gaining buy-in from key stakeholders, and developing a marketing and communication plan are crucial to the project's success. Introduction of the program and the navigators to stakeholders and all who could possibly interact with the navigation program should be targeted in the communication plan. Some outreach strategies to market the program to stakeholders include face-to-face

Figure 3-7. Virtua's Process Flow Maps

Ease of Access Nurse Navigator Process Map

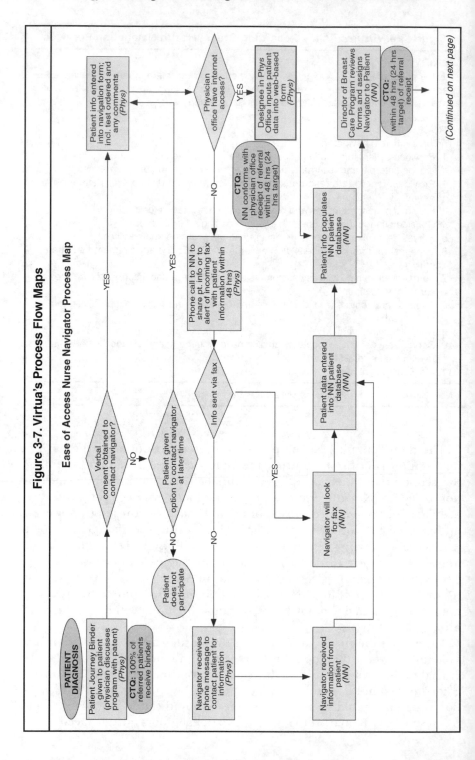

(Continued on next page)

Figure 3-7. Virtua's Process Flow Maps (Continued)

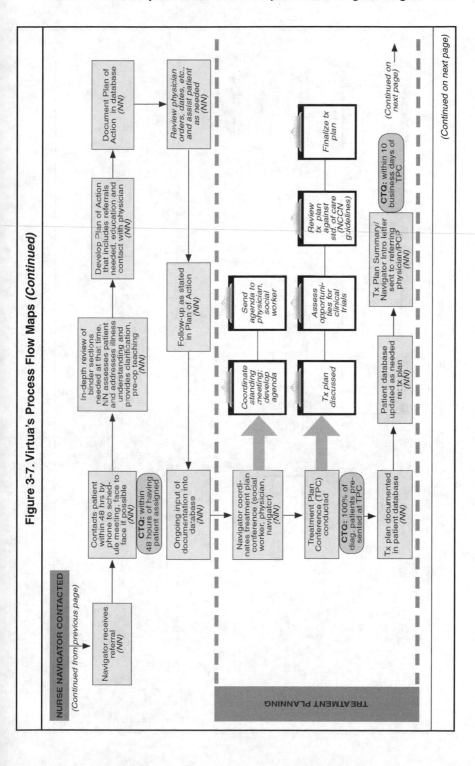

(Continued on next page)

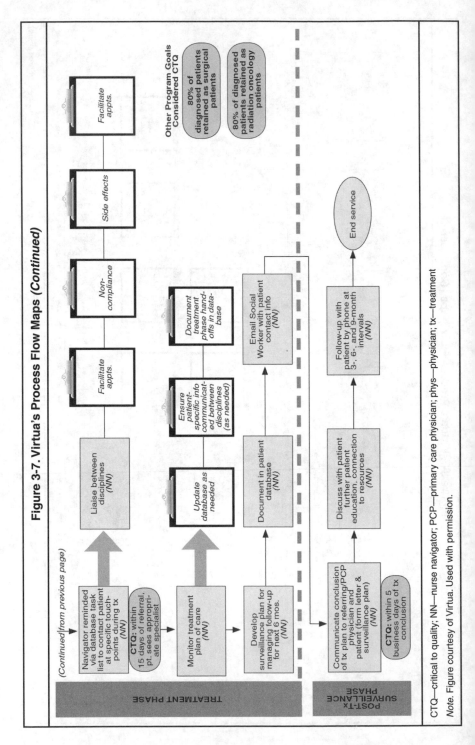

Figure 3-7. Virtua's Process Flow Maps (Continued)

CTQ—critical to quality; NN—nurse navigator; PCP—primary care physician; phys—physician; tx—treatment

Note. Figure courtesy of Virtua. Used with permission.

meetings, attendance at department meetings, and development of marketing materials. Ideally, marketing materials should be personalized, using patient success stories to illustrate services, outcomes, and patient satisfaction.

Program Components and Functions

The overarching objectives in an initiative to develop a navigation service are to (a) enhance patient access to information about cancer diagnosis, (b) facilitate timely access to healthcare services, (c) reduce delays and missed appointments, and (d) provide information on the location of appropriate social services, with the ultimate goal of improving cancer care in the community. Navigators provide education regarding available options to assist in patient decision making and ensure treatments are understood. Utilization of the navigation service considerably improves timeliness and can potentially improve quality of life (Ferrante, Chen, & Kim, 2008).

Navigator involvement may include survivorship support. The transition from active treatment to surveillance can be a stressful time for patients and families. Accustomed to constant assessment and evaluation by the healthcare team, patients, and families entering into the post-treatment phase of survivorship find the transition to be an abrupt change and can experience a sense of provider abandonment. The navigator is well-positioned to make these transitions smooth, providing a road map for the future and ensuring patients are prepared psychologically, as well as physically for a new normal. Survivorship care plans can assist patients in this transition by indicating necessary surveillance and follow-up, possible sequelae, and when and who to call for symptom management.

Despite differences in job descriptions, all navigator roles involve a holistic approach to patient care while centering on quality of life. The navigator is part of a multidisciplinary cancer team whose focus is to empower patients and humanize care. Navigators serve in many roles as educators, care facilitators, counselors, and patient advocates from providing education and psychosocial support to coordinating care across the disciplines and assisting with financial issues (Francz & Simpson, 2013). Navigators must demonstrate competence in oncology, as well as psychosocial and spiritual aspects of care for patients and families. They must have knowledge of health promotion, excellent communication skills, and the ability to form relationships, work well on a team, problem solve, and demonstrate leadership.

Upon identifying program components, actual touchpoints should be determined. These are critical times the navigator should reach out to patients. Figure 3-8 provides examples of various touchpoints, as well as actions

Figure 3-8. Virtua's Navigator Touchpoints and Actions

A. Initial Contact
- Contact patient—48 hours
- Review binder—48 hours
- Treatment plan—ongoing; initially completed with referring physician within 10 days of referral to program

B. Surgical Actions
- Follow-up pre-op testing—48 hours
- Follow-up appointment with surgeon—48 hours
- Follow-up appointment with plastic surgeon—72 hours
- Provide pre-op education—1 week prior to surgery
- Post-op follow-up—48 hours after surgery
- Post-op surgical follow-up—2 days from scheduled appointment

C. Communication Actions with Referring Physician/Primary Care Physician (PCP)
- Send program introduction letter—within 10 business days of assignment to nurse navigator
- Send letter of surveillance—within 5 business days of treatment conclusion

D. Referral Actions
- Refer to support partner—as needed
- Refer to social worker—as needed
- Refer to support group—as needed
- Refer to exercise program—as needed
- Refer to dietitian—as needed
- Refer to lymphedema/physical therapy—as needed
- Refer to Look Good Feel Better program—as needed
- Refer to American Cancer Society—as needed
- Refer to cancer genetics program—as needed
- Refer to Quit Center—as needed

E. Medical Oncology
- Initial appointment for consult—from defining surgery date
- Follow-up for initial consult—2 days after appointment date
- Follow-up first treatment—2 days after appointment date
- Follow-up final treatment—5 days after discharge

F. Radiation Oncology
- Initial appointment for consult—from defining surgery date
- Follow-up for initial consult—2 days after appointment date
- Follow-up final treatment—5 days after discharge

G. Clinical Trials
- Initial intake—ask patient if interested in learning more about eligibility for a clinical trial and offer the assistance of the research nurse
- Post pathology report—if interested, inform patient the research nurse will contact if eligible for a clinical trial

(Continued on next page)

Figure 3-8. Virtua's Navigator Touchpoints and Actions *(Continued)*
H. Surveillance Actions • Refer to social worker—5 days after discharge • Mail PCP follow-up plan—within 5 business days of treatment conclusion • Follow-up 3 months—3 months after discharge • Follow-up 6 months—6 months after discharge • Follow-up 1 year—1 year after discharge
Note. Figure courtesy of Virtua. Used with permission.

to be taken by the navigator with specific time frames assigned. Once again, meeting or exceeding patient expectations and improved quality of care are the overarching goals.

Tracking and monitoring outcomes ideally requires a technology platform or navigation software program. A database or software program serves multiple functions, including contact management, patient tracking, and outcomes reporting. The ability to monitor and track patient needs and outcomes may be accomplished with something as simple as a Microsoft Access database or may involve a commercially available navigation software program. A particularly useful function to consider when purchasing such a software program is its ability to send automated reminders to navigators when specific tasks are due. Chapter 10 further discusses navigation documentation and tracking software considerations.

Navigators and oncology program administrators receive an abundance of anecdotal information from patients, caregivers, and physicians regarding the value of navigation services. However, the development of actual program metrics is an essential piece needed to accurately measure performance. Performance targets should be established based on the unique program goals and objectives (see Table 3-1). A scorecard offers a systematic approach to organizing metrics and tracking program outcomes. Program metrics, which are further discussed in Chapter 9, could encompass quality or service goals, business goals, and customer (both internal and external) satisfaction scores.

Services goals allow program administrators to observe if specific navigator responsibilities are reaching patients within desired timeframes. Physician and patient satisfaction goals with the navigation service should align with the organization's targets for customer satisfaction. Business measures to consider include out-migration and retention metrics. Other metrics may be referrals to clinical trials, referrals to other services, volume of patients navigated, and associated downstream revenue for navigated patients. Consistent demonstration of the success and value of the navigation program will make way for program leadership to consider expanding and growing the program.

Table 3-1. Virtua's Navigation Program Metrics

Metric	Measure	Time
Service Metrics		
1. Within 48 hours, navigator will confirm receipt of referral with referring source Target: 24 hours	Number of hours between documented receipt of referral and documented acknowledgment of referral with the referring source	48 hours
2. Within 48 hours from referral, navigator will be assigned to patient Target: 24 hours	Number of hours between physician office visit date entered into database to date navigator assigned	48 hours
3. Within 48 hours of assignment, navigator will contact patient Target: 24 hours	Number of hours between documented navigator assigned and documented patient contact	48 hours
4. 100% of diagnosed patients receiving navigation service are presented at treatment planning conference within 10 business days of being assigned	Compare the number of patients whose treatment plan occurs within 10 business days of assigned to the total number of patients enrolled	10 business days
5. Within 3 weeks of definitive surgery date, patient sees appropriate oncology specialists for treatment consult	Number of business days from definitive surgery date to documented date of specialist consult appointments	15 business days
6. Within 10 business days of assignment to nurse navigator, program introduction letter is sent to referring physician/primary care physician (PCP)	Number of business days from assignment to nurse navigator information sent to referring physician/PCP	10 business days
7. Within 5 business days of treatment conclusion, letter and surveillance plan sent to referring physician/PCP	Number of business days from date of patient's treatment conclusion to documented date surveillance plan sent to referring physician/PCP	5 business days
Business Metrics		
8. 80% of diagnosed patients are retained as surgical patients	Compare total number of patients enrolled in navigation service requiring surgical intervention to the number of these patients whose surgical intervention is completed at Virtua	65%

(Continued on next page)

Table 3-1. Virtua's Navigation Program Metrics *(Continued)*

Metric	Measure	Time
9. 80% of diagnosed patients are retained as radiation oncology patients	Compare total number of patients enrolled in navigation service requiring radiation oncology services to the number of these patients whose radiation oncology service is completed at Virtua	70%
10. 100% of referred patients receive Patient Journey Binder	Navigator asks patient on first contact if they received patient binder and records in database	100%
11. Achieve mean ≥ 4.5 on a 5-point scale	Patient survey to include question regarding level of satisfaction with patient education	Mean of 4.5
12. Achieve mean ≥ 4.5 on a 5-point scale	Patient survey to include question regarding level of satisfaction with receiving information about available supportive care services	Mean of 4.5
13. Achieve mean ≥ 4.5 on 5-point scale	Patient survey to include question regarding overall satisfaction with navigator service	Mean of 4.5
14. Achieve mean ≥ 4.5 on a 5-point scale	Physician survey to include question regarding level of satisfaction with care coordination	Mean of 4.5
15. Achieve mean ≥ 4.5 on 5-point scale	Physician survey to include question regarding overall satisfaction with navigator service	Mean of 4.5

Note. Table courtesy of Virtua. Used with permission.

Common Hindrances

Working together as a team to create and shape a shared vision for the navigation program creates unity from the beginning. Obtaining physician buy-in and ongoing support is crucial for ongoing success. Understanding reasons for resistance and developing strategies to address these will aid in overcoming opposition and securing provider commitment. It may be necessary for a continued presence by navigators in physicians' offices, as well as inpatient and outpatient units, to ensure navigation services are fully understood and utilization is maximized.

Proper staffing can be difficult to justify, primarily because navigation at this point is not a reimbursable service. Medicare changes, effective January 2013, reimburse for nursing services, which transition inpatients to post–acute care and other healthcare settings. New payment codes were created for transitional care management to prevent complications and readmissions. The two Current Procedural Terminology (CPT®) codes to date that may be used for transitional care management services are 99495 and 99496. Although both require communication with the patient or caregiver within two business days of discharge (via direct contact, telephone, or electronic mechanisms), the complexity of medical decision making and the interval for the face-to-face visit are the distinguishing elements between these two codes. The 99495 CPT code is used with medical decision making of at least moderate complexity and a face-to-face visit within 14 calendar days of discharge, whereas 99496 requires high-complexity medical decision making and a face-to-face visit within 7 calendar days of discharge (American Academy of Family Physicians, 2013). These codes are only reimbursable for nurse practitioners, clinical nurse specialists, certified nurse midwives, and other primary care professionals providing the services (Shah, 2012). Considering that approximately 71% of the current National Coalition of Oncology Nurse Navigators' membership hold a bachelor, associate, or diploma degree in nursing (Francz & Simpson, 2013), reimbursement for navigation services in most healthcare systems is not likely at this time.

Once established, navigation programs must be able to prove value to the organization in order to secure ongoing support. Organizations will expect navigation programs to demonstrate a return on investment. Although measuring this can be challenging, it can be done. Thought must be given upfront about metrics to substantiate benefits of the program. This is where a thorough current state evaluation is most important. Establishing baseline data on each of the tumor sites, current out-migration statistics, market share, and patient and physician satisfaction will provide quantifiable evidence of the navigation initiatives' success. The organization's finance department can assist in approximating downstream revenue for each cancer case retained or received through the navigation program's interventions. Some strategies and considerations when attempting to assign program value and focus on specific metrics to demonstrate successes include

- Creating a formalized process to measure the impact of navigators within the healthcare system
- Establishing clearly defined goals and keeping a scorecard of progress made toward these goals
- Tracking patients who out-migrate to other healthcare systems and the associated reasons for it
- Noting patient retention and comparing program volumes over time and identifying trends

- Evaluating patient volumes for surgical, medical, and radiation oncology since the inception of the navigation program to determine if volumes have increased.

Lack of communication between the navigator and the multidisciplinary team can be one of the most stressful challenges for navigators. Open dialogue among cancer team members is extremely important to effectively communicate patients' care plans and allow navigators to properly guide patients. Navigators have reported anecdotally that at times, the patients seemed to be doing the navigating because sometimes patients were relaying to the navigator the required treatment plan information rather than the physician or care team. Weekly case conferences or individual team meetings with attending physicians can assist in alleviating this problem.

Tips for Launching and Sustaining Navigation Programs

Fortunately, ample information about the implementation and evaluation of navigation programs is available throughout oncology literature. Figure 3-9 highlights examples of practical resources, as well as evidence-based literature pertinent to navigation program development. However, given the numerous types and structures used, each organization needs to develop a navigation model that best serves the needs of individual communities and key stakeholders. After doing a complete needs assessment and gap analysis, such needs will be apparent. Regardless of the type of navigation program to be implemented, some basic tips for a successful launch include

- Aligning the navigation program to the organization's business strategy
- Obtaining organizational support for the program by building consensus with referring physicians, payers, administration, advocacy, and support networks (Schafer & Swisher, 2006)
- Identifying a physician champion who is knowledgeable about healthcare barriers, physician and patient satisfaction, and marketing to promote the positive impact of navigation (Koutnik-Fotopoulos, 2010)
- Including experts from finance, information technology, legal, and each of the oncology departments on the project development team
- Maintaining open and honest communication with all stakeholders and eliciting feedback to gain commitment (Remember that one can never communicate enough, and in the absence of communication, people will fill in the gaps with misperceptions and assumptions.)
- Developing a comprehensive job description outlining the position's exact duties and responsibilities as well as required core competencies
- Ensuring comprehensive training, including organizational, departmental, and community cultures
- Identifying organizational and community resources, which can be used to assist patients

---

Figure 3-9. Literature and Practical Resources Related to Navigation Program Development and Implementation

Program Development

Association of Community Cancer Centers. (2009). Cancer care patient navigation: Practical guide. Retrieved from http://www.accc-cancer.org/education/patientnavigation -PN2009-toc.asp

Association of Community Cancer Centers. (2009). Cancer care patient navigation: Tools for community cancer centers. Retrieved from https://www.accc-cancer.org/education/ patientnavigation-PNT2009-toc.asp

C-Change. (2009). What is cancer patient navigation? Retrieved from http://www.cancer patientnavigation.org

Freeman, H.P. (2004). A model patient navigation program: Breaking down barriers to ensure that all individuals with cancer receive timely diagnosis and treatment. *Oncology Issues, 19*(5), 44–46.

Koutnik-Fotopoulos, E. (2010). Implementing and growing a navigation program. *Journal of Oncology Navigation and Survivorship, 1,* 6–7.

Pederson, A., & Hack, T.F. (2010). Pilots of oncology health care: A concept analysis of the patient navigator role. *Oncology Nursing Forum, 37,* 55–60. doi:10.1188/10.ONF .55-60

Schafer, J., & Swisher, J. (2006). Cancer care coordination with nurse navigators. *Sg2 Health Care Intelligence.* Retrieved from http://www.sg2.com

Program Assessment and Evaluation

Campbell, C., Craig, J., Eggert, J., & Bailey-Dorton, C. (2010). Implementing and measuring the impact of patient navigation at a comprehensive community cancer center. *Oncology Nursing Forum, 37,* 61–68. doi:10.1188/10.ONF.61-68

Freund, K.M., Battaglia, T.A., Calhoun, E., Dudley, D.J., Fiscella, K., Paskett, E., ... Roetzheim, R.G. (2008). National Cancer Institute Patient Navigation Research Program: Methods, protocol, and measures. *Cancer, 113,* 3391–3399. doi:10.1002/ cncr.23960

Hopkins, J., & Mumber, M.P. (2009). Patient navigation through the cancer care continuum: An overview. *Journal of Oncology Practice, 5,* 150–152. doi:10.1200/ JOP.0943501

Koh, C., Nelson, J.M., & Cook, P.F. (2011). Evaluation of a patient navigation program. *Clinical Journal of Oncology Nursing, 15,* 41–48. doi:10.1188/11.CJON.41-48

Swanson, J.R., Strusowski, P., Mack, N., & Degroot, J. (2012). Growing a navigation program: Using the NCCCP Navigation Assessment Tool. *Oncology Issues, 27*(4), 36–45.

Varner, A., & Murph, P. (2010). Cancer patient navigation: Where do we go from here? *Oncology Issues, 25*(3), 50–53.

- Establishing an acuity system to appropriately allocate navigation resources (Swanson et al., 2012)
- Defining metrics, which can be used to substantiate value of the program (for example, improving the time to diagnosis, reducing time to initiation of cancer treatment, increasing patient satisfaction with care, and improving cost-effectiveness) (Freund et al., 2008)
- Developing a marketing strategy to garner referrals from both PCPs and specialty physicians

- Developing tracking and documentation tools to provide standardized, quantifiable data
- Eliciting ongoing feedback from patients and physicians through a standardized customer satisfaction tool (see Figure 3-10).

Expanding for Future Growth

Once established, a navigation program should be assessed annually; this is essential for program viability and future growth. Using the metrics and outcome measures established for the program, data collected can be analyzed against the baseline to determine areas needing additional attention and those requiring further development. Successes can be replicated and areas of unmet need prioritized with specific interventions and goal setting.

Tools such as the NCCCP's NAT can be used to establish a baseline assessment of the navigation program and provide a framework for expanding and advancing the program forward. For instance, when assessing the Acuity Systems (Risk Factors) category, perhaps the baseline identifies no system is available currently to assess a patient's risk factors. Using the NCCCP's NAT (Swanson et al., 2012), a goal can be established first to develop a disease-specific tool followed by the development of well-defined referral processes for identified issues when using the tool. The NAT can provide the roadmap to increase the multiple facets of patient navigation from one level of development to the next. Chapter 9 presents more detail on the NAT and program assessment.

Feedback from patients, physicians, and members of the navigation team need to be obtained and evaluated. Several survey tools are available to obtain baseline data and then at regular intervals to assess progress toward program goals. Physician and patient evaluation of the program is essential. In addition, an advisory group of key stakeholders, including frontline office staff, referring specialty and primary providers, members of the navigation team, and even patients, can be established to provide ongoing feedback to further develop and improve the program. This engagement will not only assist with assessment and improvement of services, but is also a great marketing tool.

Annually, program outcomes and metrics should be reviewed to ensure these are still reflective of progress, realistic, and valuable to the program. Progress and attainment of previously established goals should be identified and new goals established. Identification of barriers and challenges must also be assessed. Knowing the challenges assists in designing interventions to overcome or adapt to them.

Systems and structures need to be critically assessed and analyzed to ensure they are adequately supporting the navigation program and patient needs. This includes an understanding of what is and is not working well.

Figure 3-10. Navigation Patient Satisfaction Survey						
	Strongly Disagree					Strongly Agree
	0	1	2	3	4	5
1. It was easy to get through to the nurse navigator.	☐	☐	☐	☐	☐	☐
2. My calls were returned in a timely manner.		☐	☐	☐	☐	☐
3. The nurse navigator was courteous.	☐	☐	☐	☐	☐	☐
4. My navigator treated me like an individual.	☐	☐	☐	☐	☐	☐
5. My navigator was a key member of my healthcare team.	☐	☐	☐	☐	☐	☐
6. My navigator helped me get answers to my cancer care questions.	☐	☐	☐	☐	☐	☐
7. I valued working with my navigator.	☐	☐	☐	☐	☐	☐
8. My navigator answered questions in a manner I could easily understand.	☐	☐	☐	☐	☐	☐
9. My navigator provided support to my family when needed.	☐	☐	☐	☐	☐	☐
10. The support I got from my navigator helped decrease my anxiety.	☐	☐	☐	☐	☐	☐
11. The support I got from my navigator helped me to complete my treatment.	☐	☐	☐	☐	☐	☐
12. The services my navigator referred me to met my needs.	☐	☐	☐	☐	☐	☐
13. My navigator helped to expedite my care.	☐	☐	☐	☐	☐	☐
14. My navigator helped to problem-solve during my treatment.	☐	☐	☐	☐	☐	☐

15. How many times have you been in contact with your navigator?	Once ☐	2–3 times ☐	4–8 times ☐	More than 9 ☐

16. How would you rate your overall experience with your navigator?	Poor 0 ☐ 1 ☐ 2 ☐ 3 ☐ 4 ☐ 5 ☐ Excellent

17. What did you like best about having a navigator? Comments:

18. What can we do better? Comments:

If you would like a phone call to address any concerns, please check the box and provide your name and a number where you can be reached during the day.	☐

Name:	Phone number:

Note. Figure courtesy of Lehigh Valley Health Network. Used with permission.

For example, whether referrals are received in a timely manner from various departments and specialty areas should be evaluated, and whether any communication difficulties exist between specific areas and possible strategies to address these should be considered. Additionally, culturally appropriate education materials should be available and written at the patient population's comprehension level. The program marketing materials should be reviewed to determine if they meet the intended purpose.

A community assessment should be performed every three years to address healthcare disparities and barriers to care for patients. ACoS CoC (2012) will mandate community assessments in 2015. The fluidity of communities supports an interval assessment not only to identify unmet needs but, also to identify changes in cancer incidence, morbidity and mortality, and/or cultural or socioeconomic shifts within the population. The navigation program will need to reflect the changes occurring within the community and utilize that information to establish additional objectives for expansion and improvement.

Organizational priorities, as well as cancer program initiatives, need to be integrated into future goals. With difficulty in establishing a clear return on investment for navigation programs, it is imperative that the navigation program show support for organizational priorities.

Using the data collected, the team can successfully identify areas for program improvement and develop the strategies necessary to address these. Formalized tools, such as a SWOT analysis, can help guide the process by outlining successes and challenges. A SWOT analysis consists of a simple assessment of strengths, weaknesses, opportunities, and threats. Such an assessment and analysis can serve as the springboard to develop and prioritize goals and strategies to take a navigation program to the next level.

Conclusion

Navigation programs must be seen not only as a means to meet accreditation requirements, but also as a mechanism to improve patient outcomes, increase satisfaction, mitigate out-migration, contain costs, and differentiate the organization in the community. In the age of consumer-driven health care, it is necessary for healthcare systems to be innovative in navigation program development and to offer personalized services to educated consumers in a competitive market. The successful design of a navigation program includes developing services to meet customers' needs and wishes, which will ultimately improve the overall patient experience within the organization and community. A navigation program should be created not only with success in mind, but also sustainability and ease of replication for future expansion. It is important to remember that a navigation program cannot be all things to all people, rather realistic goals and expectations need to be established and constantly reinforced. Clear program objectives, which are communicated effectively, are crucial to the success of any navigation program.

References

American Academy of Family Physicians. (2013). Frequently asked questions: Transitional care management. Retrieved from http://www.aafp.org/dam/AAFP/documents/practice_management/payment/TCMFAQ.pdf

American Cancer Society. (1989). *Cancer in the poor: A report to the nation.* Atlanta, GA: Author.

American College of Surgeons Commission on Cancer. (2011, August 31). New Commission on Cancer accreditation standards gain support from four national cancer advocacy organizations: Patient-centered approach enables cancer patients to become partners in their own care [Press release]. Retrieved from http://www.facs.org/news/2011/coc-standards0811.html

American College of Surgeons Commission on Cancer. (2012). *Cancer program standards 2012: Ensuring patient-centered care* [v.1.2.1, released January 2014]. Retrieved from http://www.facs.org/cancer/coc/programstandards2012.pdf

Chowdhury, S. (2002). *Design for Six Sigma: The revolutionary process for achieving extraordinary profits.* Chicago, IL: Dearborn Trade Publishing.

Ferrante, J.M., Chen, P.-H., & Kim, S. (2008). The effect of patient navigation on time to diagnosis, anxiety, and satisfaction in urban minority women with abnormal mammograms: A randomized controlled trial. *Journal of Urban Health, 85,* 114–124. doi:10.1007/s11524-007-9228-9

Francz, S.L., & Simpson, K.D. (2013). Oncology nurse navigators: A snapshot of their educational background, compensation, and day-to-day roles and responsibilities. *Oncology Issues, 28*(1), 36–43.

Freeman, H.P. (2006). Patient navigation: A community centered approach to reducing cancer mortality. *Journal of Cancer Education, 21*(1), S11–S14.

Freund, K.M., Battaglia, T.A., Calhoun, E., Dudley, D.J., Fiscella, K., Paskett, E., ... Roetzheim, R.G. (2008). National Cancer Institute Patient Navigation Research Program: Methods, protocol, and measures. *Cancer, 113,* 3391–3399. doi:10.1002/cncr.23960

Koutnik-Fotopoulos, E. (2010). Implementing and growing a navigation program. *Journal of Oncology Navigation and Survivorship, 1*(6), 6–7. Retrieved from http://issuu.com/aonn/docs/jons_november2010

Schafer, J., & Swisher, J. (2006). Cancer care coordination with nurse navigators. *Sg2 Health Care Intelligence.* Retrieved from http://www.sg2.com

Shah, T. (2012). Lessons learned from nurse navigation. *Sg2 Health Care Intelligence.* Retrieved from http://www.sg2.com

Swanson, J.R., Strusowski, P., Mack, N., & Degroot, J. (2012). Growing a navigation program: Using the NCCCP Navigation Assessment Tool. *Oncology Issues, 27*(4), 36–45. Retrieved from http://www.accc-cancer.org/oncology_issues/articles/julaug2012/JA2012-Swanson.pdf

Vargas, R.B., Ryan, G.W., Jackson, C.A., Rodriguez, R., & Freeman, H.P. (2008). Characteristics of the original patient navigation programs to reduce disparities in the diagnosis and treatment of breast cancer. *Cancer, 113,* 426–433. doi:10.1002/cncr.23547

Wells, K.J., Battaglia, T.A., Dudley, D.J., Garcia, R., Greene, A., Calhoun, E., ... Raich, P.C. (2008). Patient navigation: State of the art or is it science? *Cancer, 113,* 1999–2010. doi:10.1002/cncr.23815

CHAPTER 4

Navigation Considerations When Working With Patients

Sharon S. Gentry, RN, MSN, AOCN®, CBCN®, CBEC, and Jean B. Sellers, RN, MSN

Introduction

Patient navigation is a concept used since 1990 to help improve patients' quality of life (QOL) and health outcomes when facing a cancer diagnosis (Dohan & Schrag, 2005; Freeman & Rodriguez, 2011). Successful navigation processes ensure that patients move rapidly through the continuum of care and healthcare system by identifying and resolving barriers to care (Dohan & Schrag, 2005).

According to the principles set forth by patient navigation pioneer Harold P. Freeman, MD, there is "a need to define the point at which navigation begins and the point at which navigation ends" (Freeman & Rodriguez, 2011, p. 3541). In today's healthcare system, it is difficult to have a consistent method with a standard beginning point of patient navigation, especially when looking at multiple portals of entry in any given system. A number of factors lead to this inability. Institutions are large and do not always have a smooth process in which patients are able to easily enter the system. Often, a cancer diagnosis will be the first experience that individuals encounter when entering a medical system. Certain communities and patient populations are vulnerable to having poorer outcomes. Underserved populations, including racial and ethnic minorities, have reduced access to care and fewer options for treatment, which make it difficult for patients to receive care (Freeman & Rodriguez, 2011).

The evolution of patient navigation has shown that, when implemented successfully, processes can improve health outcomes of patients with cancer by eliminating barriers to care and ensuring that patients receive prompt treatment (Freeman & Rodriguez, 2011; Natale-Pereira, Enard, Nevarez, & Jones, 2011). Therefore, patient-centered processes are important in order to ensure that patients have navigation support regardless of geographic location, socioeconomic status, or entry point into the healthcare system.

Changing the quality of health care and implementing patient-centered processes requires collaboration and teamwork from multidisciplinary clinics within the healthcare organization, as well as private healthcare practices and surrounding communities served. The American College of Surgeons Commission on Cancer (ACoS CoC, 2012) along with the Joint Commission, the National Committee for Quality Assurance, the Institute for Healthcare Improvement, and the American Hospital Association, has defined and revised hospital and cancer program standards to ensure that goals are patient focused. In particular, the 2015 phase-in standards driven by ACoS CoC (2012) have taken a patient-centered approach, whereby patient and family engagement is key to optimal implementation of these standards.

Patient- and Family-Centered Care

Patient-centered care requires enhanced communication among healthcare providers and has the potential to improve patient satisfaction while decreasing barriers to care (Hook, Ware, Siler, & Packard, 2012). Many institutions understand the importance of integrating the concept of patient- and family-centered care into existing delivery models. Studies have shown that including the perspectives of patients and families in the planning, delivery, and evaluation of care can improve the quality of health care and safety, as well as increase patient and provider satisfaction (Palos & Hare, 2011). These perspectives can support the institution to provide a better quality of health care, improved outcomes, wiser allocation of resources, increased patient and staff satisfaction, increased safety, and greater customer loyalty (Lusk & Fater, 2013).

Patient and family advisory boards are able to ensure that the voices of patients and families are heard (Leonhart, Bonin, & Pagel, 2008). Such input can identify opportunities to improve care, develop a collaborative atmosphere while reducing medical errors, diminish length of stay, and decrease staff turnover rates. Advisory board members can participate in a number of committees within the health system including ethics, patient safety, quality improvement, facility design, and patient education committees. Patient and family advisory board members provide an inexpensive venue to solicit input regarding patient-centered activities. Members can work with community-based organizations and health agencies to identify specific community health disparities. Unfortunately, evidence is limited as to whether this culture has been embraced within the outpatient or community settings.

ACoS CoC (2012) requires a community needs assessment to drive resource allocation for the new patient-centered standards. Patient and family advisory boards can be engaged in this assessment to identify and break down cultural barriers contributing to disparities in health and health care. This input can be extremely helpful in the development of the navigation program and other patient safety processes.

Use of a Patient-Centered Needs Assessment

Major contributors for poor outcomes can include access to care and how services are used and delivered. Delivery and access of cancer care for the poor and underserved is heightened by racial and ethnic disparities (Natale-Pereira et al., 2011). Common barriers affecting this population include the lack of available programs for screening and early detection, low levels of health literacy, failure to follow up with suspicious findings, and lack of access to care for treatment. An important outcome of the needs assessment is an understanding of the population served, healthcare disparities, available community resources, and identified gaps and barriers to care that many patients with cancer face (Palos & Hare, 2011).

As presented in Chapter 3, a comprehensive needs assessment will drive the development of navigation processes. The institution's vision, mission, and philosophy of care should be defined and communicated clearly throughout the healthcare organization, as well as to patients, families, and others in the community. As healthcare organizations determine which model of navigation to implement, it is important to have physician support and to include other departments or staff, including primary care physicians (PCPs), members of community agencies, and those who interact in the care of patients with cancer, during the program planning and role development (Advisory Board Company, 2011; Wells et al., 2008).

Patient-Centered Navigation Processes

While many cancer programs are working to develop individualized navigation processes, it is important to note that nurse navigators add value in multiple ways. Healthcare institutions have developed navigation models hoping to increase provider efficiency, enhance treatment adherence, reduce readmissions, improve care coordination, and increase patient and referring provider satisfaction (Fillion et al., 2012; Koh, Nelson, & Cook, 2011). Being able to eliminate barriers, enhance communication, and improve access to care across the continuum brings value to the nurse navigator role. The role description, along with the structure of the process, is critical to success. Additional research is necessary to determine which profession is best to assume this role, as many of the value dimensions that healthcare organizations are seeking can be achieved through less expensive navigation models that focus on lay navigators or other healthcare professionals. Collaboration among multiple professions and the outcomes of the community needs assessment will enable programs to determine the appropriate model, the navigator job description, and the services provided (Wells et al., 2008).

Patient-centered care, as defined by the Institute of Medicine (IOM), requires high-quality communication between patients and clinicians, together with support from educated patients and families. Given the complexity of cancer care, a patient- and family-centered approach to the delivery of care is critical to improve patients' physical and psychosocial outcomes, safety, and satisfaction and reduce barriers to care (IOM, 2001). Nurse and/or lay navigators are in a unique position to provide emotional support by helping patients to recognize and identify their fears and misunderstandings that accompany a cancer diagnosis (Bickell & Paskett, 2013). Although many will agree that considerable overlap exists within each navigation discipline, the oncology nurse brings the ability to assess both the clinical and psychosocial dimension (Brown et al., 2012; McMullen, 2013). This promotes an environment that is patient centered and reflected throughout the cancer continuum. The development of this trusting relationship is critical in order to reduce fear and enhance communication between patients and healthcare providers. Doing so will promote positive outcomes and a positive experience (Dohan & Schrag, 2005; McMullen, 2013; Natale-Pereira et al., 2011; Wells et al., 2008).

Access to Patient Navigation

In order to reduce the community- and population-specific barriers to care, patient navigation uses a variety of models, each designed to meet unique patient and community needs. Freeman's principles of patient navigation (see Figure 1-1 in Chapter 1) reflect the need to operate across the boundaries of current communities in order to meet the patient's needs at any given time (Freeman & Rodriguez, 2011). Navigators help individuals overcome barriers to care and navigate through the screening, treatment, survivorship, and end-of-life care continuum. The following examples of patient navigation models depict various points of entry for patients along with significant findings associated with each.

Patient Navigation Models

Freeman's model used community members, known as lay navigators, who received special training in order to better access cancer screenings for the underserved and poor populations (Freeman & Rodriguez, 2011; New-man-Horm, 2005). Patient navigators met with patients in the community to encourage breast cancer screening. The success of this model is well demonstrated by data presented in Figure 4-1. The dramatic improvements noted from 1990 to 2011 were attributed to the provision of free and low-cost mammograms along with breast health examinations and patient navigation processes.

Horner et al. (2013) designed a nurse navigation program based on the patient-centered model of care described in the Institute of Medicine's report, *Cancer Care for the Whole Patient: Meeting Psychosocial Health Needs* (Adler & Page, 2008). It was designed to test the effectiveness of patients receiving navigation services from oncology nurse navigators. Patients were assigned to a nurse navigator upon diagnosis at the healthcare facility. The nurse navigators received special training by a psychologist who reviewed psychosocial competencies, including communication strategies, interpersonal skills, depression assessment, and strategies to use when addressing depression. This training helped the navigators improve their skills in caring for patients with cancer.

Hook et al. (2012) explored a community-based model of nurse navigation for patients in a rural setting to identify and resolve barriers to care while providing additional support and education. Navigation services were offered to newly diagnosed patients with breast cancer at a rural physician clinic. The process was implemented at the beginning of the diagnostic workup and extended until the completion of treatment. More than 450 patients were navigated during a three-year period. The services were provided by telephone, clinic consultations, and hospital visits. The patient satisfaction surveys indicated that the patients were highly satisfied with the nurse navigation services; specifically, 97% felt better prepared as a result of the navigator's guidance and provision of education.

Pedersen and Hack (2011) performed an analysis of the British Columbia Patient Navigation Model. This model was developed as a means to prevent fragmentation in the care of patients with cancer and identified gaps in the delivery of cancer care for the community. Patient navigation was initiated at

---

Figure 4-1. Harlem Breast Cancer Data

1990 (N = 606 patients with breast cancer)	2011 (N = 325 patients with breast cancer)
• 6% of women presented with stage 1 breast cancer • 49% of women presented with stage 3 or 4 • Five-year survival: 39%	• 41% of women presented with stage 0 or 1 • 21% had stage 3 or 4 • Five-year survival: 70%

Note. Based on information from Freeman & Rodriguez, 2011.

the onset of these gaps, which were identified as (a) the time of initial diagnosis, (b) the completion of active treatment, and (c) the beginning of palliative care. Program planners felt that these three groups of patients would require the most supportive care.

Seek and Hogle (2007) identified a community nurse navigation model using a nurse practitioner to evaluate patients with lung cancer. The nurse navigator became involved when patients presented with a biopsy or were suspected to have non-small cell lung cancer. The navigator ensured that all diagnostic tests were performed prior to the multidisciplinary lung cancer clinic. Once the treatment plan was agreed upon, the summary was forwarded to all healthcare professionals involved in the patient's care. The nurse navigator reviewed the summary in detail with the patient and caregiver to ensure their understanding of the plan of care. Prior to the implementation of this model, patients experienced an average wait time of one to three months from diagnosis to initiation of treatment. After implementation of the model, this time decreased to two weeks. The patients reported being completely satisfied with the services received at the multidisciplinary lung cancer clinic but expressed dissatisfaction with not having the nurse navigator's services continue once care was assigned to a primary physician.

Results of the National Cancer Institute (NCI) Patient Navigation Research Program (PNRP) were published in the October 2012 issue of *Cancer Epidemiology, Biomarkers and Prevention*. Trained patient navigators, including nurses, case managers, community health workers, social workers, and lay individuals, assessed patients in a given healthcare or community environment and demonstrated the ability to reduce the time from abnormal cancer finding to diagnosis, which in turn ensured that treatment was started sooner (Battaglia et al., 2012; Fiscella et al., 2012; Hoffman et al., 2012; Markossian, Darnell, & Calhoun, 2012; Paskett et al., 2012). The results clearly demonstrated the economic value of linking patients who present with abnormal findings from breast, cervical, prostate, or colorectal cancer examinations with navigators. The navigators in each study were connected with patients early in the process and reduced the time from an abnormal screening to a definitive diagnosis in underserved populations. Although it was agreed that not all patients require the skills of a navigator, those who have the potential to be high risk or who may demonstrate noncompliance with follow-up tended to benefit the most, and navigation of these patients has the potential to save the most money for the health system (Byers, 2012).

Lorhan et al. (2013) developed a patient navigation model using volunteers recruited from the existing healthcare volunteer program. Training sessions were developed to ensure that volunteers knew and understood navigation roles and responsibilities. The sessions included information related to developing communication skills, addressing barriers to care, and increasing knowledge regarding access to care and education. The program demonstrated the importance of lay patient navigators and the ability to provide supportive care to patients at the time of diagnosis. This program was different from Freeman's model in that the focus was not on the screening portion of the continuum of care but rather was initiated at the time of a cancer diagnosis. The lay navigator received the referral and contacted the patient by telephone to determine the patient/family situation. The second contact was made with the patient on the day of the oncology appointment. At that time, the navigator obtained more data related to health system barriers to care and provided orientation to the cancer center. The third contact was made one week after the first oncology appointment via a telephone call to see if the patient had any additional questions or experienced any barriers to care. Positive results from both patients and navigators indicated that this model was able to successfully meet the needs of patients.

The University of North Carolina Cancer Network's Lay Navigation Model (UNC Lineberger Comprehensive Cancer Center, n.d.-b) was initiated by members of the community, healthcare organization, and county commissioners who requested a program in which patients with cancer would receive additional supportive care during treatment. The program was a collaboration between the volunteer program at a local hospital and an academic medical center 240 miles away. A training manual was developed that included a description of the lay navigator's role, a basic understanding of cancer and health literacy, principles of infection control and patient safety, aspects of effective communication, and setting professional boundaries. Lay navigators were volunteers recruited from the community and were required to complete hospital orientation, which included background checks, Health Insurance Portability and Accountability Act (HIPAA) training, infection and safety control, health literacy education, cancer education, and communication skills and training. A full-time volunteer coordinator collaborated with the nurse navigator to ensure that patient referrals were carefully matched with lay navigators based upon identified needs. Referrals into the program came from local PCPs, community care clinics, healthcare organizations, public health departments, and other agencies, as well as patient self-referral. The identified goals from both healthcare organizations was to provide necessary skills and training to ensure that lay navigators had the support and confidence to deliver safe care within the scope of the defined role and job description. The types of support given to patients included transportation, respite care, meal preparation, social outings, emotional support, and the provision of information about local resources. Navigator visits were provided in a variety of settings including patients' homes, physicians' offices, and at other agreed-upon locations. A key element to the program's success was the ongoing training of the lay navigators.

The current healthcare system is in need of change. Navigation services eliminate barriers to care to enable patients to move rapidly across the care continuum. The role of the navigator must be defined in order to set the standard for competencies, training, and certification (Dohan & Schrag,

2005) and to prevent navigators from becoming a catchall for nonrelated navigation tasks such as administrative or clerical duties. Navigation programs must be patient centered and include representation from healthcare organizations, as well as the communities to be served. This will ensure that navigation processes derive value for the organization and that patients have access to necessary care regardless of the portal of entry (Byers, 2012).

Patient Workflow

The navigation workflow is bidimensional in nature: patient centered and healthcare system oriented (Fillion et al., 2012). Considering the needs of patients along with system characteristics promotes continuity of care. Nurse navigators may work in the outreach/screening part of the care continuum and oversee nonclinical staff to increase cancer screening rates (Cascella & Keren, 2012; Koh et al., 2011; Lagrosa, 2011) or may interact with patients at diagnosis, navigating them throughout the treatment phase and the transition into survivorship or end-of-life care (Arias, 2012; Eley, Rogers-Clark, & Murray, 2008; Wilcox & Bruce, 2010). No matter where the role exists in the care continuum, nurse navigators possess oversight of the comprehensive care needs, provide education and advocacy for patients, link patients to networks of professional and community resources, and act as a distinct, constant contact to enhance psychosocial care (Doll et al., 2007).

Enhanced patient care and smooth workflow among systems is a major objective of patient navigation programs. To understand current processes and identify where systems can be improved, it is critical for navigators to view the healthcare system through the eyes of the patient and document the operational workflow to gain a perspective on ineffective processes and communication gaps.

A flow diagram captures how navigators work with a patient population embedded in the system of care. It gives a visual outline of patient entry points, specific patient interventions, where referrals are made to others in the healthcare system, interrelationships of community programs, and where the process ends. Blaseg (2009) described the Billings Clinic workflow from referral sources through discharge by using a flowchart with specific navigator tasks and contact points (see Figure 4-2). This process is supported by a fishbone diagram to visualize multidisciplinary team contributions that promote increased patient satisfaction and high-quality patient-centered care (see Figure 4-3).

Shockney (2011) described the use of a linear flowchart as a prerequisite to navigate patients. Figure 4-4 depicts a patient flow process in breast care, but the general flow process principles can be applied to any disease-specific or high-risk population. Documentation of care processes needs to be detailed in regard to who provides care for the patient, where services are performed, when and how various aspects of care are completed, and why each

Figure 4-2. Billings Clinic's Care Navigation Referral Process

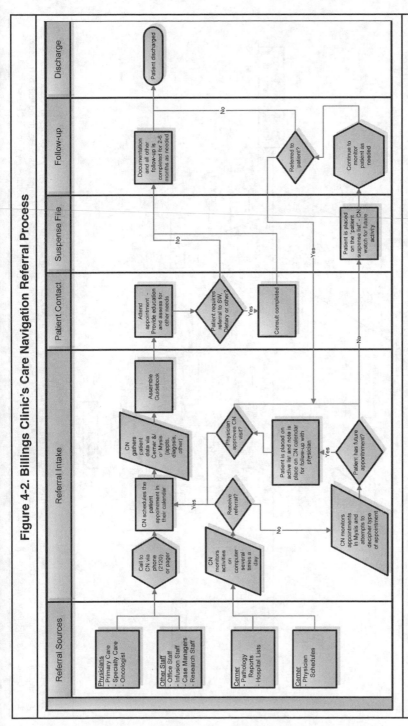

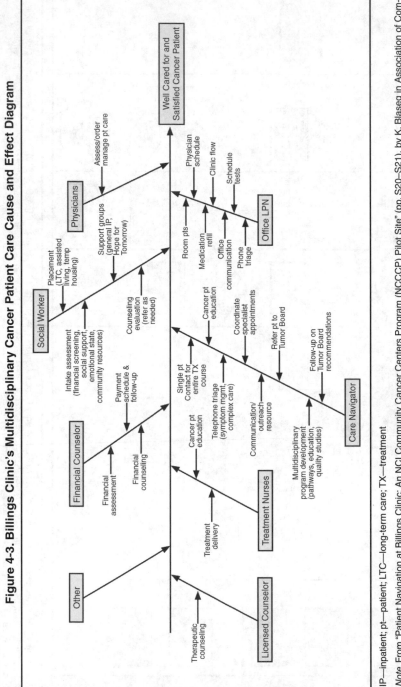

Figure 4-3. Billings Clinic's Multidisciplinary Cancer Patient Care Cause and Effect Diagram

IP—inpatient; pt—patient; LTC—long-term care; TX—treatment

Note. From "Patient Navigation at Billings Clinic: An NCI Community Cancer Centers Program (NCCCP) Pilot Site" (pp. S20–S21), by K. Blaseg in Association of Community Cancer Centers, *Cancer Care Patient Navigation: A Call to Action,* 2009, Rockville, MD: Author. Copyright 2009 by Billings Clinic. Reprinted with permission from *Cancer Care Patient Navigation: A Practical Guide for Community Cancer Centers,* a publication of the Association of Community Cancer Centers.

Figure 4-4. Johns Hopkins' Breast Center Flowchart Depicting Patient Flow Process

Process Being Performed	Avg. Number of Days to Next Step	Comments
Recruitment of patient to have screening mammogram		
Screening mammogram performed		
Screening mammogram read by radiologist		
Patient informed of abnormal results		
Patient scheduled for diagnostic mammogram/US		
Referring physician notified		
Patient scheduled for biopsy/ educated re: procedure		
Biopsy performed in breast imaging setting		
Biopsy results available from pathology		
Referring physician informed of results being breast cancer		
Patient informed that pathology results are cancer		
Surgical consultation scheduled		
Patient seen by a breast surgeon for consultation		
MRI requested and ordered (if needed)		
Results of MRI known and reviewed by surgeon		
Plastic surgery consultation arranged (due to MRI findings)		

(Continued on next page)

Figure 4-4. Johns Hopkins' Breast Center Flowchart Depicting Patient Flow Process *(Continued)*

Process Being Performed	Avg. Number of Days to Next Step	Comments
Breast cancer surgery scheduled		
Preop teaching scheduled		
Preop tests and H&P scheduled		
Surgery performed (mast with DIEP flap for example)		
Pathology available for surgery		
Receptors from pathology available from surgery		
Oncotype DX® ordered (if appropriate)		
Patient returns for postop visit		
Patient scheduled for medical oncology consultation (if needed)		
Patient seen by medical oncologist (if appropriate)		
Patient has staging workup (if needed)		
Results of staging workup available and reviewed by oncologist		
Patient receives teaching about chemotherapy regimen		
Patient begins chemotherapy regimen • Cycle I		
• Cycle II		
• Cycle III		
• Cycle IV		

(Continued on next page)

Figure 4-4. Johns Hopkins' Breast Center Flowchart Depicting Patient Flow Process *(Continued)*		
Process Being Performed	**Avg. Number of Days to Next Step**	**Comments**
Patient scheduled for radiation oncology consultation (if needed)		
Patient seen by radiation oncologist (if needed)		
Education about radiation therapy conducted		
Simulation for radiation therapy scheduled		
Simulation for radiation performed		
Radiation therapy begins		
Radiation therapy completed		
Patient scheduled to see medical oncologist for hormonal therapy		
Patient begins hormonal therapy		
Patient monitored for adherence to hormonal therapy		
Patient scheduled for follow-up appts/tests as needed		
DIEP—deep inferior epigastric perforators; H&P—history and physical; MRI—magnetic resonance imaging; US—ultrasound		
Note. Figure courtesy of Lillie Shockney, RN, BS, MAS, Johns Hopkins Breast Center. Used with permission.		

element is needed. Such documentation of processes reveals the efficiency of care delivered and exposes opportunities for improvement in processes. Shockney's (2010) institution reduced the time to chemotherapy initiation by two weeks as a result of assessing breast care workflow and adjusting the timing of the postsurgical medical oncologist appointment. In the old workflow, patients' medical oncology consultations were scheduled after the first postoperative surgeons' visits, thus creating several weeks of delay in establishing further treatment plans. A revised workflow was developed whereby scheduling of the medical oncology consultations now happens at the time surgery is scheduled and occurs within two weeks after surgery.

Hunnibell et al. (2012) described the value of this same process in assessing the time between procedures, referrals, and time to definitive treatment involved in lung cancer care. Through flow mapping, the authors identified "bottlenecks of the processes and opportunities for improvement," as well as "information about system and patient-related barriers that contributed to delays in timely treatment" (p. 31).

Figure 4-5 depicts an oncology nurse navigator workflow model designed by the Oncology Nursing Society's Nurse Navigator Special Interest Group, which can be applied to patients with a suspicious or confirmed diagnosis of cancer. The model uses the nursing process to direct the patient from diagnosis/pretreatment through survivorship or end-of-life care. It promotes communication among team members, patient advocacy, and informed decision making.

Outlining the workflow from the patient perspective allows navigators to see care processes and delivery through a consumer lens. Depending upon the navigator's focus within the cancer continuum, the starting point may not be at the front door of a clinic as the patient arrives for the screening, examination, or consultation. Rather, processes may start prior to this at outreach sites or wherever patients are recruited for screening.

Cascella and Keren (2012) outlined culturally appropriate outreach and navigation for breast cancer screening in Connecticut's highest area for breast cancer mortality using unique venues such as job training programs, parent groups, programs for the homeless, and a church's food pantry. The program promoted nurse and lay navigation in an underserved area to increase screening. The nurse navigator oversaw trained bilingual outreach survivors who encouraged women to participate in breast screening and acted as peer role models. To increase community awareness, the program promoted care through culturally appropriate newspapers and community web-based calendars, which further led to several radio interviews. The institution's newsletter also included information about the program. Patients were scheduled for care at the point of contact in the community and followed to see if scheduled appointments were kept (see Figure 4-6). Participants received financial counseling to access other benefits, such as Medicaid and supplementary state programs. In addition, navigators assisted women in connecting with PCPs for regular health care.

When looking at process flow, navigators need to be aware of transportation and facility barriers. This includes ensuring that directions to the care facility are clear and that facility signage directs patients to the correct floor or room. Culturally appropriate information in the waiting area specific for clinic patrons should be present. The Oncology Nursing Society website has links to a Diversity Champions toolkit, as well as articles and other resources to help navigators with diversity and cultural awareness (Oncology Nursing Society, n.d.). Navigators possessing the skills of cultural competence can improve patient communication, increase trust in the relationship, sup-

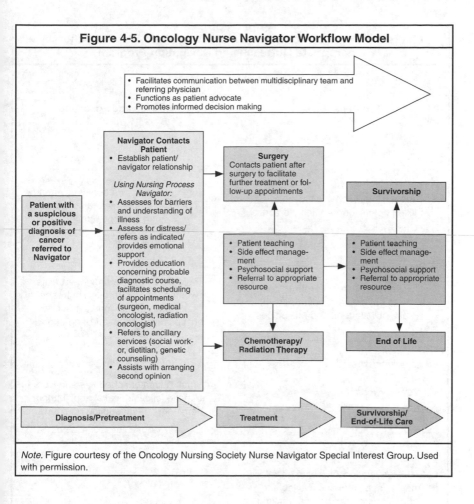

Figure 4-5. Oncology Nurse Navigator Workflow Model

- Facilitates communication between multidisciplinary team and referring physician
- Functions as patient advocate
- Promotes informed decision making

Patient with a suspicious or positive diagnosis of cancer referred to Navigator

Navigator Contacts Patient
- Establish patient/navigator relationship

Using Nursing Process Navigator:
- Assesses for barriers and understanding of illness
- Assess for distress/refers as indicated/provides emotional support
- Provides education concerning probable diagnostic course, facilitates scheduling of appointments (surgeon, medical oncologist, radiation oncologist)
- Refers to ancillary services (social worker, dietitian, genetic counseling)
- Assists with arranging second opinion

Surgery
Contacts patient after surgery to facilitate further treatment or follow-up appointments

Survivorship

- Patient teaching
- Side effect management
- Psychosocial support
- Referral to appropriate resource

- Patient teaching
- Side effect management
- Psychosocial support
- Referral to appropriate resource

Chemotherapy/Radiation Therapy

End of Life

Diagnosis/Pretreatment → **Treatment** → **Survivorship/End-of-Life Care**

Note. Figure courtesy of the Oncology Nursing Society Nurse Navigator Special Interest Group. Used with permission.

port emotional and spiritual health, and demonstrate respect to the patient (Campinha-Bacote, 2011).

It is important to evaluate flow processes with consideration for those who may have mobility, visual, or other impairments. Iezzoni, Kilbridge, and Park (2010) shared comments from patients with mobility impairments who reflected upon past experiences in healthcare facilities. Patients described difficulty when accessing doors, attempting to complete screening examinations, and getting on examination tables. The Centers for Disease Control and Prevention (2012) has suggestions for accessibility to healthcare facilities for people with disabilities. The site has practical suggestions for outpatient clinics and healthcare facilities to consider. This list could be a tool for nurse navigators to use when assessing patient flow. The Center for Universal Design and the North Carolina Office on Disability and Health (2007) published a report, *Removing Barriers to Health Care*, which discussed univer-

Figure 4-6. Workflow for Mujer-a-Mujer/Woman-to-Woman Culturally Appropriate Outreach and Navigation Program

Program Setup	Outreach and Follow-up
Identify outreach sites; develop talking points for outreach workers	Nurse educator and survivors attend outreach programs and schedule women for appointments
Develop and distribute recruitment flyers to patients and volunteers via e-blast, newsletters, and MD offices	Patient outreach coordinator tracks women referred through outreach programs, sends reminders, and notifies nurse educator of no-shows
Vet survivors; train in one-on-one sessions	Nurse educator schedules survivors to make follow-up calls, appointment reminders, rescheduling no-shows
Establish relationships with MDs for making appointments available to outreach program; develop tracking database	
Develop and distribute promotional materials to internal and external media outlets	

Note. From "Mujer a Mujer/Woman to Woman: Using a Unique Venue for Culturally Appropriate Outreach and Navigation in an Underserved Area to Increase Screening," by S. Cascella and J. Keren, 2012, *Journal of Oncology Navigation and Survivorship, 3*(2), p. 21. Copyright 2012 by the Academy of Oncology Nurse Navigators, Inc. Reprinted with permission.

sal design and the Americans With Disabilities Act requirements for health-care providers. The report stressed that not all healthcare barriers are physical and included basic rules of disability etiquette, which are invaluable to navigators.

Referrals and Portals of Entry

Entry Points

Workflows that have the point of entry at a specific diagnostic test may be restricted to a single entry point. Arias (2012) used the breast biopsy at a breast center as the entry point, and referrals were made by physicians only. At the entry point, the nurse navigator interacted with all members of the healthcare team working with the patient to promote interdisciplinary care.

If pathology reports drive the point of contact, the clinical skills and disease knowledge of the navigator allow a decision to be made to either call the patient or schedule an appointment for a one-on-one discussion with the appropriate healthcare professional based upon direction by the physician. For example, a gastrointestinal nurse navigator can comfortably call patients with negative colon workups but might direct patients with a positive cancer pathology report to be scheduled for a personal consultation with an advanced practice nurse or physician.

Desimini et al. (2011) described this point of contact as a major influence in keeping patients in the system for further care. Specifically, outmigration of patients with breast cancer dropped from 240 to 28 in one year at the Henrico Doctors' Hospital in Virginia when a nurse navigator started contacting patients for return diagnostics. The nurse navigator educated patients on the pathologic findings, followed up on further scheduling needs, responded immediately to the perceived needs of patients, and assessed for barriers to follow-up care.

As part of the interdisciplinary team, the navigator connects with patients and often continues to follow them throughout treatment. Blais (2008), Koh et al. (2011), and Seek and Hogle (2007) supported multiple points of entry for patients into navigation programs. Campbell, Craig, Eggert, and Bailey-Dorton (2010) started with single physician referrals but quickly expanded to multiple entry points from self-referrals, caregivers, and staff based on the philosophy that all patients could profit from navigation. Blaseg (2009) identified four entry portals: (a) physicians, (b) other staff from the facility, (c) hospital reports such as laboratory and admission lists, and (d) physician schedules. Additional patient entry points may include referrals from community agencies, survivors, or caregivers. Pathology reports are consistent entry points for navigators, especially because patients who are initially diagnosed outside the healthcare facility must have the pathologist review and confirm the diagnosis before beginning definitive treatment.

No matter where the entry point or points lie in the system of care, offering navigation to everyone is ideal (Freeman & Rodriguez, 2011). When specific populations, such as uninsured, low-income, or non–English speaking individuals, are singled out, nurse navigators should be aware that navigation services may be drawing attention to the selected group. The goal is to not make patients feel more disadvantaged or noticeable in an unfamiliar or new system of care. Campbell et al. (2010) found that nurse navigation benefited patients from all economic situations and races. Interestingly, although nurse navigators mainly worked with underprivileged patients, a specific population, navigation services were offered to all patients in the system.

Nurse navigators need to have an awareness of system and community agencies in order to address identified barriers. Exploring the community and healthcare system to identify available resources will allow navigators to readily reveal gaps in care or support. For example, in rural areas, nurse navigators may identify transportation and lodging as barriers to care with limited community resources available.

Diagnostic Contact

When nurse navigators are present when the diagnosis is explained, they can begin an assessment of patients' coping and psychosocial skills. Additionally, if caregivers are present, navigators can observe the family dynamics. Education on the disease process, as well as next steps, will begin. With a patient-centered focus on personalized care, the navigator can make appropriate referrals to other providers on the team. Genetics assessment is a priority if the outcome might influence the surgical decision. With a later stage or large tumor, the medical oncologist appointment takes precedence for possible neoadjuvant therapy. Assessment for clinical trial participation begins with referrals to the research team if appropriate. The nurse navigators explain each clinical decision to the patients and caregivers, along with assessment of the patients' expectations and understanding. Navigators are an intermediary to share the personalized clinical information and patients' choices with the other healthcare team members.

The time between diagnosis and the first treatment is a stepping stone for patients and caregivers into the world of cancer care. Multiple decisions are made in this phase, which requires the clinical knowledge and skills of an oncology nurse. A key role of nurse navigators is to validate patients' understanding regarding the diagnosis and proposed treatments. Understanding patients' needs and expectations is critical to ensure that appropriate information is provided for patients to effectively participate in informed treatment decision making. Fillion et al. (2006) documented comments from patients and families who experienced a nurse navigator that revealed appreciation for timely and understandable information provided by navigators. In the same study, other nurses emphasized the improvements in patient education, and physicians described patients as being better prepared for visits. Wilcox and Bruce (2010) described in detail individualized education packets provided at first navigation contact with new patients. The main focus for education at this phase of care is information about the disease, treatment options, possible effects of the treatment decisions, and supportive resources. Patients should have the tools to make informed decisions, whether from written material, computer-aided teaching, or video. Wilcox and Bruce (2010) asserted that

> as patients suddenly find themselves thrown into a whirlwind of what seems like an endless sea of information and medical terminology, a navigator becomes a consistent "go-to" resource to assist patients in making sense of what they are being told by the medical team, thereby reducing the risk of crisis. (p. 22)

Wagner et al. (2010) asked a group of patients about information gaps. The patients perceived the navigators to bridge this gap as counselors with clinical knowledge, educational resources, and skills that empowered the patients to be more involved.

Clinical Trial Screening

Clinical trial participation is part of both the patient-centered dimension and the health system–oriented aspect of navigation. Nurse navigators are in a key position to advocate for clinical trials and to assess patient understanding of responsibilities. Presentation of information to patients from a nurse navigator who has knowledge in clinical trials should include key points such as the benefits and risks for the patient or future patients and an explanation of unfamiliar terms. Expected commitment from the patient involving time, travel, or diagnostics, such as radiology or blood work, as well as any compensation, needs to be discussed with patients (Shockney, 2008). Nurse navigators often collaborate with clinical research nurses and physicians to identify those patients who may be appropriate for a specific trial (Holmes, Major, Lyonga, Alleyne, & Clayton, 2012).

Schwaderer and Itano (2007) recognized the potential to increase clinical trial enrollment during the development and implementation of a navigator program by removing barriers to care so that patients could complete the prescribed treatment. The NCI Community Cancer Centers Program used a minority matrix and nurse navigation to improve accrual to clinical trials (Gonzalez et al., 2011). Keys included the trusting relationships between navigators and caregivers that developed as navigators addressed other aspects of care. Navigators were able to introduce the concept of a clinical trial at an earlier stage of care and treatment decision making. This allowed patients to be more open to this idea, and in turn, navigators had an affirmative influence on physicians referring to clinical trials.

Holmes et al. (2012) specifically designed a nurse navigation program to increase African American patient participation in clinical trials in the community setting. Within two years, this population enrollment increased from 3% to 7%, which was credited to a single nurse navigator. Furthermore, 86% of the African American eligible patients were enrolled in at least one protocol, and researchers found that patients who had a positive encounter with one trial were more likely to enroll in an additional clinical trial. It is interesting to note that an assessment from the navigator revealed that access and understanding of trials were not the main limiting factors to enrolling in a clinical trial for patients; rather, the main factor was a lack of appropriate clinical trials for a patient's clinical case.

Multidisciplinary Clinics/Tumor Board Conferences

Nurse navigators play an important role in the coordination of multidisciplinary clinics and/or tumor board conferences, which are a part of the continuity of care for patients. Education about the consultative process is critical to help patients and caregivers understand the process. Without appropriate guidance and information, patients may view this multidisciplinary process as a negative event, fearing that the cancer is more advanced if the case needs to be presented to a special team. However, with proper education, patients can recognize this as a chance to get several expert opinions on the best care for the clinical situation and individual tumor characteristics.

Ançel (2012) discussed the importance of patient-centered information that includes the individual patients' needs along with accurate patient assessment by the nurse for the team presentation. The humanization of navigated care allows personalized education for each patient (Fillion et al., 2012). Patients can experience a greater feeling of control, improved compliance by understanding why tests are needed, and realistic expectations with clear communication. The interdisciplinary interaction between navigators and healthcare team members improves the coordination of care for patients. Messier (2010) described the following benefits of multidisciplinary meetings.

- All disciplines have an opportunity to influence decisions on the patient's care.
- Evidence-based guidelines are promoted and agreed on for the patient's benefit.
- Personal interactions are conducted among colleagues.
- Patient education can be enhanced.

Oncology nurse navigators, along with other team members, can present new patient cases, patients with multifaceted symptoms, or patients requiring follow-up such as those with metastatic disease facing several treatment options (Plante & Joannette, 2009). Navigators often triage patient referrals to the multidisciplinary team for discussion and schedule the necessary staging studies prior to the clinic visit or discussion (Hunnibell et al., 2012; Wilcox & Bruce, 2010). With the increasing numbers of patients diagnosed with cancer, nurse navigators must have the clinical knowledge and skills to identify appropriate cases for review. Nurse navigators use clinical knowledge to efficiently guide the number of cases that can be reasonably presented in the given time frame. Obtaining outside medical records, pathology results, or scans should be delegated to an appropriate administrative assistant. Seek and Hogle (2007) discussed an evidence-based model implemented for patients with lung cancer, which can be applied to patients with other cancer diagnoses. This model used a nurse practitioner as a navigator to coordinate follow-up care, provide a point of ongoing contact for questions and education, and initiate referrals to appropriate supportive staff such as social workers or dietitians to proactively prepare for the planned treatment. Wilcox and Bruce (2010) discussed the role of nurse navigators in educating patients after the multidisciplinary clinic on the chosen treatment and communicating to the treatment staff the information reviewed. Figure 4-7 depicts the role of the nurse navigator in a multidisciplinary clinic.

Swanson et al. (2012) described the development of a multidisciplinary assessment tool for community cancer centers to implement when creating or expanding a multidisciplinary care model. Nurse navigators and physicians were identified as two key roles crucial to successful multidisciplinary cancer care. The roles of experienced nurse navigators in multidisciplinary care were described as opening communication among team members, guiding patients through the care planning overview, coordinating patients' schedules, and addressing patients' follow-up needs. The central contact role of nurse navigators was emphasized if patients could not see all care professionals on the same day or on-site. The expectation was for nurse navigators to guide patients through the care process at multiple visits to care providers or to coordinate the care with the use of multiple sites.

Treatment

Continuity of care continues as navigators repeatedly touch base with patients in the treatment phase, whether treatment consists of chemotherapy, radiation therapy, surgery, hormonal therapy, or immunotherapy. Fillion et al. (2012) defined continuity of care as part of the health system–oriented dimension of nurse navigation. It is task focused, with navigators assisting patients to move from diagnosis to active treatment, "mapping the continu-

Figure 4-7. Role of the Nurse Navigator in Multidisciplinary Clinics

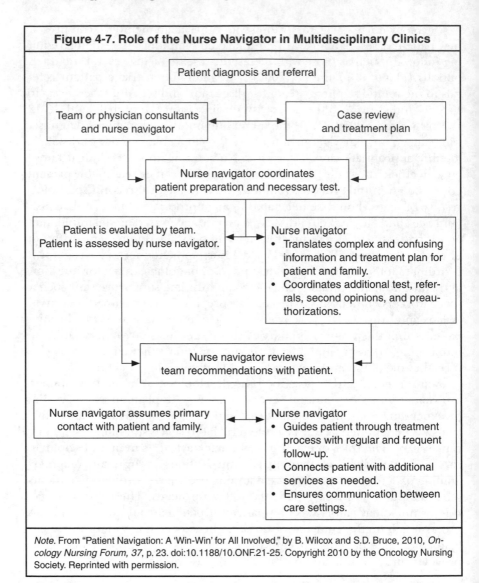

Note. From "Patient Navigation: A 'Win-Win' for All Involved," by B. Wilcox and S.D. Bruce, 2010, *Oncology Nursing Forum, 37*, p. 23. doi:10.1188/10.ONF.21-25. Copyright 2010 by the Oncology Nursing Society. Reprinted with permission.

um of cancer care, explaining treatments and care plans while minimizing uncertainty . . . [to] increase participation of patients in their own care as well as decrease barriers to cancer care adherence" (Fillion et al., 2012, p. E62). The consistent relationship during the care trajectory results in an acquisition of accrued knowledge of the patient and links this knowledge to future care. Benefits of continuity include a sense of predictability, coherence in care, increased feelings of confidence, and growth of trust in the navigator who provides regular personal contact. This ongoing relationship allows for reevaluation of patients' and caregivers' needs, including educational, psychosocial, or physical care, as patients progress through the continuum of care.

The treatment phase consists of multiple healthcare providers, internal support personnel, and countless procedures. Nurse navigators can proactively prepare and guide patients through treatment completion (Psooy, Schreuer, Borgaonkar, & Caines, 2004). Horner et al. (2013) pointed out that this proactive care at regularly scheduled encounters distinguishes navigators from the oncology clinic nurses who reactively respond to patients' questions or concerns. Nurse navigators use clinical knowledge of treatments, side effects, and complications to prepare patients for possible effects that can directly affect patient outcomes (Case, 2011). Patients' needs evolve as care progresses along the continuum, warranting the need for continued reassessment (Wagner et al., 2010). Community or healthcare resources introduced at the beginning of navigation may need to be suggested or offered again.

Lymphedema evaluation can be part of the workflow as navigators proactively attempt to decrease treatment complications. With the system knowledge of the treatment plans for patients, a referral to the physical therapy department or rehabilitative care unit can reduce the risk of lymphedema, as well as promote further patient education on this chronic condition. All patients at high risk for lymphedema should be offered a consult with a trained lymphedema specialist when risk is identified. At-risk individuals include patients with breast cancer who have had more than four lymph nodes removed or who will be receiving radiation therapy to dense lymph node areas (National Lymphedema Network Medical Advisory Committee, 2012). This care pattern can also be applied to gynecologic, head and neck, and radiation patients who have treatment focused on a dense lymph node area. Fu, Ryan, and Cleland (2012) investigated the knowledge of oncology nurses regarding lymphedema and practice patterns of lymphedema care. Oncology nurse navigators had the highest perceived knowledge in lymphedema risk reduction and were more likely to provide education for this effect. These participants also had the highest perceived competence to address risk reduction of lymphedema. Nurse navigators were confident in educating high-risk patients about risk factors to avoid and prevention of lymphedema. Fu et al. (2012) encouraged navigators to continue this practice, as early identification of lymphedema can allow prompt treatment and have a positive impact on survivors' QOL.

When research supports that patients can have a survival benefit with diet modifications, exercise, tobacco avoidance or cessation, and other health-promoting activities, nurse navigators can introduce these ideas along the treatment continuum as teachable moments arise. One evidence-based example involves offering all patients with triple-negative breast cancer a dietitian consultation to discuss a low-fat diet based on the analysis by Chlebowski et al. (2006). The same could be applied to patients with stage III colon cancer based on a study of dietary patterns in this subgroup, which showed less recurrence and mortality with a prudent diet (lower-fat diet characterized by high intake of fruits, vegetables, whole grains, legumes, poultry, and fish) compared to a Western diet (characterized by high intake of refined grains, processed and red meats, fat, desserts, and high-fat dairy products) (Meyerhardt et al., 2007).

Rehabilitative Services

With an increasing aging population, a rapidly growing number of cancer survivors, and the need for patients to use resources after treatment, cancer rehabilitation is outpacing other disease rehabilitation studies (Ugolini et al., 2012). No published studies on nurse navigation and cancer rehabilitation are available at this time, but evidence-based research has been completed, showing the benefits of rehabilitation in patients with cancer. As nurse navigators coordinate and proactively prepare patients for care, cancer rehabilitation can be a part of the nurse navigator workflow across the care continuum.

To support the use of rehabilitation services for patients, ACoS CoC (2012) eligibility requires that rehabilitation services be offered on-site or by referral in the local community. Health insurers cover cancer rehabilitation when impairment is documented and the treatment is delivered by healthcare professionals who are licensed or certified in rehabilitation medicine (Silver, 2013).

Most healthcare professionals think of cancer rehabilitation as lymphedema treatment or as occupational therapy and physical therapy for the acute treatment of inpatients. However, rehabilitation can address cognitive impairment, mood, fatigue, and distress (Banks et al., 2010; Cramp & Byron-Daniel, 2012; Hanna, Avila, Meteer, Nicholas, & Kaminsky, 2008; Von Ah, Jansen, Allen, Schiavone, & Wulff, 2011). Banks et al. (2010) conducted a large questionnaire study of more than 80,000 men and women older than age 45 to evaluate distress in cancer survivors, which supported the use of rehabilitative care in the cancer continuum. Psychological distress in cancer survivors was found to be related more to the level of disability rather than the cancer diagnosis.

Rehabilitation assessment can start at the diagnostic phase of care. For example, if a patient with breast cancer has limited right shoulder mobility and will be having a right lumpectomy, referral to the rehabilitation team is appropriate because arm positioning for surgery or radiation may be limited. Mayo et al. (2011) showed that physical functioning could be improved by working preoperatively with patients with colorectal cancer scheduled for abdominal surgery. The outcome measure was functional walking capacity. The term *prehabilitation* was used to describe the approach of providing rehabilitation before the patient undergoes a physiologically stressful event such as surgery. The improvement prior to surgery was carried over to the postoperative phase as participants recovered functional capacity quicker than control subjects after surgery and perceived themselves as healthier and more energetic. Li et al. (2013) confirmed prehabilitation benefits in another study of patients with colorectal cancer with interventions focused on walking, anxiety reduction, and nutrition counseling. The prehabilitation patients had better walking capacity at four weeks after surgery. At eight weeks, 81% of the therapy patients had healed compared to 40% of the control group. Increasing evidence supports the referral of patients undergoing chemotherapy to rehabilitation for exercise to improve functional capacity. Adamsen et al. (2009) used cardiovascular exercise, resistance training, relaxation, and massage in a group of patients with various cancers being treated for advanced disease. They reported improved aerobic capacity, muscular strength, and physical and functional activity. In addition, participants noted improved emotional well-being and vitality. Research also has shown that it is feasible and safe for patients with inoperable lung cancer undergoing chemotherapy to complete a six-week structured exercise and relaxation training program (Quist et al., 2012). In this study, patients saw improvement in walking distance, muscle strength, and emotional well-being.

Granda-Cameron et al. (2010) described an interdisciplinary model for a cachexia clinic that treated patients at high risk for or experiencing cancer cachexia with cancer treatment. Physical rehabilitation was a part of the clinic to increase muscle strength and tone, to safely increase patients' activity levels, to increase endurance, and to educate families on how to assist patients with rehabilitation. Nurse navigators referring patients to a dietitian for cachexia also should consider adding rehabilitation services as well.

Even in patients receiving palliative care, cancer rehabilitation needs to be addressed. Oldervoll et al. (2005) demonstrated that palliative care patients were willing to participate in a structured exercise program. The group met twice a week for six weeks, and 54% of severely ill patients completed the program. Patients with advanced non-small cell lung cancer performed weight training and aerobic exercise twice weekly for eight weeks and experienced a significant improvement in lung cancer symptoms. QOL did not decrease, nor did fatigue increase during the study. However, the withdrawal rate was high due to deterioration in health status, with 44% completing the program.

The care continuum includes a place for rehabilitation services coordinated by nurse navigators. *Cancer Rehabilitation and Survivorship: Transdisciplinary Approaches to Personalized Care* (Lester & Schmitt, 2011) contains a wealth of information for nurse navigators interested in cancer rehabilitation and survivorship. The majority of studies reviewed herein to support cancer rehabilitation discussed positive QOL effects of rehabilitation, such as vitality, energy, strength, and emotional well-being. If nurse navigators promoted the increased adoption of cancer rehabilitation, quality can be enriched for patients throughout the care continuum. The benefits gained in functional capacity will keep the patients functioning at a higher level throughout life.

Palliative Care

Opportunity exists for nurse navigators to promote the integration of palliative care into oncology services, as well as to promote the awareness of palliative care. Hauser et al. (2011) hypothesized that navigators can assess for symptoms such as pain, dyspnea, and depression; take subsequent action to notify patients' healthcare providers for uncontrolled symptoms; and empower patients and families to address goals of care through open communication with the healthcare team. Navigators can successfully influence the use of palliative care and transition to hospice care by engaging in proactive conversations with patients about goals of care and advance care planning. Navigators can assist with the transition from the hospital to the home or other long-term care locations and use knowledge of medical aspects of care and the healthcare system to supplement patients' care with palliative services. Hauser et al. (2011) stressed that navigator training should include knowledge of symptoms and how to screen for these, education about palliative care and advance care planning, how to discuss goals of care or advance care planning, and methods to access palliative and hospice care for patients.

Research shows a lack of understanding regarding the meaning of palliative care. The *2011 Public Opinion Research on Palliative Care* (Center to Advance Palliative Care) used both qualitative and quantitative research methods with consumers and healthcare providers to identify barriers to palliative care use, the most common of which included a lack of awareness regarding palliative care terminology and availability of palliative care services. The term *palliative care* often had no meaning to consumers or else was associated only with end-of-life care. Physicians equated palliative care to hospice care, with the overall goal being comfort. From this research, a revised definition of palliative care was established (Center to Advance Palliative Care, 2011):

> Palliative care is specialized medical care for people with serious illnesses. This type of care is focused on providing patients with relief from the symptoms, pain, and stress of a serious illness— whatever the diagnosis.
> The goal is to improve quality of life for both the patient and the family. Palliative care is provided by a team of doctors, nurses, and other specialists who work with a patient's other doctors to provide an extra layer of support. Palliative care is appropriate at

any age and at any stage in a serious illness, and can be provided
together with curative treatment. (p. 7)

This new definition has had a positive impact on consumers' understanding of the concept, as well as favorably influencing use of these services when needed.

To promote the use of palliative care by healthcare professionals, the American Society of Clinical Oncology released a provisional clinical opinion calling for the integration of palliative care into standard oncology care (Smith, Temin, et al., 2012). The statement reflected the Center to Advance Palliative Care's (2011) definition by recognizing it as specialized medical care for people with serious illness, no matter what the diagnosis, and provided by a team of specialists. It stressed that symptom relief can be provided at any stage of illness and described palliative care as an extra layer of support provided to physicians and promoted its use along with curative treatment to improve QOL and survival.

Von Roenn, Voltz, and Serrie (2013) called for increasing education about palliative care to promote the integration into oncology practice and suggested early training in physician residency programs. This same idea could apply to any healthcare professional training. One resource for healthcare professionals is the Education in Palliative and End-of-Life Care (EPEC®) curriculum (EPEC, n.d.). The curriculum incorporates interactive techniques based on adult education theory and includes 16 modules, which can be completed in-person or by distance learning. Another resource is the Education in Palliative and End-of-Life Care for Oncology (EPEC™-O) training available free of charge through the NCI (2013). This program contains 15 modules and 3 plenary sessions completed in a self-study or CD-ROM format. EPEC-O programs specific to American Indian, Alaska Native, and African American cultural considerations also exist.

Von Roenn et al. (2013) reviewed clinical studies to identify barriers for integrating palliative care into oncology practice. Findings supported the public opinion research (Center to Advance Palliative Care, 2011) in that healthcare professionals perceived palliative care as symptom control provided during terminal care and did not feel that such a service was conducive to newly diagnosed patients or those undergoing active treatment. One study of patients with lung cancer found that fewer than 25% of patients were referred to palliative care because the physicians were concerned it would alarm patients and families (Smith, Nelson, et al., 2012). These findings support healthcare providers' lack of understanding of palliative care and reluctance to communicate palliative considerations to patients.

Goldsmith, Ferrell, Wittenberg-Lyles, and Ragan (2013) stated, "Palliative care prioritizes patient pain and symptom management, emphasizes communication with patients and their families, and establishes coordination of care" (p. 163). Furthermore, they described a communication model that oncology nurses can use as a resource to enhance communication skills for challenging palliative care discussions. The COMFORT curriculum represents an acronym for Communication, Orientation and opportunity, Mindful presence, Family, Openings, Relating, and Team. It is based on the National Consensus Project for Quality Palliative Care (2009) clinical practice guidelines. Case examples involving the eight domains of quality palliative care exemplify the communication techniques needed to promote quality oncology palliative care. With a patient- and family-centered focus, this holistic model for narrative clinical communication is a resource for nurse navigators who are transitioning patients into palliative care in the oncology setting.

Palliative care offers cost savings to the healthcare organization, and nurse navigators are in positions to support this economical care strategy. Gade et al. (2008) randomized seriously ill patients to either usual care or palliative care service plus usual care. The study was conducted at three sites for Kaiser Permanente. The palliative care service, consisting of a palliative care physician, nurse, social worker, and chaplain, assessed patients during hospitalizations and created outpatient plans of care inclusive of PCPs. Total healthcare costs were lower in the patients receiving the palliative service because they had fewer intensive care unit stays and readmissions. Interestingly, the palliative service patients reported greater satisfaction with the care experience and communication. Furthermore, these patients were able to perform more activities of daily living upon hospital discharge than the usual care group. Hospice admissions were equal between the groups, but the palliative care group had longer stays in hospice. Morrison et al. (2008) also showed hospital cost savings with a palliative care consult team. Patients who received palliative care were matched to a usual care patient. The study involved eight hospitals, and data were analyzed over a three-year period. Findings revealed that the palliative care patients had lower hospital costs because of decreased intensive care expenses and lower laboratory and pharmacy utilization.

Patient-Centered Medical Homes

As patient-centered medical homes develop in oncology to increase the quality of care, decrease cost, and increase patient satisfaction, nurse navigators may have more defined patient contact points. The patient-centered medical home (PCMH) model evolved in primary care to address fragmented care delivery in a system with high costs and poor health-related outcomes (Cronholm et al., 2013; Eagle & Sprandio, 2011). The Agency for Healthcare Research and Quality (n.d.) defined five attributes of the model.

• Comprehensive care: PCMHs attempt to meet patients' physical and mental healthcare needs, including prevention and wellness, acute care, and chronic care. The team approach of multiple care providers is acknowledged.

- Patient-centered care: PCMHs recognize patients' unique needs, culture, values, and preferences and acknowledge the family as a core member of the care team.
- Coordinated care: PCMHs focus on coordination of care among the entire healthcare system, especially during transitions between sites of care. Open communication is built among caregivers, family members, the healthcare team, community agencies, and supportive services.
- Accessible care: PCMHs center on more efficient time frames, such as a shorter wait for care, around-the-clock care, and enhanced communication via email and telephone calls.
- Quality and safety: PCMHs encourage the use of evidence-based medicine and clinical decision support tools to guide shared decision making with patients and families, demonstrating to payers the value of quality care and patient satisfaction.

Cronholm et al. (2013) described factors influencing the transformation process when the focus was on improving diabetic care. The setting involved 25 PCP practices in southeastern Pennsylvania in which 118 interviews were performed with the multidisciplinary staff involved in the practice transformation. A key factor was the requirement of teams to focus on proactive, comprehensive patient care. Healthcare professionals described anticipating patients' problems and encouraging patients to be invested and empowered in care decisions and delivery. Staff acclimated to self-examination of practice as clinical data and quality improvement scores showed whether outcomes were met. This fostered more accountability and a collaborative approach to help patients receive care for their chronic disease. The change created tension as new roles emerged when the practice shifted to team-based care. Frustrations arose as some members were asked to move away from traditional clinician-centered care and share responsibilities with other team members.

Hudson et al. (2012) used the PCMH as a conceptual framework in a qualitative study to explore patients' understanding of survivorship care and motivation to seek care or resources for survivorship. The authors recruited patients with early breast or prostate cancer from five community hospitals in New Jersey. In-depth telephone or in-person interviews were conducted with a semistructured script to assess how survivors transitioned out of active treatment, who was providing survivorship care, and survivors' satisfaction with care. Three types of survivor experiences were recognized from the interviews: (a) Low-activated patients were identified as those with modest follow-up understanding and limited resources; this group was unprepared for follow-up and displayed little motivation to seek care or use resources. (b) The highly activated patients with modest follow-up understandings and moderate resources demonstrated limited understanding for cancer follow-up and relied on the healthcare team to direct care; this group did express motivation and measures to ensure that follow-up care was received. (c) The highly activated patients with detailed follow-up understanding and moderate-high resources reported the most detailed expectations for follow-up care and sought out information on care to discuss with the healthcare team. Hudson et al. (2012) suggested that PCMH structures must be flexible to adapt to different types of patients and varied capacities to engage in shared decision making and patient-centered care. Patient engagement for self-management in chronic disease management and the healthcare team's ability to activate patients in care must be considered when applying the PCMH model. Furthermore, they suggested behavioral training for providers and members of the PCMH community to enhance communication with patients.

Care coordination across the healthcare system is a required aspect of the PCMH and calls for open communication among the entire healthcare team. Nurse navigators coordinate care and promote communication between patients and the healthcare team. Eagle and Sprandio (2011) pioneered this model of care in oncology by using services that oncology offices were already providing, such as care coordination, treatment planning, telephone triage, in-office chemotherapy, and transition services to palliative care and hospice. The Oncology Patient-Centered Medical Home model exceeded current office practices by standardizing processes in the oncology practice, measuring guideline adherence and outcomes, and tracking rates of emergency department use and hospitalization. The use of improved coordination, open access, and avoidance of potential patient complications led to lower healthcare system costs. Sprandio (2010) described an approach that used clinically trained nurses to monitor symptoms and intervene early. He reported that patients were engaged in care and empowered to report concerns before an emergency department or clinic visit became necessary. Despite an increase in patient volume, emergency department visits decreased by 50% with the use of telephone triage with symptom management algorithms.

In 2013, the oncology breast navigators at Novant Health Derrick L. Davis Cancer Center identified an opportunity to decrease emergency department use (Novant Health Derrick L. Davis Cancer Center, 2013). A telephone triage system was developed as part of the breast nurse navigation workflow to contact patients three days after implementation of a new regimen. For example, chemotherapy patients were called after initiation of a new regimen to assess for delayed nausea and vomiting. Patients expressed appreciation for this support during the telephone calls. The nurse navigator reinforced the prescribed nausea and vomiting medication plan. If the assessment revealed that the plan was not working, the patient was put back in contact with the appropriate clinical staff, thereby avoiding an emergency department visit.

Defining and Identifying High-Risk Populations

Whether nurses navigate by tumor site or by a designated system entry site, certain high-risk patients will be identified in the workflow as the navigation process evolves. These patients require more of the navigators' time and focus because of physical, social, or psychological needs. Some examples of high-risk populations are patients with high-acuity tumors, such as breast, pancreatic, gynecologic, head and neck, glioblastoma, or lung. These patients require a large amount of acute care for treatment and rehabilitation, including therapy such as physical, speech, or lymphedema therapy or sexual health counseling. Patients with advanced-stage disease upon initial diagnosis may need more support in adjusting to the cancer diagnosis and comprehending the idea of controlling the disease and increasing QOL with symptom control. Psychological needs can involve patients dealing with emotional or mental disorders, having difficulty coping with the diagnosis, or having difficulty adapting to the demands of cancer care. The Billings Clinic created an acuity scale based on the variables the cancer diagnosis and patients collectively bring to the table (see Table 4-1). Although the scale is not scientifically validated and is more often used to analyze workload, it gives guidance on identifying high-risk patients with intense needs and the navigation time commitment (Blaseg, 2009).

Byers (2012) discussed patient navigation in degrees when referring to screening navigation, stating it is "best timed for those patients who are at high-risk for noncompliance or for those who show early indications of noncompliance" (p. 1618). Nurses have recognized this principle of care for years. It is a workflow dynamic called the Pareto effect, more commonly referred to as the 80/20 rule (Vardaman, Cornell, & Clancy, 2012). Simply stated, 20% of patients use approximately 80% of healthcare resources, or, applied to nurse navigation, 20% of patients will use 80% of the navigator's time. Interestingly, during an analysis of outcome variables in a nurse navigator program, Koh et al. (2011) found an inverse relationship between patient satisfaction and the time that nurse navigators spent with patients, in that navigators spent more time with patients who were the least satisfied with their care.

One lesson learned in a randomized controlled study of oncology nurse navigation was that acuity of patients' disease did not correlate with patients' anguish in coping with the disease (Horner et al., 2013). It was the holistic picture of personal coping, economic state, support, and previous care experiences that caused worry to patients. These are all psychosocial elements that nurse navigators should assess. The development of an ongoing relationship between the nurse navigator and the patient allows a profound understanding of the patient that affects clinical decision making for personalized care.

Table 4-1. Billings Clinic's Patient Navigation Acuity Scale	
Acuity Scale	Description
0	No navigation
0.5	Meet patient if referral received; Initial guidance/education/coordination as needed; Typically no follow-up required
1	Meet patients upon diagnosis; Initial guidance/education/coordination; Typically no follow-up required
1.5	Meet patient upon diagnosis; Coordination of multimodality treatment; Typically ongoing guidance/education for 3–4 months
2	Meet patients upon diagnosis; Coordination of multimodality treatment; Moderate intensity of needs; Typically ongoing guidance/education for 5–6 months or more
2.5	Meet patients upon diagnosis; Coordination of multimodality treatment; High intensity of needs, often inpatient hospitalizations associated with care Typically ongoing guidance/education for 6–12 months or more
4	Meets patient upon diagnosis; Coordination of multimodality treatment; High intensity of needs, often associated with care coordination outside of facility; Typically ongoing guidance/education for 6–12 months or more

Note. From "Patient Navigation at Billings Clinic: An NCI Community Cancer Centers Program (NCCCP) Pilot Site" (p. S24), by K. Blaseg in Association of Community Cancer Centers, *Cancer Care Patient Navigation: A Call to Action,* 2009, Rockville, MD: Author. Copyright 2009 by Billings Clinic. Reprinted with permission from *Cancer Care Patient Navigation: A Practical Guide for Community Cancer Centers,* a publication of the Association of Community Cancer Centers.

Patient workflow in a healthcare system does not proceed in a linear process such as in a mechanical factory. Instead, it is a complex adaptive system made up of interdependent parts, and the parts interact at different times in distinctive ways in the system (Vardaman et al., 2012). Add to this multifaceted system a unique individual responding to the diagnosis of cancer. Each individual response is different because of the cognitive appraisal of how cancer will influence well-being. Meaning is attached to cancer as patients judge the situation from their individual perspective (Fitch, 2008). What may be useful for one person to cope and move forward with care may be different for another individual. Nurse navigators enter and match care interventions to individual needs, desired objectives, and methods of coping. Case (2011) defined this as *safe passage*: "The nurse uses expert clinical judgment, systems thinking, and advocacy to identify complications early or promote adherence to appropriate treatment in the complex, vulnerable patient" (p. 38). When navigated patients were asked about their perceptions regarding quality of cancer care, the patients reported that nurse navigators existed in two worlds—an insider to the healthcare system and a caring companion (Carroll et al., 2010). The patients entrusted the nurse navigators with personal knowledge of their overall life situation and saw them as insiders to the healthcare system. Examples given were addressing administrative challenges, providing a sense of security, and being a resource with telephone calls or clinical visits (Carroll et al., 2010). The trust that develops between patients and nurse navigators can extend to the larger healthcare system. It reflects the bidimensional nature of the nurse navigator workflow—patient centered and health system oriented.

Interfacing With Primary Care Providers

Nurse navigators' communication skills must include the ability to communicate effectively with all healthcare team members, including PCPs. This will ensure that patients, upon returning to their communities, will continue to have continuity of care. PCPs are an integral part of the healthcare team and play an important role during treatment and into survivorship. Patients' comorbid conditions, such as diabetes, heart disease, gastroesophageal reflux, and hypertension, must be monitored during the cancer care continuum just as they were before the cancer diagnosis and treatment, and nurse navigators can act as a conduit to ensure that communication regarding any comorbidities is shared among all members of the healthcare team.

Consultation and/or progress notes are often used as a means to communicate with PCPs in the community or healthcare system. Models of navigation should be designed to automatically forward providers' and/or navigators' notes to PCPs. Navigators can explain the PCP's role in relation to the cancer care team to ensure that patients understand the PCP's roles and responsibilities in ongoing medical care, as well as the responsibilities of other healthcare team members. This ongoing communication by navigators can minimize role confusion for patients and their family or caregivers.

Desimini et al. (2011) analyzed the financial impact of a nurse navigation program, looking at patients with breast cancer from suspicious findings to 12 months after diagnosis. A four-year downstream analysis revealed an increase in surgical procedures, chemotherapy infusions, radiation therapy, and diagnostic testing during the first three years of the program. Higher patient retention rates and service volume increases were attributed to PCP referral patterns and acceptance of navigation services resulting from continued PCP involvement with patients.

Communication Training for Patient-Centered Care

A variety of communication skills training programs have been developed for oncology providers. Sheldon (2005) identified the importance of having effective communication skills training for healthcare providers in order to enhance patient-provider communication. She reviewed 21 communication training research studies published between 1982 and 2004. Although program length varied, the confidence and communication skills of providers improved in 19 of the 21 studies. Sheldon identified the most important skill for healthcare providers as the ability to use open-ended questions when performing patient assessments and respond in an empathetic manner, especially when working with distressed and emotional patients.

Other studies have found value in additional communication training for oncology nurses, as this facilitates a patient-centered communication style. Communication training includes training to communicate with providers and patients about disease management and psychosocial aspects of care. Communication as well as QOL was found to improve when patient's everyday needs were included in the planning of identified goals of care (Langewitz et al., 2010; Wittenberg-Lyles, Goldsmith, & Ferrell, 2013).

While it is essential for the healthcare team to communicate effectively with patients, it is equally important for patients to be able to communicate with the healthcare team in order to freely share feelings, anxieties, and any dissatisfaction with care. Nurse navigators are well positioned to provide such training, coaching, and empowerment to patients. Mishel et al. (2009) identified the importance of communication skills training for men newly diagnosed with early-stage prostate cancer. This training improved doctor-patient communication and empowered patients to manage uncertainty and participate in decisions to minimize decisional regret.

Patient-Centered Barriers to Care

Studies have defined numerous barriers that patients encounter when trying to navigate the healthcare system (Freeman & Rodriguez, 2011; Palos & Hare, 2011). Freeman and Rodriguez (2011) identified five common barriers to care for the uninsured and underinsured population: (a) financial, (b) communication, (c) medical system, (d) transportation, and (e) emotional difficulties. Korber, Padula, Gray, and Powell (2011) conducted a qualitative study using telephone interviews and focus groups to identify common barriers to care as identified by patients with breast cancer in a navigation program. Participants acknowledged barriers such as difficulty absorbing a lot of information in a short period of time, not understanding how to manage symptoms, lack of emotional support, inability to have treatment tailored to individual needs, and the challenge of understanding team member roles and available resources. When Bowles et al. (2008) interviewed professionals with experience in healthcare and patient advocacy, several issues emerged as preventing patients from receiving high-quality, patient-centered care. These included a failure to have a clear process for helping patients navigate the system, failure of patients to receive multidisciplinary care, poor follow-up and communication, and failure to empower patients to be active in the decision-making process. Interesting to note, each of these studies indicated that having navigators included in care processes would have eliminated many struggles experienced by patients and institutions and would have provided social support critical for positive outcomes.

Building on providing patient-centered care, nurse navigators use knowledge and skills to assess and manage symptoms and risk behaviors to identify potential barriers to care in patients with a past, current, or potential diagnosis of cancer. During the assessment, critical data will be gathered to help identify barriers that may affect patient care (Pedersen & Hack, 2011). Documentation processes should be integrated into the existing medical record in order to prevent duplication. Using the nursing process, the navigator can efficiently gather valuable information. Critical questions related to living situation, means of contact, and past medical history and healthcare utilization will alert nurse navigators to tailor interventions to avoid future potential problems. Such information may help with the patient's adherence to the plan of care, as an understanding of the patient's cultural and health literacy barriers may enable the patient to more openly discuss and share fears. Forming a partnership among navigators, patients, and caregivers will enable positive information sharing with the ultimate goal of improving patients' and caregivers' QOL and knowledge of existing resources (Kornblith et al., 2006).

Addressing Distress and Psychosocial Needs

Distress encompasses the emotional, physical, and psychological aspects of facing a cancer diagnosis and treatment (Gosselin, Crane-Okada, Irwin, Tringali, & Wenzel, 2011). Early research identified distress as the sixth vital sign and asserted that all patients with cancer should routinely be screened for distress during treatment (Bultz & Johansen, 2011; Carlson, Waller, & Mitchell, 2012). Although patients can identify and report anxiety (Carlson et al., 2012), distress can have multiple meanings and thus can be difficult for patients to define, given its subjective meaning and difficulty to clearly articulate. According to Bultz and Holland (2006), the National Comprehensive Cancer Network (NCCN) used the word *distress* "to describe the psychological, social and spiritual (nonphysical) aspects of care because it carries no stigmatizing connotations and because patients feel comfortable with it" (p. 312). In 2007, the Institute of Medicine released *Cancer Care for the Whole Patient: Meeting Psychosocial Health Needs* (Adler & Page, 2008), a report identifying the seriousness of unmet psychosocial needs faced by patients with cancer and their families. One recommendation was for cancer programs to include distress screening as part of the assessment. Building upon this, ACoS CoC (2012) requires accredited cancer programs to develop a process for distress screening by 2015. The CoC specifies that patients must be screened for distress at least once during a pivotal visit, such as upon diagnosis, a pre- or post-op surgical visit, consultation with an oncologist, initiation of chemotherapy or radiation therapy, and transition into either survivorship or hospice care.

A failure to acknowledge and measure distress can lead to poorer outcomes, including decreased patient adherence (Blair, 2012). However, many cancer centers struggle with implementation and therefore have not fully incorporated screening (Bultz & Johansen, 2011). Significant issues need to be considered before distress screening is implemented, including the principal purpose of screening, staff roles and responsibilities, available resources to meet identified needs, and screening interfaces with existing processes and the medical record. It is critical to ensure that organizational and community resources are in place prior to implementation of distress screening. While many feel that navigators help to ensure that this assessment takes place, it is important to recognize that the identification and treatment of distress requires a multidisciplinary approach (Blair, 2012). Furthermore, those assigned to screen for distress must be trained and knowledgeable in how to appropriately respond, which requires time, planning, and administrative support to ensure success (Gosselin et al., 2011).

Distress Screening

Screening for distress is an important component to include when providing high-quality cancer care. Patients have expressed a desire and expectation for needs to be identified and addressed. Many barriers to care experienced by patients can contribute to distress. Fortunately, nurse navigators can play a significant role in reducing distress and allowing patients to feel as though their concerns have been heard and addressed (Swanson & Koch, 2010).

Hammonds (2012) found that nurse navigators in a university outpatient clinic were able to easily identify patients at risk for distress when using the NCCN Distress Thermometer. Although many cancer programs have migrated to the community setting, inclusion of psychosocial programs have not been a part this trend (Bultz & Holland, 2006). Failure to address distress can negatively affect how patients perceive the healthcare system (Satin, Linden, & Phillips, 2009). According to Bultz and Holland (2006), fewer than 5% of patients with psychological distress are identified or receive needed care. Studies have shown depression to be a common psychological symptom experienced by patients with cancer (Blair, 2012). If left untreated or undiagnosed, distress may affect QOL. Many studies confirm that distress is often overlooked and that many patients do not receive appropriate screening or treatment (Mitchell, Hussain, Grainger, & Symonds, 2011; Satin et al., 2009). Bultz and Holland (2006) found unrecognized depression and anxiety can lead to increased use of emergency departments in an attempt to get relief from distress-related symptoms. This places additional financial burdens on not only the patient but the healthcare system as well.

Holland and Reznik (2005) recognized the importance of distress screening during survivorship. The cancer experience can have a life-changing impact on many individuals, including the need to accept loss, lack of control in some situations, and fear of recurrence.

Horner et al. (2013) outlined the development of a nurse navigator training program built upon the psychosocial skills included in nursing curriculums. Training topics included empathic and motivational communication strategies, assessment of depression, and the development of creative strategies to address distress. This training gave the nurse navigators confidence in using the NCCN Distress Thermometer to screen patients and in providing the appropriate intervention.

Untreated psychological distress could be associated with increased incidence of suicide rates among patients with cancer. When screening for distress, nurse navigators must be aware that patients who are already experiencing depression and anxiety are at an increased risk for suicide (Cooke, Gotto, Mayorga, Grant, & Lynn, 2013). Fang et al. (2012) found that the risk of completed suicide is higher in the days after a cancer diagnosis and remains high throughout the year; thus, this is an important time to screen for distress. Misono, Weiss, Fann, Redman, and Yueh (2008) found that patients diagnosed with certain cancers, including lung, stomach, and head and neck, had the highest suicide rates. Cooke et al. (2013) identified a number of risk factors for healthcare team members to be aware of: (a) having a family history with attempted or successful suicide, (b) disease progression, (c) lack of social support, (d) difficulty with symptom management, and (e) ongoing depression. However, the authors felt that few patients are being assessed or screened for thoughts of suicide (Cooke et al., 2013). Effective psychosocial care, consisting of a multidisciplinary team approach, has been shown to positively influence patient outcomes and QOL (Misono et al., 2008).

Tools to Measure Distress

Many health professionals report uncertainty regarding which tool to use to accurately measure distress (Mitchell, Kaar, Coggan, & Herdman, 2008).

Multiple reasons have been cited including lack of time, limited resources, and a deficiency of authority to successfully implement the process throughout the health system (Fulcher & Gosselin-Acomb, 2007). Several tools have been developed and validated to measure distress, with advantages and disadvantages associated with each; however, consensus seems to indicate that using a short tool may increase the ability to identify more patients who are experiencing anxiety (Grassi et al., 2011).

The NCCN Distress Thermometer was developed in 2007 as a visual analog tool for patients to indicate their distress level (NCCN, 2012). Potential sources of distress are listed for patients to self-identify. This single-page tool can facilitate conversations between patients and healthcare providers to better elicit what is contributing to patient concerns and how these issues can be effectively resolved. According to the NCCN guidelines, patients should be screened during the initial visit and then as clinically indicated throughout treatment. Further evaluation is needed for distress levels of 4 or greater with subsequent referrals as appropriate.

Fulcher and Gosselin-Acomb (2007) piloted the NCCN Distress Thermometer in a radiation oncology clinic, finding that insurance and financial problems were the most common practical concerns, whereas worry was the most common emotional concern. Swanson and Koch (2010) used the NCCN Distress Thermometer with an adult oncology inpatient unit. Patients were screened a minimum of three to four times per admission with reductions in distress scores noted for patients age 65 and younger, as well as rural patients working with the nurse navigator. Tuinman, Gazendam-Donofrio, and Hoekstra-Weebers (2008) conducted a study using the NCCN Distress Thermometer and noted the importance of having verbal conversations to clarify and identify other barriers that patients may not have disclosed. Jacobsen et al. (2005) identified the need for additional research to ensure minority and low-literacy populations are able to complete the tool independently. Furthermore, it has been suggested that use of this tool should become a routine part of survivorship care with all PCPs and healthcare clinics (Holland & Reznik, 2005).

Although many consider the NCCN Distress Thermometer to be the standard tool for distress screening, a universally accepted screening tool has yet to be determined (Mitchell et al., 2008). Another tool commonly used to measure QOL is the Functional Assessment of Cancer Therapy–General (FACT-G). This tool has been validated and used in a variety of settings. The FACT-G consists of 27 items and four domains of well-being: physical, social/family, emotional, and functional (Fiscella et al., 2011). The questions address specific issues related to cancer including treatment, side effects, and symptoms. Because the QOL focus for patients living with advanced cancer may change as goals become centered on comfort rather than increasing survival, a shortened QOL tool for palliative care, the FACIT-Pal-14, is in the early stages of development. It is based on the FACT-G tool and consists of 14 questions specific to the palliative care population (Zeng et al., 2013).

The *SupportScreen* is a HIPAA-compliant, touch-screen computerized screening tool that allows patients to identify distress while alerting the healthcare team of such. This tool has been extensively used by the City of Hope, a comprehensive cancer center located in Duarte, California, and in a community-based demonstration project conducted by the Cancer Support Community to validate its use in the community setting. Clark et al. (2012) asserted that the *SupportScreen* is a best-practice approach to determining level of distress and tailoring appropriate support for patients based on individual preferences.

The University of North Carolina Cancer Network incorporated psychosocial training provided by a licensed psychologist and advanced practice nurses into its outreach navigation program (UNC Lineberger Comprehensive Cancer Center, n.d.-a). Education was offered by appropriate staff via video conferencing to ensure that nurse navigators were comfortable assessing for distress, providing emotional support, and making appropriate referrals. Protocols and policies were established that outlined distress screening using the NCCN tool, upon initial diagnosis, at the start of treatment, two weeks after treatment, at the end of treatment or transition to survivorship, and with recurrence or disease progression, as well as during palliative care. Nurse navigators have reported that some patients in rural communities have expressed difficulty in understanding and completing the NCCN tool. Thus, the tool is verbally reviewed by the nurse navigators during their assessments, thereby identifying distress levels and problems sooner.

Several cancer programs have demonstrated the use of nurse navigators in addressing distress; however, many continue to struggle with how to meet this important standard. Using non–health professionals and standardized questions, Kornblith et al. (2006) conducted a study to measure distress levels in older patients. Patients who had been diagnosed with advanced-stage breast, prostate, or colorectal cancer and were older than age 65 were called each month for six months by trained telephone monitors. Patients who scored above the cutoff level received a follow-up telephone call by an oncology nurse. Specific educational material was provided as indicated by disease and educational needs reported during the telephone conversations. Psychological distress, physical problems, and social support were measured using agreed-upon validated tools, and those who scored above the cutoff level were referred to an oncology nurse for further evaluation and possible referral. Overall conclusions found that patients who had received both telephone support and educational materials reported less anxiety, depression, and overall distress. It was thought that this could easily be replicated in other cancer centers as a cost-effective way to measure distress.

Patient-centered workflow processes with regard to distress screening must be incorporated into existing processes and not seen as an extra burden in order to be truly effective. The ability to assess QOL, inclusive of distress and anxiety screening, has been identified as a critical component of patient navigation (Fiscella et al., 2011). Having this information enables nurse navigators to support patients and caregivers while navigating the complexities and barriers that exist within institutions and communities (Palos & Hare, 2011).

Care Transitions

With the first introduction of the nurse navigator role to patients, an expectation should be set as to how long one will journey with the patient (Freeman & Rodriguez, 2011). The job description of the nurse navigator determines the role boundaries and responsibilities. By knowing the terms of the navigator commitment, the patient can be prepared to transition to another healthcare team member's care across the continuum of care. In some healthcare systems, one navigator may provide care from outreach to survivorship, whereas in other systems, different navigators provide care along the continuum. For example, the navigator in the outreach area, who promotes early detection through routine cancer screening, might explain that the role will continue until a screening examination is completed. If a malignancy is confirmed from the screening, the outreach navigator would introduce the patient to a navigator working in the treatment area. After treatment is completed, another transition may occur if a different navigator addresses the long-term survivorship care needs. The patient thus understands who will be involved throughout the continuum of care. The nurse navigator communicates any pertinent patient information and care issues to the healthcare team. Based upon the community assessment driving the navigation program, each healthcare system will establish a unique nurse navigation process to meet the distinct needs of patient care coordination. Just like a workflow diagram, a "team you will meet" timeline could be established and show what each member of the oncology team will be responsible for and anticipated time of involvement. This proactive navigation principle reinforces teamwork within the system and visualizes seamless care.

Shockney (2011) described the "worried well" as patients who have depended on navigators' nursing expertise and continue to call for small things after the navigation period has ended, taking up sizeable amounts of time. A clear explanation of scope of responsibilities helps patients understand the end of the nurse navigation processes and who should be contacted for future concerns. By setting distinct boundaries around the navigation role, nurse navigators use their time most efficiently and direct these individuals to the appropriate healthcare team members.

Survivorship Care

The National Coalition for Cancer Survivorship (n.d.) defines a survivor as someone from the time of diagnosis and for the balance of life. After active treatment with surgery, chemotherapy, or radiation therapy, patients may feel a sense of abandonment by the oncology team. The Institute of Medicine report *From Cancer Patient to Cancer Survivor: Lost in Transition* (Hewitt, Greenfield, & Stovall, 2006) recommended that patients should have an explanation and summary of treatment received and a follow-up care plan in order to progress into survivorship care. This report is the basis for the ACoS CoC's Survivorship Care Plan standard, which is to be phased in by all accredited healthcare systems by 2015. This patient-centered care standard ensures that a process is in place for all patients upon completion of cancer treatment to be provided with a comprehensive care summary and follow-up plan (ACoS CoC, 2012).

Nurse navigators can incorporate the healthcare system's survivorship care into initial discussions with the patient regarding the continuum of care from diagnosis to survivorship. This proactive preparation may enhance the transition when it is time to bridge the patient into the survivorship phase of care. Nurse navigators can be instrumental committee members in the development of survivorship care tools and processes such as the treatment summary, follow-up care plan, and communication to PCPs. Grant, Economou, and Ferrell (2010) suggested that nurses assess and evaluate available resources for survivorship care including prevention, surveillance, interventions, and coordination/communication. Nurse navigators have a holistic view of the population's needs and available resources to identify gaps in survivorship services, thus serving as a valuable task force member when planning survivorship processes for the healthcare system. Chapter 7 discusses survivorship navigation in more detail.

End-of-Life Care

In certain cases, the work of nurse navigators in the treatment continuum will continue as the patient approaches the end of life. Nurse navigators should promote the use of hospice services by recognizing short survival windows and understanding that patients may have end-of-life tasks to complete. Examples of these tasks might include composing a will or living will or fulfilling closure needs with caregivers, family, and friends. Nurse navigators can help patients transition to hospice and ensure that patients and families have end-of-life care resources. However, clear boundaries need to be defined for the role of navigators once hospice is involved to prevent duplication of services and confusion of roles.

Fischer, Sauaia, and Kutner (2007) identified a model using a bilingual and bicultural lay navigator to work with seriously ill Latinos at the end of life, hypothesizing that patient navigation services would increase referrals for advance directives, decrease reports of pain, and increase hospice referrals. Lay navigators received additional training regarding hospice, advance care planning, and pain management and then made five home visits to address the three end-of-life topics. A control group was used who received only written information on the three topics. Although results are not yet published, this model could be applicable to other outreach navigation programs to address disparities in end-of-life care.

Identified barriers facing patients at the end of life are the same as those facing patients throughout the disease process: challenges with the healthcare system, financial concerns, health literacy needs, and discrimination (Fischer et al., 2007). Nurse navigators at Roswell Park Cancer Institute in Buffalo, New York, recognized barriers for patients at the end of life and established processes whereby individuals in need of assistance in creating a will or settling custody issues had access to a legal team through a special grant (Lally, 2008).

Patient Feedback

To determine what comes next in a nurse navigation program, feedback from the population served is critical. The impact of navigation on the population served and the organization is important to measure for program evaluation. In the workflow of nurse navigators, a consistent time should be designated for completion of the patient survey. Whatever instrument is used to capture the voice of the patient, the quantitative or qualitative data should be presented to key stakeholders of the navigation program. Recurring themes can lead to opportunities for improvement, modifications in the navigator role, or changes in the delivery of care in the system. This can propel the program forward with a patient-centered focus. Further information on patient feedback and program metrics is covered in Chapter 9, and additional examples of patient satisfaction tools are included in Chapters 3 and 8.

Conclusion

Nurse navigators are in a position to promote patient-centered care as healthcare systems partner with communities to design the navigation model that best meets the needs of key stakeholders and patients. Navigators meet patients at multiple portals of entry. The workflow of nurse navigators will continue to be bidimensional in nature with a patient-centered and health system orientation. Nurse navigators empower patients to move forward on the journey with the confidence and resources needed to make decisions for care. When the focus of navigation remains on the patient, the work of the nurse navigator threads among the various multidisciplinary team members and weaves a path of seamless care for patients.

References

Adamsen, L., Quist, M., Andersen, C., Møller, T., Herrstedt, J., Kronborg, D., ... Rørth, M. (2009). Effect of a multimodal high intensity exercise intervention in cancer patients undergoing chemotherapy: Randomised controlled trial. *BMJ, 339,* b3410. doi:10.1136/bmj.b3410

Adler, N.E., & Page, A.E. (Eds.). (2008). *Cancer care for the whole patient: Meeting psychosocial health needs.* Washington, DC: National Academies Press.

Advisory Board Company. (2011). *Maximizing the value of patient navigation: Lessons for optimizing program performance* (Publication No. 21759). Retrieved from http://www.advisory.com/Research/Oncology-Roundtable/Studies/2011/Maximizing-the-Value-of-Patient-Navigation

Agency for Healthcare Research and Quality. (n.d.). Patient centered medical home resource center: Defining the PCMH. Retrieved from http://pcmh.ahrq.gov/page/defining-pcmh

American College of Surgeons Commission on Cancer. (2012). *Cancer program standards: Ensuring patient-centered care* [v.1.2.1, released January 2014]. Retrieved from http://facs.org/cancer/coc/programstandards2012.html

Ançel, G. (2012). Information needs of cancer patients: A comparison of nurses' and patients' perceptions. *Journal of Cancer Education, 27,* 631–640. doi:10.1007/s13187-012-0416-2

Arias, J. (2012). Patient navigation: Blending imaging and oncology in breast cancer. *Journal of Oncology Navigation and Survivorship, 3*(1), 16–21. Retrieved from http://issuu.com/aonn/docs/jons-feb2012

Banks, E., Byles, J.E., Gibson, R.E., Rodgers, B., Latz, I.K., Robinson, I.A., ... Jorm, L.R. (2010). Is psychological distress in people living with cancer related to the fact of diagnosis, current treatment or level of disability? Findings from a large Australian study. *Medical Journal of Australia, 193*(Suppl. 5), S62–S67. Retrieved from https://www.mja.com.au/journal/2010/193/5/psychological-distress-people-living-cancer-related-fact-diagnosis-current

Battaglia, T.A., Bak, S.M., Heeren, T., Chen, C.A., Kalish, R., Tringale, S., ... Freund., K.M. (2012). Boston Patient Navigation Research Program: The impact of navigation on time to diagnostic resolution after abnormal cancer screening. *Cancer Epidemiology, Biomarkers and Prevention, 21,* 1645–1654. doi:10.1158/1055-9965.EPI-12-0532

Bickell, N.A., & Paskett, E.D. (2013). Reducing inequalities in cancer outcomes: What works? *American Society of Clinical Oncology Educational Book, 2013,* 250–254. doi:10.1200/EdBook_AM.2013.33.e250

Blair, E.W. (2012). Understanding depression: Awareness, assessment, and nursing intervention. *Clinical Journal of Oncology Nursing, 16,* 463–465. doi:10.1188/12.CJON.463-465

Blais, D. (2008). Nurse navigation: Supporting patients and their families through the healthcare system. *Alberta RN, 64*(7), 19.

Blaseg, K. (2009). Patient navigation at Billings Clinic: An NCI Community Cancer Centers Program (NCCCP) pilot site. In Association of Community Cancer Centers, *Cancer care patient navigation: A call to action* (pp. S15–S24). Retrieved from http://accc-cancer.org/education/pdf/PN2009/s15.pdf

Bowles, E.J.A., Tuzzio, L., Wiese, C.J., Kirlin, B., Greene, S.M., Clauser, S.B., & Wagner, E.H. (2008). Understanding high-quality cancer care: A summary of expert perspectives. *Cancer, 112*, 934–942. doi:10.1002/cncr.23250

Brown, C.G., Cantril, C., McMullen, L., Barkley, D.L., Dietz, M., Murphy, C.M., & Fabrey, L.J. (2012). Oncology Nurse Navigator Role Delineation Study: An Oncology Nursing Society report. *Clinical Journal of Oncology Nursing, 16*, 581–585. doi:10.1188/12. CJON.581-585

Bultz, B.D., & Holland, J.C. (2006). Emotional distress in patients with cancer: The sixth vital sign. *Community Oncology, 3*, 311–314. doi:10.1016/S1548-5315(11)70702-1

Bultz, B.D., & Johansen, C. (2011). Screening for distress, the 6th vital sign: Where are we, and where are we going? *Psycho-Oncology, 20*, 569–571. doi:10.1002/pon.1986

Byers, T. (2012). Assessing the value of patient navigation for completing cancer screening. *Cancer Epidemiology, Biomarkers and Prevention, 21*, 1618–1619. doi:10.1158/1055-9965.EPI -12-0964

Campbell, C., Craig, J., Eggert, J., & Bailey-Dorton, C. (2010). Implementing and measuring the impact of patient navigation at a comprehensive community care center. *Oncology Nursing Forum, 37*, 61–68. doi:10.1188/10.ONF.61-68

Campinha-Bacote, J. (2011). Delivering patient-centered care in the midst of a cultural conflict: The role of cultural competence. *Online Journal of Issues in Nursing, 16*(2), Manuscript 5. doi:10.3912/OJIN.Vol16No02Man05

Carlson, L.E., Waller, A., & Mitchell, A.J. (2012). Screening for distress and unmet needs in patients with cancer: Review and recommendations. *Journal of Clinical Oncology, 30*, 1160–1177. doi:10.1200/JCO.2011.39.5509

Carroll, J.K., Humiston, S.G., Meldrum, S.C., Salamone, C.M., Jean-Pierre, P., Epstein, R.M., & Fiscella, K. (2010). Patients' experiences with navigation for cancer care. *Patient Education and Counseling, 80*, 241–247. doi:10.1016/j.pec.2009.10.024

Cascella, S., & Keren, J. (2012). Mujer a mujer/woman to woman: Using a unique venue for culturally appropriate outreach and navigation in an underserved area to increase screening. *Journal of Oncology Navigation and Survivorship, 3*(2), 20–26. Retrieved from http://issuu. com/theoncologynurse/docs/jons_april_12_final

Case, M.A.B. (2011). Oncology nurse navigator: Ensuring safe passage. *Clinical Journal of Oncology Nursing, 15*, 33–40. doi:10.1188/11.CJON.33-40

Center for Universal Design & North Carolina Office on Disability and Health. (2007). Removing barriers to health care: A guide for healthcare professionals. Retrieved from http://fpg.unc. edu/sites/fpg.unc.edu/files/resources/other-resources/NCODH_RemovingBarriers ToHealthCare.pdf

Centers for Disease Control and Prevention. (2012, October 12). Disability and health: Accessibility. Retrieved from http://www.cdc.gov/ncbddd/disabilityandhealth/accessibility.html

Center to Advance Palliative Care. (2011). *2011 public opinion research on palliative care: A report based on research by public opinion strategies.* Retrieved from http://www.capc.org/tools -for-palliative-care-programs/marketing/public-opinion-research/2011-public-opinion -research-on-palliative-care.pdf

Chlebowski, R.T., Blackburn, G.L., Thomson, C.A., Nixon, D.W., Shapiro, A., Hoy, M.K., ... Elashoff, R.M. (2006). Dietary fat reduction and breast cancer outcome: Interim efficacy results from the Women's Intervention Nutrition Study. *Journal of the National Cancer Institute, 98*, 1767–1776. doi:10.1093/jnci/djj494

Clark, P.G., Bolte, S., Buzaglo, J., Golant, M., Daratsos, L., & Loscalzo, M. (2012). From distress guidelines to developing models of psychosocial care: Current best practices. *Journal of Psychosocial Oncology, 30*, 694–714. doi:10.1080/07347332.2012.721488

Cooke, L., Gotto, J., Mayorga, L., Grant, M., & Lynn, R. (2013). What do I say? Suicide assessment and management [Online exclusive]. *Clinical Journal of Oncology Nursing, 17*, E1–E7. doi:10.1188/13.CJON.E1-E7

Cramp, F., & Byron-Daniel, J. (2012). Exercise for the management of cancer-related fatigue in adults. *Cochrane Database of Systematic Reviews, 2012*(11). doi:10.1002/14651858.CD006145. pub3

Cronholm, P.F., Shea, J.A., Werner, R.M., Miller-Day, M., Tufano, J., Crabtee, B.F., & Gabbay, R. (2013). The patient centered medical home: Mental models and practice culture driving the transformation process. *Journal of General Internal Medicine, 28*, 1195–1201. doi:10.1007/s11606-013-2415-3

Desimini, E.M., Kennedy, J.A., Helsley, M.F., Shiner, K., Denton, C., Rice, T.T., ... Lewis, M.G. (2011). Making the case for nurse navigators—Benefits, outcomes, and return on investment. *Oncology Issues, 26*(5), 26–33. Retrieved from http://pages.nxtbook.com/nxtbooks/accc/oncologyissues_20110910/offline/accc_oncologyissues_20110910.pdf

Dohan, D., & Schrag, D. (2005). Using navigators to improve care of underserved patients: Current practices and approaches. *Cancer, 104*, 848–855. doi:10.1002/cncr.21214

Doll, R., Barroetavena, M.C., Ellwood, A.-L., Fillion, L., Habra, M.E., Linden, W., & Stephen, J. (2007). The cancer care navigator: Toward a conceptual framework for a new role in oncology. *Oncology Exchange, 6*(4), 28–33. Retrieved from http://www.oncologyex.com/gif/archive/2007/vol6_no4/6_continuing_care_4.pdf

Eagle, D., & Sprandio, J. (2011). A care model for the future: The oncology medical home. *Oncology, 25*, 571, 575–576. Retrieved from http://www.cancernetwork.com/practice-policy/care-model-future-oncology-medical-home

Eley, R.M., Rogers-Clark, C., & Murray, K. (2008). The value of a breast care nurse in supporting rural and remote cancer patients in Queensland. *Cancer Nursing, 31*(6), E10–E18. doi:10.1097/01.NCC.0000339246.60700.cf

EPEC. (n.d.). Education in Palliative and End-of-Life Care (EPEC®). Retrieved from http://www.epec.net/epec_core.php

Fang, F., Fall, K., Mittleman, M.A., Sparén, P., Ye, W., Adami, H.-O., & Valdimarsdóttir, U. (2012). Suicide and cardiovascular death after a cancer diagnosis. *New England Journal of Medicine, 366*, 1310–1318. doi:10.1056/NEJMoa1110307

Fillion, L., Cook, S., Veillette, A.-M., Aubin, M., de Serres, M., Rainville, F., ... Doll, R. (2012). Professional navigation framework: Elaboration and validation in a Canadian context [Online exclusive]. *Oncology Nursing Forum, 39*, E58–E69. doi:10.1188/12.ONF.E58-E69

Fillion, L., de Serres, M., Lapointe-Goupil, R., Bairati, I., Gagnon, P., Deschamps, M., ... Demers, G. (2006). Implementing the role of patient-navigator nurse at a university hospital centre. *Canadian Oncology Nursing Journal, 16*, 11–17, 5–10.

Fiscella, K., Ransom, S., Jean-Pierre, P., Cella, D., Stein, K., Bauer, J.E., ... Walsh, K. (2011). Patient-reported outcome measures suitable to assessment of patient navigation. *Cancer, 117*(Suppl. 15), 3603–3617. doi:10.1002/cncr.26260

Fiscella, K., Whitley, E., Hendren, S., Raich, P., Humiston, S., Winters, P., ... Epstein, R. (2012). Patient navigation for breast and colorectal cancer treatment: A randomized trial. *Cancer Epidemiology, Biomarkers and Prevention, 21*, 1673–1681. doi:10.1158/1055-9965.EPI-12-0506

Fischer, S.M., Sauaia, A., & Kutner, J.S. (2007). Patient navigation: A culturally competent strategy to address disparities in palliative care. *Journal of Palliative Medicine, 10*, 1023–1028. doi:10.1089/jpm.2007.0070

Fitch, M.I. (2008). Supportive care framework. *Canadian Oncology Nursing Journal, 18*, 6–14.

Freeman, H.P., & Rodriguez, R.L. (2011). History and principles of patient navigation. *Cancer, 117*(Suppl. 15), 3539–3542. doi:10.1002/cncr.26262

Fu, M.R., Ryan, J.C., & Cleland, C.M. (2012). Lymphedema knowledge and practice patterns among oncology nurse navigators. *Journal of Oncology Navigation and Survivorship, 3*(4), 8–15. Retrieved from http://issuu.com/theoncologynurse/docs/jons_august_2012_web

Fulcher, C.D., & Gosselin-Acomb, T.K. (2007). Distress assessment: Practice change through guideline implementation. *Clinical Journal of Oncology Nursing, 11*, 817–821. doi:10.1188/07. CJON.817-821

Gade, G., Venohr, I., Conner, D., McGrady, K., Beane, J., Richardson, R.H., ... Della Penna, R. (2008). Impact of an inpatient palliative care team: A randomized control trial. *Journal of Palliative Medicine, 11*, 180–190. doi:10.1089/jpm.2007.0055

Goldsmith, J., Ferrell, B., Wittenberg-Lyles, E., & Ragan, S.L. (2013). Palliative care communication in oncology nursing. *Clinical Journal of Oncology Nursing, 17*, 163–167. doi:10.1188/13. CJON.163-167

Gonzalez, M., Berger, M., Bryant, D., Ellison, C., Harness, J., Krasna, M., ... Wilkinson, K. (2011). Using a minority matrix and patient navigation to improve accrual to clinical trials. *Oncology Issues, 26*(2), 59–60. Retrieved from http://ncccp.cancer.gov/files/CT_Minority_Matrix_MARCH_APRIL_2011-508.pdf

Gosselin, T.K., Crane-Okada, R., Irwin, M., Tringali, C., & Wenzel, J. (2011). Measuring oncology nurses' psychosocial care practices and needs: Results of an Oncology Nursing Society psychosocial survey. *Oncology Nursing Forum, 38*, 729–737. doi:10.1188/11.ONF.729-737

Granda-Cameron, C., DeMille, D., Lynch, M.P., Huntzinger, C., Alcorn, T., Levicoff, J., ... Mintzer, D. (2010). An interdisciplinary approach to manage cancer cachexia. *Clinical Journal of Oncology Nursing, 14*, 72–80. doi:10.1188/10.CJON.72-80

Grant, M., Economou, D., & Ferrell, B.R. (2010). Oncology nurse participation in survivorship care. *Clinical Journal of Oncology Nursing, 14*, 709–715. doi:10.1188/10.CJON.709-715

Grassi, L., Rossi, E., Caruso, R., Nanni, M.G., Pedrazzi, S., Sofritti, S., & Sabato, S. (2011). Educational intervention in cancer outpatient clinics on routine screening for emotional distress: An observational study. *Psycho-Oncology, 20*, 669–674. doi:10.1002/pon.1944

Hammonds, L.S. (2012). Implementing a distress screening instrument in a university breast cancer clinic: A quality improvement project. *Clinical Journal of Oncology Nursing, 16*, 491–494. doi:10.1188/12.CJON.491-494

Hanna, L.R., Avila, P.F., Meteer, J.D., Nicholas, D.R., & Kaminsky, L.A. (2008). The effects of a comprehensive exercise program on physical function, fatigue, and mood in patients with various types of cancer. *Oncology Nursing Forum, 35*, 461–469. doi:10.1188/08.ONF.461-469

Hauser, J., Sileo, M., Araneta, N., Kirk, R., Martinez, J., Finn, K., ... Rodrigue, M.K. (2011). Navigation and palliative care. *Cancer, 117*(Suppl. 15), 3585–3591. doi:10.1002/cncr.26266

Hewitt, M., Greenfield, S., & Stovall, E. (Eds.). (2006). *From cancer patient to cancer survivor: Lost in transition.* Washington, DC: National Academies Press.

Hoffman, H.J., LaVerda, N.L., Young, H.A., Levine, P.H., Alexander, L.M., Brem, R., ... Patierno, S.R. (2012). Patient navigation significantly reduces delays in breast cancer diagnosis in the District of Columbia. *Cancer Epidemiology, Biomarkers and Prevention, 21*, 1655–1663. doi:10.1158/1055-9965.EPI-12-0479

Holland, J.C., & Reznik, I. (2005). Pathways for psychosocial care of cancer survivors. *Cancer, 104*(Suppl. 11), 2624–2637. doi:10.1002/cncr.21252

Holmes, D.R., Major, J., Lyonga, D.E., Alleyne, R.S., & Clayton, S.M. (2012). Increasing minority patient participation in cancer clinical trials using oncology nurse navigation. *American Journal of Surgery, 203*, 415–422. doi:10.1016/j.amjsurg.2011.02.005

Hook, A., Ware, L., Siler, B., & Packard, A. (2012). Breast cancer navigation and patient satisfaction: Exploring a community-based patient navigation model in a rural setting. *Oncology Nursing Forum, 39*, 379–385. doi:10.1188/12.ONF.379-385

Horner, K., Ludman, E.J., McCorkle, R., Canfield, E., Flaherty, L., Min, J., ... Wagner, E.H. (2013). An oncology nurse navigator program designed to eliminate gaps in early cancer care. *Clinical Journal of Oncology Nursing, 17*, 43–48. doi:10.1188/13.CJON.43-48

Hudson, S.V., Miller, S.M., Hemler, J., McClinton, A., Oeffinger, K.C., Tallia, A., & Crabtree, B.F. (2012). Cancer survivors and patient-centered medical home. *Translational Behavioral Medicine, 2*, 322–331. doi:10.1007/s13142-012-0138-3

Hunnibell, L.S., Rose, M.G., Connery, D.M., Grens, C.E., Hampel, J.M., Rosa, M., & Vogel, D.C. (2012). Using nurse navigation to improve timeliness of lung cancer care at a veterans hospital. *Clinical Journal of Oncology Nursing, 16*, 29–36. doi:10.1188/12.CJON.29-36

Iezzoni, L.I., Kilbridge, K., & Park, E.R. (2010). Physical access barriers to care for diagnosis and treatment of breast cancer among women with mobility impairments. *Oncology Nursing Forum, 37,* 711–717. doi:10.1188/10.ONF.711-717

Institute of Medicine. (2001). *Crossing the quality chasm: A new health system for the 21st century.* Washington, DC: National Academies Press.

Jacobsen, P.B., Donovan, K.A., Trask, P.C., Fleishman, S.B., Zabora, J., Baker, F., & Holland, J.C. (2005). Screening for psychological distress in ambulatory cancer patients: A multicenter evaluation of the Distress Thermometer. *Cancer, 103,* 1494–1502. doi:10.1002/cncr.20940

Koh, C., Nelson, J.M., & Cook, P.F. (2011). Evaluation of a patient navigation program. *Clinical Journal of Oncology Nursing, 15,* 41–48. doi:10.1188/11.CJON.41-48

Korber, S.F., Padula, C., Gray, J., & Powell, M. (2011). A breast navigator program: Barriers, enhancers, and nursing interventions. *Oncology Nursing Forum, 38,* 44–50. doi:10.1188/11.ONF.44-50

Kornblith, A.B., Dowell, J.M., Herndon, J.E., Engelman, B.J., Bauer-Wu, S., Small, E.J., … Holland, J.C. (2006). Telephone monitoring of distress in patients aged 65 years or older with advanced stage cancer: A Cancer and Leukemia Group B study. *Cancer, 107,* 2706–2714. doi:10.1002/cncr.22296

Lagrosa, D. (2011). Breast patient navigation program hopes to reduce disparities among Hispanic/Latina women. *Journal of Oncology Navigation and Survivorship, 2*(3), 20–21. Retrieved from http://issuu.com/aonn/docs/jons_may2011

Lally, R.M. (2008). They have a dream: Nurses work to reduce cancer disparities in their communities. *ONS Connect, 23*(6), 10–14. Retrieved from http://www.nxtbook.com/nxtbooks/ons/connect_200806/index.php?startid=10

Langewitz, W., Heydrich, L., Nübling, M., Szirt, L., Weber, H., & Grossman, P. (2010). Swiss Cancer League communication skills training programme for oncology nurses: An evaluation. *Journal of Advanced Nursing, 66,* 2266–2277. doi:10.1111/j.1365-2648.2010.05386.x

Leonhart, K.K., Bonin, D., & Pagel, P. (2008, April). *Guide for developing a community-based patient safety advisory council* (AHRQ Publication No. 08-0048). Retrieved from http://www.ahrq.gov/professionals/quality-patient-safety/patient-safety-resources/resources/patient-safety-advisory-council/patient-safety-advisory-council.pdf

Lester, J.L., & Schmitt, P. (Eds.). (2011). *Cancer rehabilitation and survivorship: Transdisciplinary approaches to personalized care.* Pittsburgh, PA: Oncology Nursing Society.

Li, C., Carli, F., Lee, L., Charlebois, P., Stein, B., Liberman, A.S., … Feldman, L.S. (2013). Impact of a trimodal prehabilitation program on functional recovery after colorectal cancer surgery: A pilot study. *Surgical Endoscopy, 27,* 1072–1082. doi:10.1007/s00464-012-2560-5

Lorhan, S., Cleghorn, L., Fitch, M., Pang, K., McAndrew, A., Applin-Poole, J., … Wright, M. (2013). Moving the agenda forward for cancer patient navigation: Understanding volunteer and peer navigation approaches. *Journal of Cancer Education, 28,* 84–91. doi:10.1007/s13187-012-0424-2

Lusk, J.M., & Fater, K. (2013). A concept analysis of patient-centered care. *Nursing Forum, 48,* 89–98. doi:10.1111/nuf.12019

Markossian, T.W., Darnell, J.S., & Calhoun, E.A. (2012). Follow-up and timeliness after an abnormal cancer screening among underserved, urban women in a patient navigation program. *Cancer Epidemiology, Biomarkers and Prevention, 21,* 1691–1700. doi:10.1158/1055-9965.EPI-12-0535

Mayo, N.E., Feldman, L., Scott, S., Zavorsky, G., Kim, D.J., Charlebois, P., … Carli, F. (2011). Impact of preoperative change in physical function on postoperative recovery: Argument supporting prehabilitation for colorectal surgery. *Surgery, 150,* 505–514. doi:10.1016/j.surg.2011.07.045

McMullen, L. (2013). Oncology nurse navigators and the continuum of cancer care. *Seminars in Oncology Nursing, 29,* 105–117. doi:10.1016/j.soncn.2013.02.005

Messier, N. (2010). The navigator's role in coordinating multidisciplinary clinics and tumor boards. *Journal of Oncology Navigation and Survivorship, 1*(6), 21. Retrieved from http://issuu.com/aonn/docs/jons_november2010

Meyerhardt, J.A., Niedzwiecki, D., Hollis, D., Saltz, L.B., Hu, F.B., Mayer, R.J., … Fuchs, C.S. (2007). Association of dietary patterns with cancer recurrence and survival in patients with stage III colon cancer. *JAMA, 298,* 754–764. doi:10.1001/jama.298.7.754

Mishel, M.H., Germino, B.B., Lin, L., Pruthi, R.S., Wallen, E.M., Crandell, J., & Blyler, D. (2009). Managing uncertainty about treatment decision making in early stage prostate cancer: A randomized clinical trial. *Patient Education and Counseling, 77,* 349–359. http://dx.doi.org/10.1016/j.pec.2009.09.009

Misono, S., Weiss, N.S., Fann, J.R., Redman, M., & Yueh, B. (2008). Incidence of suicide in persons with cancer. *Journal of Clinical Oncology, 26,* 4731–4738. doi:10.1200/JCO.2007.13.8941

Mitchell, A.J., Hussain, N., Grainger, L., & Symonds, P. (2011). Identification of patient-reported distress by clinical nurse specialists in routine oncology practice: A multicenter UK study. *Psycho-Oncology, 20,* 1076–1083. doi:10.1002/pon.1815

Mitchell, A.J., Kaar, S., Coggan, C., & Herdman, J. (2008). Acceptability of common screening methods used to detect distress and related mood disorders—Preferences of cancer specialists and non-specialists. *Psycho-Oncology, 17,* 226–236. doi:10.1002/pon.1228

Morrison, R.S., Penrod, J.D., Cassel, J.B., Caust-Ellenbogen, M., Litke, A., Spragen, L., & Meier, D.E. (2008). Cost savings associated with US hospital palliative care consultation programs. *Archives of Internal Medicine, 168,* 1783–1790. doi:10.1001/archinte.168.16.1783

Natale-Pereira, A., Enard, K.R., Nevarez, L., & Jones, L.A (2011). The role of patient navigators in eliminating health disparities. *Cancer, 117*(Suppl. 15), 3543–3552. doi:10.1002/cncr.26264

National Cancer Institute. (2013, June 26). EPEC™-O palliative care education materials: EPEC™-O self-study. Retrieved from http://www.cancer.gov/cancertopics/cancerlibrary/epeco

National Coalition for Cancer Survivorship. (n.d.). History of NCCS. Retrieved from http://www.canceradvocacy.org/about-us/our-history

National Comprehensive Cancer Network. (2012, October 11). *NCCN Clinical Practice Guidelines in Oncology: Distress management* [v.2.2013]. Retrieved from http://www.nccn.org/professionals/physician_gls/pdf/distress.pdf

National Consensus Project for Quality Palliative Care. (2009). *Clinical practice guidelines for quality palliative care* (2nd ed.). Retrieved from http://www.nationalconsensusproject.org/Guideline.pdf

National Lymphedema Network Medical Advisory Committee. (2012, May). Position statement of the National Lymphedema Network: Lymphedema risk reduction practices. Retrieved from http://lymphnet.org/pdfDocs/nlnriskreduction.pdf

Newman-Horm, P.A. (2005). *C-Change. Cancer patient navigation.* Washington, DC: C-Change.

Novant Health Derrick L. Davis Cancer Center. (2013). *Annual breast nurse navigation cancer committee report.* Winston-Salem, NC: Author.

Oldervoll, L.M., Loge, J.H., Paltiel, H., Asp, M.B., Vidvei, U., Hjermstad, M.J., & Kaasa, S. (2005). Are palliative cancer patients willing and able to participate in a physical exercise program? *Palliative and Supportive Care, 3,* 281–287. doi:10.1017/S1478951505050443

Oncology Nursing Society. (n.d.). Diversity and cultural competency. Retrieved from http://www2.ons.org/Membership/Diversity

Palos, G.R., & Hare, M. (2011). Patient, family caregivers, and patient navigators: A partnership approach. *Cancer, 117*(Suppl. 15), 3592–3602. doi:10.1002/cncr.26263

Paskett, E.D., Katz, M.L., Post, D.M., Pennell, M.L., Young, G.S., Seiber, E.E., … Murray, D.M. (2012). The Ohio Patient Navigation Research Program: Does the American Cancer Society patient navigation model improve time to resolution in patients with abnormal screening tests? *Cancer Epidemiology, Biomarkers and Prevention, 21,* 1620–1628. doi:10.1158/1055-9965.EPI-12-0523

Pedersen, A.E., & Hack, T.F. (2011). The British Columbia Patient Navigation Model: A critical analysis. *Oncology Nursing Forum, 38*, 200–206. doi:10.1188/11.ONF.200-206

Plante, A., & Joannette, S. (2009). Montérégie Comprehensive Cancer Care Centre: Integrating nurse navigators in Montérégie's oncology teams: The process. Part 2. *Canadian Oncology Nursing Journal, 19*, 72–77. Retrieved from http://www.cano-acio.ca/~ASSETS/DOCUMENT/Member%20Communications/CONJ%2019.2.pdf

Psooy, B.J., Schreuer, D., Borgaonkar, J., & Caines, J.S. (2004). Patient navigation: Improving timeliness in the diagnosis of breast abnormalities. *Canadian Association of Radiologists Journal, 55*, 145–150.

Quist, M., Rørth, M., Langer, S., Jones, L.W., Laursen, J.H., Pappot, H., … Adamsen, L. (2012). Safety and feasibility of a combined exercise intervention for inoperable lung cancer patients undergoing chemotherapy: A pilot study. *Lung Cancer, 75*, 203–208. doi:10.1016/j.lungcan.2011.07.006

Satin, J.R., Linden, W., & Phillips, M.J. (2009). Depression as a predictor of disease progression and mortality in cancer patients: A meta-analysis. *Cancer, 115*, 5349–5361. doi:10.1002/cncr.24561

Schwaderer, K.A., & Itano, J.K. (2007). Bridging the healthcare divide with patient navigation: Development of a research program to address disparities. *Clinical Journal of Oncology Nursing, 11*, 633–639. doi:10.1188/07.CJON.633-639

Seek, A.J., & Hogle, W.P. (2007). Modeling a better way: Navigating the healthcare system for patients with lung cancer. *Clinical Journal of Oncology Nursing, 11*, 81–85. doi:10.1188/07.CJON.81-85

Sheldon, L.K. (2005). Communication in oncology care: The effectiveness of skills training workshops for healthcare providers. *Clinical Journal of Oncology Nursing, 9*, 305–312. doi:10.1188/05.CJON.305-312

Shockney, L.D. (2008). Talking to patients about participating in clinical trials. In L.D. Shockney (Ed.), *The John Hopkins breast cancer handbook for health care professionals* (pp. 269–275). Burlington, MA: Jones and Bartlett.

Shockney, L.D. (2010). Evolution of patient navigation. *Clinical Journal of Oncology Nursing, 14*, 405–407. doi:10.1188/10.CJON.405-407

Shockney, L.D. (2011). *Becoming a breast cancer nurse navigator.* Burlington, MA: Jones and Bartlett.

Silver, J. (2013, April). *The next frontier in survivorship care.* Presentation delivered for Mind-Stream Education Oncology Nurse Navigation Executive Leadership Forum, Orlando, FL.

Smith, C.B., Nelson, J.E., Berman, A.R., Powell, C.A., Fleischman, J., Salazar-Schicchi, J., & Wisnivesky, J.P. (2012). Lung cancer physicians' referral practices for palliative care consultation. *Annals of Oncology, 23*, 382–387. doi:10.1093/annonc/mdr345

Smith, T.J., Temin, S., Alesi, E.R., Abernethy, A.P., Balboni, T.A., Basch, E.M., …Von Roenn, J.H. (2012). American Society of Clinical Oncology provisional clinical opinion: The integration of palliative care into standard oncology care. *Journal of Clinical Oncology, 30*, 880–887. doi:10.1200/JCO.2011.38.5161

Sprandio, J.D. (2010). Oncology patient-centered medical home and accountable cancer care. *Community Oncology, 7*, 565–572. doi:10.1016/S1548-5315(11)70537-X

Swanson, J., & Koch, L. (2010). The role of the oncology nurse navigator in distress management of adult inpatients with cancer: A retrospective study. *Oncology Nursing Forum, 37*, 69–76. doi:10.1188/10.ONF.69-76

Swanson, P.L., Strusowski, P., Asfeldt, T., De Groot, J., Hegedus, P.D., Krasna, M., & White, D. (2012). Expanding multidisciplinary care in community cancer centers: An MDC assessment tool developed by the NCCCP. In Association of Community Cancer Centers, *The NCCCP Monograph: Enhancing access, improving the quality of care, and expanding research in the community setting* (pp. 40–44). Retrieved from http://accc-cancer.org/publications/NCI-CCCProgram.asp

Tuinman, M.A., Gazendam-Donofrio, S.M., & Hoekstra-Weebers, J.E. (2008). Screening and referral for psychosocial distress in oncologic practice. *Cancer, 113*, 870–878. doi:10.1002/cncr.23622

Ugolini, D., Neri, M., Cesario, A., Bonassi, S., Milazzo, D., Bennati, L., … Pasqualetti, P. (2012). Scientific production in cancer rehabilitation grows higher: A bibliometric analysis. *Supportive Care in Cancer, 20*, 1629–1638. doi:10.1007/s00520-011-1253-2

UNC Lineberger Comprehensive Cancer Center. (n.d.-a). Comprehensive Cancer Support Program: Mental health services. Retrieved from http://unclineberger.org/ccsp/programs/mental-health-services

UNC Lineberger Comprehensive Cancer Center (n.d.-b). Nurse navigation. Retrieved from http://unclineberger.org/unc-cancer-network/educationandoutreach

Vardaman, J.M., Cornell, P.T., & Clancy, T.R. (2012). Complexity and change in nurse workflows. *Journal of Nursing Administration, 42*, 78–82. doi:10.1097/NNA.0b013e3182433677

Von Ah, D., Jansen, C., Allen, D.H., Schiavone, R.M., & Wulff, J. (2011). Putting Evidence Into Practice: Evidence-based interventions for cancer and cancer treatment-related cognitive impairment. *Clinical Journal of Oncology Nursing, 15*, 607–615. doi:10.1188/11.CJON.607-615

Von Roenn, J.H., Voltz, R., & Serrie, A. (2013). Barriers and approaches to the successful integration of palliative care and oncology practice. *Journal of the National Comprehensive Cancer Network, 11*(Suppl. 1), S11–S16. Retrieved from http://www.jnccn.org/content/11/suppl_1/S-11.long

Wagner, E.H., Bowles, E.J.A., Greene, S.M., Tuzzio, L., Wiese, C.J., Kirlin, B., & Clauser, S.B. (2010). The quality of cancer patient experience: Perspectives of patients, family members, providers and experts. *Quality and Safety in Health Care, 19*, 484–489. doi:10.1136/qshc.2010.042374

Wells, K.J., Battaglia, T.A., Dudley, D.J., Garcia, R., Greene, A., Calhoun, E., … Raich, P.C. (2008). Patient navigation: State of the art or is it science? *Cancer, 113*, 1999–2010. doi:10.1002/cncr.23815

Wilcox, B., & Bruce, S.D. (2010). Patient navigation: A "win-win" for all involved. *Oncology Nursing Forum, 37*, 21–25. doi:10.1188/10.ONF.21-25

Wittenberg-Lyles, E., Goldsmith, J., & Ferrell, B. (2013). Oncology nurse communication barriers to patient-centered care. *Clinical Journal of Oncology Nursing, 17*, 152–158. doi:10.1188/13.CJON.152-158

Zeng, L., Bedard, G., Cella, D., Thavarajah, N., Chen, E., Zhang, L., … Chow, E. (2013). Preliminary results of the generation of a shortened quality-of-life assessment for patients with advanced cancer: the FACIT-Pal-14. *Journal of Palliative Medicine, 16*, 509–515. doi:10.1089/jpm.2012.0595

CHAPTER 5

Breast Cancer Navigation

Barbara Francks, RN, BSN, OCN®, CBCN®, Mary Lou Iverson, RN, MN, OCN®, and Jackie Miller, RN, BSN, OCN®

Introduction

Breast cancer is the most common cancer in women (American Cancer Society, 2014). The journey of a patient with breast cancer typically starts with screening and continues on to a positive diagnosis and potentially complicated course of treatment. This emotionally overwhelming and often bewildering situation presents many challenges for newly diagnosed patients with breast cancer, such as learning medical terminology and jargon, maneuvering in an unknown healthcare facility, adjusting work schedules to meet treatment demands, explaining the diagnosis and treatment details to family and friends, and shifting financial resources. Patients with breast cancer have reported feelings of fear, loneliness, depression, anger, anxiety, and distrust. Patient navigation is one strategy that has proven successful in supporting patients (Advisory Board Company, 2007; Freeman, 2012).

The concept of patient navigation was founded by Harold P. Freeman, MD, in 1990; he identified navigation services that helped reduce health disparities in breast cancer treatment and mortality for African American women in Harlem, New York City (Freeman, 2012). From that point, cancer navigation programs have rapidly evolved because of benefits to survival and the need for multiple oncology specialists and multimodality treatments (Robinson-White, Conroy, Slavish, & Rosenzweig, 2010). Since their introduction in 1990, breast cancer navigation programs have produced favorable outcomes in reducing barriers and eliminating gaps in care for patients with breast cancer (Hendren et al., 2011; Horner et al., 2013; Stanley et al., 2013). The complexity of breast cancer treatment, as well as patient volumes, may justify the need for a breast cancer nurse navigator to focus on improvements in timeliness of care and patient outcomes (Schafer & Swisher, 2006). Today, breast cancer nurse navigation has become a valued service and a standard for cancer program accreditation (National Accreditation Program for Breast Centers, 2013).

Essential Qualities of a Breast Cancer Navigator

Breast cancer management can be complex and challenging for newly diagnosed patients. Adding to the complexity is the reality that patients with breast cancer are notably diverse in demographic and ethnic backgrounds, financial circumstances, coping skills, support systems, and contributing comorbidities. Patients have identified compassionate guidance and accurate education regarding breast cancer as essential to successfully traversing the breast cancer continuum (Korber, Padula, Gray, & Powell, 2011). With this in mind, breast cancer nurse navigators will optimally have experience in breast cancer care and in-depth knowledge of breast cancer treatment guidelines, as well as a solid understanding of cancer treatments, to be able to successfully navigate patients. Wide-ranging nursing experience and education allow breast cancer nurse navigators to approach patients with confidence while maintaining professional and supportive relationships. Moreover, a thorough understanding of each of the roles on the multidisciplinary team and good rapport with these individuals will facilitate seamless referrals and timely access to care for patients with breast cancer.

Overview of Breast Cancer Navigation

Breast cancer navigation can begin and end at various points throughout the cancer continuum and should be based on the specific program objectives, as well as patient and community needs. Often, breast cancer navigation begins with access to and implementation of breast cancer screening and diagnostic procedures. Navigators have been very successful in engaging participation in screening programs, particularly among those experiencing healthcare disparities (Brown et al., 2012; Campbell, Craig, Eggert, & Bailey-Dorton, 2010; Chatman & Green, 2011; Freeman & Rodriguez, 2011; Hendren et al., 2011; McDonald, 2011). Barriers that impede access to screening and follow-up procedures result in increased incidence of advanced breast cancer.

From the time a patient finds a breast lump or is informed of an abnormal mammogram, a sense of urgency typically ensues. Timeliness of follow-up studies or consultation with appropriate physicians is critical. Research has shown that patient navigation significantly reduces delays in breast cancer diagnosis (Hoffman et al., 2012), whereby navigated women reach diagnostic resolution significantly faster than those not navigated. While successful breast diagnostic navigation can decrease the time to diagnosis (Markossian, Darnell, & Calhoun, 2012), expediently reaching a definitive diagnosis of breast cancer after screening also can improve outcomes and overall survival for those with early-stage breast cancer (Stanley et al., 2013).

In centers where mammography screening occurs throughout the community, programs must determine how to identify patients who require breast navigation services. For example, a patient may have a breast biopsy performed at an imaging center and then be referred back to the ordering physician or to a breast surgeon. Outreach communication should be conducted with imaging centers, primary care physicians, and gynecologists to promote available navigation services and pathways for initiating patient referrals. Such efforts conducted periodically will establish strong working relationships and demonstrate accessibility, as well as commitment, to meeting the needs of external providers and staff.

In addition to facilitating access to screening and timely resolution of abnormal findings, breast cancer nurse navigators help patients understand the purpose of procedures and comprehend the meaning of pathology results. This education provides the opportunity to establish rapport and trusting relationships with patients, which sets the stage for the continuum of navigation and assists in alleviating initial fears and stressors. Moreover, breast cancer nurse navigators may help with patient retention by connecting patients with necessary specialists for diagnostic and staging workups, treatment planning, and evaluations, thereby preventing outmigration. Desimini et al. (2011) found the use of a breast cancer navigator and implementation of a multidisciplinary clinic model to be effective strategies in improving both patient retention and quality of care.

Navigation is essential during breast cancer treatment because of the complexities involved with multiple providers and multifaceted treatment trajectories (Robinson-White et al., 2010). The treatment course for patients with breast cancer may include surgical interventions involving mastectomy or lumpectomy, sentinel or axillary node biopsies, and possible reconstruction; systemic treatments such as adjuvant or neoadjuvant chemotherapy, targeted therapies, and hormonal therapy; and possible radiation therapy for localized control (Meade & Dowling, 2012).

The Breast Cancer Nurse Navigator Role

To recognize and understand the comprehensive needs of newly diagnosed patients with breast cancer and where navigation efforts should be focused, breast cancer nurse navigators should first walk the entire patient process from the time of an abnormal mammogram through the cancer trajectory into surveillance, hospice, palliative care, or end of life. This activity facilitates an overall awareness of the multifaceted pathway that patients encounter and provides a basis for navigators to determine how patient-centered care can best be achieved within the oncology program.

Patient Education

From the time of an abnormal mammogram, patients diagnosed with breast cancer are bombarded with information and required to make life-altering decisions. Fear and anxiety can add to feelings of being overwhelmed and unable to cope. Patients become quickly vulnerable and may remove themselves from the decision-making process, relying on the healthcare team to decide on the course of treatment. Education from a reliable and experienced source is key to helping patients assume an active role in the treatment planning process and gain control of the situation. Three strategies that breast cancer nurse navigators might use for improved patient education are as follows.

- Assessing patients' desire for education. Although breast cancer nurse navigators are responsible to provide information, education efforts are most effective when patients are open to being active participants in the learning process.
- Assessing language barriers, providing information in the language easiest for patients to learn in (using translator services when needed), and using a variety of teaching modalities such as brochures, pictures, verbal instruction, CDs/DVDs, web-based learning modules, and group learning opportunities as appropriate. A recent Cisco report asserted that "in general, multimodal learning has been shown to be more effective than traditional, unimodal learning. Adding visuals to verbal (text and/or auditory) learning can result in significant gains in basic and higher-order learning" (Metiri Group, 2008, p. 14).
- Providing small quantities of information with each patient interaction. As an expert in the care of patients with breast cancer, breast cancer nurse navigators can determine the appropriate time points to introduce various pieces of education so as not to overwhelm patients with too much information during initial visits. It is important for navigators to allow patients to guide the educational sessions and ask questions. Furthermore, establishing a time limit for educational sessions can help to ensure that patients do not experience information overload.

Breast cancer nurse navigators play a pivotal role in fostering empowerment and providing patients with information intended to enhance abilities to make appropriate healthcare choices (American Medical Association, 2011). To illustrate this point, consider the significant advances in breast cancer treatment. Historically, radical mastectomy was the gold-standard treatment for breast cancer. Although this procedure improved survival, especially for those diagnosed with early-stage disease, the consequences were disfigurement and significant emotional toll. Then, in 1976, Bernard Fisher published information on the systemic theory, suggesting that breast-conserving surgery followed by radiation and chemotherapy may be as effective as mastectomy (Travis, 2005), and breast conservation has since become the mainstay of surgical treatment for early-stage breast cancer. However, patients still have decisions to make regarding surgical options, which can be overwhelming. Patients with breast cancer are often first overcome by the cancer diagnosis and then shortly thereafter have to make decisions that may affect survival.

Guiding patients through the breast cancer maze involves educating, reinforcing, and supporting them through the provision of specific information regarding treatment options. As such, navigators must have good communication with the multidisciplinary team to be aware of specific treatment options presented given patients' individual circumstances. This, however, can be a challenge in community settings where navigators may not have direct access to the treating physicians. In such situations, navigators must be assertive in establishing a means of communication with physician teams to obtain clarification on physician-provided information.

Patients with breast cancer expect breast cancer nurse navigators to be knowledgeable and informed about treatment options. The navigator's role in decision making is specifically to further educate, reinforce, and empower patients to discuss with the treatment team the options that are most appealing. As liaisons to the healthcare team, breast cancer nurse navigators help to communicate and clarify information to physicians and patients regarding care. Although clinical data are important for physicians in determining optimal choices for patients, it is essential that a holistic, individualized, patient-centered approach be applied to take into account patient preferences, values, and cultural considerations (Barry & Edgman-Levitan, 2012). Navigators often can shed light on these aspects, having spent significant time with patients and families, and can provide the physician team with pertinent information. Breast cancer nurse navigators can become more effective health coaches by helping patients to be well informed, being actively engaged in the process, and determining which matters are of greatest concern.

Confident, informed decision making is critical to patients as they move through the cancer continuum. For example, a woman may express a desire for lumpectomy but indicate not being comfortable with the thought of receiving radiation. The breast cancer nurse navigator can coordinate a consultation with a radiation oncologist to answer questions and allay concerns. In some situations, decisions may clearly follow a preferred course of treatment, and patient preference may not be as paramount. For example, a physician may recommend a mastectomy for a patient with multicentric ductal carcinoma in situ because a lumpectomy would not produce acceptable cosmetic results. Nevertheless, in most cases of early-stage breast cancer, patient involvement in decision making will be expected and breast cancer nurse navigators should be prepared to assist patients with this process.

The use of breast cancer education and decision-making tools can be helpful. Breast cancer nurse navigators can organize options in the form of a decision tree and assist patients in evaluating options by reviewing each step of the process. Patients with breast cancer given the choice of breast-conserving surgery versus mastectomy can be assisted by breast cancer nurse navigators to understand the rationale, advantages, and disadvantages of each option. The navigator can help patients explore goals and should include families in the education process as appropriate.

Advocating and Coordinating Multidisciplinary Care

Advocating for access to care is a critical role of breast cancer nurse navigators. Many patients lack the necessary resources (e.g., financial, educational, emotional) to receive optimal care in a timely manner. Examples of barriers to care can include lack of health insurance, financial limitations, housing and transportation issues, limited family support, and language or literacy concerns. Nurse navigators assist patients to overcome barriers to care by providing resources and initiating referrals to ancillary support services for additional assistance. It is important to note that the role of navigators is to advocate and empower patients and families to seek out available resources, not to enable and assume this responsibility for them.

Coordination of care among the various healthcare providers and ancillary services is crucial in the seamless journey of patients with breast cancer. Breast cancer nurse navigators act as a conduit for communication and synchronization of treatments for patients, multidisciplinary providers, and ancillary services. Table 5-1 depicts the possible timing of various ancillary support services commonly engaged with this patient population.

Multidisciplinary clinics are an effective approach to organizing the treatment course for breast cancer. This model brings together multiple providers in a cost-efficient and comprehensive approach to patient evaluation during a single visit or within a short span of time. The multidisciplinary team approach to care ensures communication among all disciplines and is essential in providing quality care to patients with breast cancer.

Breast cancer nurse navigators can play a central role in coordinating multidisciplinary clinics by assessing patients' needs, scheduling appointments, accompanying patients to consultations, and educating patients and family members about treatment options and resources, as well as serving as another set of ears for patients. After completion of all consultations, providers communicate with each other to establish the most effective plan of care (Advisory Board Company, 2008) and then often look to the breast cancer nurse navigator to organize a schedule for initiating the desired treatment plan in a timely manner.

Breast cancer nurse navigators frequently attend and facilitate interdisciplinary case conferences, which are commonly referred to as *tumor boards*. At

Table 5-1. Timing of Ancillary Services Used With Breast Cancer Management	
Service	When to Refer
Lymphedema specialist	Before (ideally) or after lymph node sampling or with development of any signs of lymphedema
Dietitian	Before the initial chemotherapy treatment or with any concerns regarding weight or healthy eating
Social worker	With identification of any psychosocial needs, financial concerns, coping concerns, or assistance needed related to travel or lodging
Financial counselor	Before chemotherapy or radiation for preauthorization of services and for any concerns about finances, lack of insurance, or insurance coverage
American Cancer Society programs	Individualized according to the patient needs
Wig boutique	Before alopecia develops
Survivorship programs	At the end of active treatment
Fertility specialist	With the determination of the chemotherapy regimen for any woman younger than age 40 or man younger than age 50

these conferences, medical oncologists, radiation oncologists, breast cancer surgeons, reconstructive surgeons, radiologists, pathologists, genetic counselors, social workers, dietitians, advanced practice nurses, pharmacists, research staff, financial counselors, lymphedema therapists, and breast cancer nurse navigators discuss patient cases to determine the most appropriate course of treatment for each patient. Furthermore, breast cancer nurse navigators can be instrumental in advocating for care coordination by suggesting challenging cases that require intense communication between disciplines in developing a coordinated approach to treatment planning. By the end of each case presentation, consensus is reached regarding the patient's treatment plan (Advisory Board Company, 2007).

Breast cancer nurse navigators advocate for compliance with standards of care and evidence-based guidelines. This includes National Comprehensive Cancer Network guidelines, clinical trial and research opportunities, and genetic and genomic testing. Furthermore, navigators can reduce physician workload by helping to coordinate treatment plans, assisting with communication involving various members of the healthcare team, and facilitating transitions between care settings.

Reinforcing Information Regarding Clinical Trials

Breast cancer nurse navigators are critical to the research process and can positively influence clinical trial accrual by collaborating with research teams in an effort to educate patients about breast protocols and opportunities for enrollment. Navigators should establish strong, collegial working relationships with the clinical research team. Two strategies that breast cancer nurse navigators can use to assist in increasing clinical trial accruals are ensuring that a clinical research nurse is present at breast cancer conferences and partnering with the clinical research nurse on quality initiatives within the cancer program. Depending on the scope of responsibilities, breast cancer nurse navigators also may participate in institutional review boards or suggest new clinical trials and protocols for consideration. Expanding the role of breast cancer nurse navigators to include knowledge of clinical trials improves the value of navigation programs, fosters a team approach to care, and ultimately benefits patients (AccrualNet™, 2013).

Facilitating Genetic Counseling Referrals

Knowledge about the clinical application of genetics helps navigators to identify patients at risk and advocate for access to cancer predisposition genetic counseling, testing, and risk-reduction strategies for high-risk individuals and families. Breast cancer nurse navigators have been shown to successfully identify patients eligible for breast cancer risk assessment and provide education regarding the benefits of such (Mays et al., 2012).

Genetic risk assessment and testing can affect treatment decision making and should be conducted early in breast cancer diagnosis when gathering a family history (Everett & Senter, 2013). The breast cancer nurse navigator may be one of the first individuals to interact with a patient and identify a potential hereditary syndrome, at which time a genetic counseling referral should be initiated. Navigators may address myths associated with genetic testing and discrimination, as well as answer questions about insurance coverage (Radford, 2012). Breast cancer nurse navigators can expedite the referral process, ensure that patients receive counseling before testing, and communicate this information to the physician team.

Preparing Patients for Surgery

Providing an opportunity for breast cancer nurse navigators to meet face-to-face with patients with breast cancer before surgery fosters relationship building and trust with patients, as well as affords an opportunity to convey insightful information regarding pre- and postoperative expectations.

Although surgeons may have provided detailed information about the procedure, patients do not absorb all of this and can benefit from additional reinforcement. It can be effective for breast cancer nurse navigators to ask patients to recall what was discussed at the surgical planning appointment and then build upon that information. This may include reinforcing sentinel lymph node injection, biopsy, and possible axillary lymph node dissection, as well as drain care.

Patients undergoing a mastectomy without reconstruction will need information regarding resources for postmastectomy bras and temporary prostheses. This information helps prepare patients both emotionally and physically. According to the National Accreditation Program for Breast Centers (2013) standards, patients choosing mastectomy should be offered a preoperative referral to a reconstructive plastic surgeon. Such referral can be coordinated and expedited by breast cancer nurse navigators.

Specific education that breast cancer nurse navigators can provide includes an overview of the care pathway, as well as admission and discharge procedures. Furthermore, it is important to discuss postoperative pain and provide pain management strategies, including the prevention of constipation. Navigators can instruct patients on lymphedema prevention and exercises, knowing that reinforcement will be needed postoperatively. Follow-up by the breast cancer nurse navigator after surgery, whether in the hospital or at home by telephone, provides continuity of support and encouragement into recovery.

Preparing Patients for Breast Reconstruction

Although breast reconstructive surgery is secondary in relation to survival, it should be considered an important part of the breast cancer treatment plan. The two main decisions for patients choosing reconstructive breast surgery are (a) which option for reconstruction and (b) when to have reconstruction. Navigators can help educate patients about the types of reconstruction available and the timing considerations associated with immediate versus delayed reconstruction. Reconstructive surgery may require additional surgeries, frequent follow-ups, and several months before final results are realized. Education is essential to ensure that patients are realistic in their expectations and outcomes.

Preparing Patients for Chemotherapy and Radiation

Patients with breast cancer who require chemotherapy and/or radiation are often overwhelmed with the information received. As such, patients sometimes consent to treatment without fully understanding the risks and benefits. Education and frequent reinforcement of key concepts is important in minimizing patients' anxieties and clarifying misconceptions (Stark & House, 2000). Breast cancer nurse navigators are in an ideal position to reinforce education from the oncologists, provide guidance with regard to symptom management measures, discuss patients' concerns, and direct any unanswered questions to the appropriate healthcare professional.

Once consensus is reached regarding the treatment plan, breast cancer nurse navigators can coordinate necessary treatment schedules and make further referrals as appropriate. As patients travel through the treatment course, navigators often check in during key touchpoints and remain available to assist if any difficulties arise.

Navigating Patients With Advanced Breast Cancer

Supporting patients with advanced breast cancer is perhaps one of the most challenging aspects of breast cancer nurse navigators' roles. There is a delicate balance of treatment, symptom management, and emotional support. Most discussion and research surrounding navigation services primarily focus on interventions with early-stage patients. The navigation requirements of patients with metastatic disease are distinctly different, and further development of this perspective is needed.

The desire for emotional support varies with each patient. Assessing patients' need to discuss concerns and feelings is critical because patients who are dissatisfied with emotional support are more likely to be anxious and depressed. Patients' needs for support can fluctuate throughout the cancer journey, and breast cancer nurse navigators are pivotal in determining when increased support is indicated by taking the time to listen to patients' concerns and answering questions. Patients in need of additional emotional support can benefit from social work, support group, and clergy referrals.

Providing patients with information on advance directives and living wills can be a sensitive issue for patients with advanced breast cancer. Ideally, information on treatment preferences and healthcare proxy is given to all patients upon initial diagnosis. However, despite many patients having the desire to make independent healthcare decisions, few actually follow through with a written advance directive (Emanuel, Barry, Stoeckle, Ettelson, & Emanuel, 1991). This may be the result of patients' understanding of the prognosis being imperfect and a tendency to overestimate the probability of long-term survival (Weeks et al., 1998). In addition, the healthcare team may be reluctant to discuss patients' concerns at length. As such, the role of breast cancer nurse navigators can include providing appropriate forms and information resources, as well as being available to listen to patients' concerns and questions. Navigators can coach and support patients who are reluctant to talk with the healthcare team about difficult treatment decisions.

Breast Cancer Survivorship Navigation

Navigators have an opportunity to work collaboratively with patients and physicians to improve care provided beyond breast cancer treatment. After patients have completed active treatment, typically a five-year surveillance plan is established under the care of either the medical oncologist or a primary care physician. Breast cancer nurse navigators can play an essential role in providing survivorship information to patients and primary care physicians at the end of treatment. Research by Ness et al. (2013) identified that cancer survivors continue to experience difficulties associated with the cancer diagnosis and treatment for many years. Patients may find that physical, emotional, and financial concerns continue because cancer treatment and survivorship each present unique challenges. Fatigue, neuropathy symptoms, changes in fertility and sexuality, osteoporosis, and lymphedema are potential side effects that can be debilitating and negatively affect quality of life for breast cancer survivors.

By offering information about treatment-related late and long-term side effects, support groups, education regarding signs of disease recurrence and the possibility of future cancers, health screening recommendations, and a summary of treatment received, navigators help survivors focus on wellness and encourage them to enter the post-treatment phase with a sense of control and confidence (Meade & Dowling, 2012). After receiving survivorship information, patients are often receptive to incorporating healthy lifestyle changes and are empowered to be active participants in the surveillance phase of breast cancer management (Nissen, Tsai, Blacs, Swenson, & Koering, 2013).

Case Example

Sue is a 57-year-old woman who presented to the clinic for a mammogram, which revealed suspicious findings. Two days later, Sue returned for an ultrasound-guided biopsy of the left breast. At that time, Sue met with Alice, the breast diagnostic navigator. Alice introduced herself and the role of the breast diagnostic navigator, which centered on ensuring patient education and support during the resolution of abnormal findings and diagnostic evaluation. After Sue's procedure, Alice confirmed Sue's contact information and instructed her that she would call as soon as results were available. Alice tracked the biopsy, and results revealed a grade 2–3 invasive ductal cancer in the left breast. Additionally, the pathology indicated positive estrogen and progesterone receptors, whereas HER2/neu status was not amplified. Alice called Sue to provide information on the cancer diagnosis and pathology specifics along with anticipatory guidance with regard to the next steps in the cancer journey. Alice scheduled Sue with a surgeon, and then informed Sue that her role as the breast diagnostic navigator was finished, but that Janet, the breast cancer treatment navigator, would be in contact to further coordinate the multidisciplinary clinic consultations. Alice then notified Janet of Sue's breast cancer diagnosis and scheduled consultation with the surgeon. Janet scheduled medical oncology and radiation oncology consults on the same day as the surgical consultation, and then contacted Sue by phone to introduce the role of the breast cancer treatment navigator and schedule of multidisciplinary consultations.

Janet attended the multidisciplinary consultations with Sue and her husband. Each provider examined Sue and discussed potential individualized treatment options; the providers then conferred with each other to reach agreement and formalize the treatment plan. During these appointments, Janet assessed Sue and her husband for specific needs. She provided education about breast cancer using National Cancer Institute and American Cancer Society booklets and informed them on when and how to contact the healthcare team. Janet measured Sue's arms and recorded this information in the electronic medical record (EMR); these baseline measurements provide valuable information in the event that Sue develops lymphedema in the future. After the multidisciplinary consultations, Janet gave Sue a brief written summary of the evaluations and the proposed treatment. She also sent a copy of this written summary along with copies of the dictated consultations and diagnostic reports to Sue's referring provider.

Based on Janet's assessment of Sue, a referral was made to the genetic counselor because six close family relatives were previously diagnosed with breast cancer. Janet made referrals to the oncology social worker and financial counselor, as Sue had no insurance, lived three hours from the clinic, and had a very limited income. Furthermore, Janet notified the research nurse to request a review of clinical trials to determine patient eligibility. After receiving negative *BRCA* results, Sue chose to have a mastectomy with sentinel node biopsy. Janet offered a referral to a reconstructive surgeon but Sue declined this; thus, Janet worked with the surgeon's office staff to schedule Sue for a mastectomy in two days.

Surgical pathology showed clear margins, tumor size of 3.4 cm, and two of two positive sentinel lymph nodes. Janet then scheduled Sue to be seen again by the medical and radiation oncologists for further treatment decisions. Janet accompanied Sue to these appointments, wherein the medical oncologist recommended an aggressive chemotherapy regimen. Janet coordinated appointments for an echocardiogram, blood work, port placement, and a return appointment for chemotherapy initiation. The radiation oncologist indicated a desire to evaluate Sue after chemotherapy for deep-inspiratory breath-hold radiation therapy.

Along with educating Sue about the particular chemotherapy regimen, Janet scheduled appointments for Sue with the dietitian, lymphedema specialist, wig stylist, and infusion center. These appointments were entered onto a calendar, which Janet provided to Sue along with an explanation of the rationale for each. While Sue proceeded with chemotherapy, Janet tracked her course through the EMR and visited Sue periodically during infusion appointments.

After Sue completed chemotherapy, Janet scheduled a return visit with the radiation oncologist who suggested a course of whole breast radiation using the deep-inspiratory breath-hold technique. Janet worked closely with the radiation technicians to coordinate the radiation schedule. As with chemotherapy, Janet tracked Sue throughout the course of radiation treatment and checked in periodically to identify and assist with any barriers or challenges experienced. Following completion of the course of radiation, Janet scheduled Sue for follow-up with the medical oncologist.

The medical oncologist ordered hormonal therapy and indicated that Sue should return in one month. After the one month follow-up visit, which confirmed Sue was tolerating the hormonal therapy, Sue entered the post-treatment surveillance period, where Janet provided her with a treatment summary and survivorship care plan, which detailed the surveillance schedule, potential late and long-term side effects, signs of recurrence, and available community resources. At this time, Janet explained the conclusion of navigation processes but reassured Sue that she was still just a telephone call away should questions, concerns, or needs arise in the future.

Conclusion

As the specialty of breast cancer navigation progresses, further evidence-based practice will likely be defined, which will refine navigation models of care coordination and care delivery. The role of a breast cancer navigator provides experienced oncology nurses with an opportunity to apply and practice the art of nursing science in an autonomous setting where they can advocate for patients, actively participate in the development and implementation of best practices, and interact as a valued member of the entire healthcare team. With the guidance of a breast cancer nurse navigator, patients with breast cancer who are coping with emotional and physical difficulties can successfully traverse the breast cancer continuum despite the barriers that impede the efficacious management of a breast cancer diagnosis, treatment, and survivorship.

References

AccrualNet™. (2013). Guest expert: Eileen Dimond: Are your patient navigator colleagues participating in clinical trials accrual? It might be time to consider a new paradigm. Retrieved from https://accrualnet.cancer.gov/communities/conversation/guest_expert_eileen_dimond _are_your_patient_navigator_colleagues_participating_in_clinical_trials

Advisory Board Company. (2007). *Developing a nurse navigator program for oncology services.* Retrieved from https://www.advisory.com/Research/Marketing-and-Planning-Leadership -Council/Original-Inquiry/2007/05/Developing-a-Nurse-Navigator-Program-for-Oncology -Services

Advisory Board Company. (2008). *Elevating the patient experience: Building successful patient navigation, multidisciplinary care, and survivorship programs.* Washington, DC: Author.

American Cancer Society. (2014). *Cancer facts and figures 2014.* Retrieved from http://www. cancer.org/research/cancerfactsstatistics/cancerfactsfigures2014

American Medical Association. (2011). *Report 7 of the Council on Medical Service (I-11).* Retrieved from http://www.ama-assn.org/resources/doc/cms/i11-cms-report7.pdf

Barry, M.J., & Edgman-Levitan, S. (2012). Shared decision making—The pinnacle of patient-centered care. *New England Journal of Medicine, 366,* 780–781. doi:10.1056/ NEJMp1109283

Brown, C.G., Cantril, C., McMullen, L., Barkley, D.L., Dietz, M., Murphy, C.M., & Fabrey, L.J. (2012). Oncology nurse navigator role delineation study: An Oncology Nursing Society report. *Clinical Journal of Oncology Nursing, 16,* 581–585. doi:10.1188/12.CJON.581-585

Campbell, C., Craig, J., Eggert, J., & Bailey-Dorton, C. (2010). Implementing and measuring the impact of patient navigation at a comprehensive community cancer center. *Oncology Nursing Forum, 37,* 61–68. doi:10.1188/10.ONF.61-68

Chatman, M.C., & Green, R.D. (2011). Addressing the unique psychosocial barriers to breast cancer treatment experienced by African-American women through integrative navigation. *Journal of National Black Nurses Association, 22*(2), 20–28.

Desimini, E.M., Kennedy, J.A., Helsley, M.F., Shiner, K., Denton, C., Rice, T.T., … Lewis, M.G. (2011). Making the case for nurse navigators—Benefits, outcomes, and return on investment. *Oncology Issues, 26*(5), 26–33. Retrieved from http://pages.nxtbook.com/nxtbooks/ accc/oncologyissues_20110910/offline/accc_oncologyissues_20110910.pdf

Emanuel, L.L., Barry, M.J., Stoeckle, J.D., Ettelson, L.M., & Emanuel, E.J. (1991). Advance directives for medical care—A case for greater use. *New England Journal of Medicine, 324,* 889–895. doi:10.1056/NEJM199103283241305

Everett, J., & Senter, L. (2013). Molecular genetics in the community setting: Positioning your cancer program for success. *Oncology Issues, 28*(2), 26–31. Retrieved from http://www.accc -cancer.org/oncology_issues/articles/marapr13/MA13-Everett.pdf

Freeman, H.P. (2012). The origin, evolution, and principles of patient navigation. *Cancer Epidemiology, Biomarkers and Prevention, 21,* 1614–1617. doi:10.1158/1055-9965.EPI-12-0982

Freeman, H.P., & Rodriguez, R.L. (2011). History and principles of patient navigation. *Cancer, 117*(Suppl. 15), 3539–3542. doi:10.1002/cncr.26262

Hendren, S., Chin, N., Fisher, S., Winters, P., Griggs, J., Mohile, S., & Fiscella, K. (2011). Patients' barriers to receipt of cancer care, and factors associated with needing more assistance from a patient navigator. *Journal of the National Medical Association, 103,* 701–710. Retrieved from http://www.ncbi.nlm.nih.gov/pmc/articles/PMC3713073

Hoffman, H.J., LaVerda, N.L., Young, H.A., Levine, P.H., Alexander, L.M., Brem, R., … Patierno, S.R. (2012). Patient navigation significantly reduces delays in breast cancer diagnosis in the District of Columbia. *Cancer Epidemiology, Biomarkers and Prevention, 21,* 1655–1663. doi:10.1158/1055-9965.EPI-12-0479

Horner, K., Ludman, E.J., McCorkle, R., Canfield, E., Flaherty, L., Min, J., … Wagner, E.H. (2013). An oncology nurse navigator program designed to eliminate gaps in early cancer care. *Clinical Journal of Oncology Nursing, 17,* 43–48. doi:10.1188/13.CJON.43-48

Korber, S.F., Padula, C., Gray, J., & Powell, M. (2011). A breast navigator program: Barriers, enhancers, and nursing interventions. *Oncology Nursing Forum, 38,* 44–50. doi:10.1188/11. ONF.44-50

Markossian, T.W., Darnell, J.S., & Calhoun, E.A. (2012). Follow-up and timeliness after an abnormal cancer screening among underserved, urban women in a patient navigation pro-

gram. *Cancer Epidemiology, Biomarkers and Prevention, 21,* 1691–1700. doi:10.1158/1055-9965
.EPI-12-0535

Mays, D., Sharff, M.E., DeMarco, T.A., Williams, B., Beck, B., Sheppard, V.B., ... Tercyak, K.P.
(2012). Outcomes of a systems-level intervention offering breast cancer risk assessments
to low-income underserved women. *Familial Cancer, 11,* 493–502. doi:10.1007/s10689-012
-9541-7

McDonald, C. (2011). A first-hand look at the role of the breast cancer nurse navigator. *Care
Management, 17*(6), 11–13, 27–28. Retrieved from http://www.jcaremanagement.com/pdf_
nonmember/6CM_dec2011_jan2012.pdf

Meade, E., & Dowling, M. (2012). Early breast cancer: Diagnosis, treatment and survivorship.
British Journal of Nursing, 21(17), S4–S8, S10.

Metiri Group. (2008). *Multimodal learning through media: What the research says.* Retrieved from
http://www.cisco.com/web/strategy/docs/education/Multimodal-Learning-Through
-Media.pdf

National Accreditation Program for Breast Centers. (2013). *2013 breast center standards manual.*
Retrieved from http://napbc-breast.org/standards/2013standardsmanual.pdf

Ness, S., Kokal, J., Fee-Schroeder, K., Novotny, P., Satele, D., & Barton, D. (2013). Concerns
across the survivorship trajectory: Results from a survey of cancer survivors. *Oncology Nursing
Forum, 40,* 35–42. doi:10.1188/13.ONF.35-42

Nissen, M.J., Tsai, M.L., Blaes, A.H., Swenson, K.K., & Koering, S. (2013). Effectiveness of treatment summaries in increasing breast and colorectal cancer survivors' knowledge about
their diagnosis and treatment. *Journal of Cancer Survivorship: Research and Practice, 7,* 211–
218. doi:10.1007/s11764-012-0261-7

Radford, C. (2012). Christi Radford on the nurse navigator's role in genetic counseling. Retrieved from http://www.onclive.com/conference-coverage/nconn-2012/Cristi-Radford
-on-the-Nurse-Navigators-Role-in-Genetic-Counseling

Robinson-White, S., Conroy, B., Slavish, K.H., & Rosenzweig, M. (2010). Patient navigation in breast cancer: A systemic review. *Cancer Nursing, 33,* 127–140. doi:10.1097/
NCC.0b013e3181c40401

Schafer, J., & Swisher, J. (2006). Cancer care coordination with nurse navigators. *Sg2 Health Care
Intelligence.* Retrieved from http://www.sg2.com

Stanley, S., Arriola, K.J., Smith, S., Hurlbert, M., Ricci, C., & Escoffery, C. (2013). Reducing
barriers to breast cancer care through Avon patient navigation programs. *Journal of Public
Health Management and Practice, 19,* 461–467. doi:10.1097/PHH.0b013e318276e272

Stark, D.P.H., & House, A. (2000). Anxiety in cancer patients. *British Journal of Cancer, 83,* 1261–
1267. doi:10.1054/bjoc.2000.1405

Travis, K. (2005). Bernard Fisher reflects on a half-century's worth of breast cancer research.
Journal of the National Cancer Institute, 97, 1636–1637. doi:10.1093/jnci/dji419

Weeks, J.C., Cook, E.F., O'Day, S.J., Peterson, L.M., Wenger, N., Reding, D., ... Phillips, R.S.
(1998). Relationship between cancer patients' predictions of prognosis and their treatment
preferences. *JAMA, 279,* 1709–1714. doi:10.1001/jama.279.21.1709

CHAPTER 6

Cancer Site–Specific Navigation

Penny Daugherty, RN, MS, OCN®, Nicole G. Messier, RN, BSN, Frank dela Rama, RN, MS, AOCNS®, Heather Stern, RN, BSN, OCN®, Susan J. Keen, BSN, RN, OCN®, CTTS, and Karyl D. Blaseg, RN, MSN, OCN®

Introduction

The initial patient navigation model developed by Freeman used lay navigators with the intent of reducing the time from identification of an abnormal finding during a breast examination and mammogram to diagnosis and definitive treatment of breast cancer among patients seen in an urban hospital setting (Freeman & Rodriguez, 2011). As successes were demonstrated, models evolved in which oncology nurses and other healthcare professionals were engaged as navigators to focus specifically on the medical and healthcare system aspects of access to and coordination of care. Although coordination of timely and efficient care continues to be a primary objective of the patient navigation paradigm, as the specialty has developed, the role of oncology nurse navigators has transformed and now often incorporates further disease site–specific services including education, symptom management, and psychosocial support as patients move through the continuum of care (Shockney, 2010). As such, individualized disease-specific patient navigation models have emerged based upon disease, treatment modalities, and proclivity for recurrence rather than a directed emphasis on disease-free survivorship, which was the focus of the original breast cancer patient navigation concept.

This chapter examines oncology nurse navigation through the lens of management of a number of site-specific cancers, including prostate, bladder, gynecologic, gastrointestinal, head and neck, and thoracic. While patient navigation programs share many common traits regardless of the type of cancer, each cancer site presents unique and specific patient-related and healthcare system–associated challenges for oncology nurse navigators.

Navigating Patients With Gastrointestinal Cancers

Cancer treatment for many gastrointestinal (GI) tumors is complex and often requires multimodality treatment with chemotherapy, radiation therapy, and surgery. Nurse navigators with specialized knowledge and expertise in GI oncology care can enhance coordination of services and communication between patients and cancer specialists.

While patients with breast cancer are often navigated through the system with precision, the story can be vastly different for patients with a new diagnosis of gastric or esophageal cancer. It is not uncommon for patients who have been diagnosed with GI cancers to experience delays of several weeks before all imaging studies and necessary consultations are completed because of the many specialists involved. This can be especially true at large, regional institutions, which might treat patients from large geographic areas. For example, Fletcher Allen Health Care in Burlington, Vermont, is a regional referral center for Vermont and upstate New York; therefore, a large percent of the patients travel more than two hours to seek treatment at the institution. Prior to implementation of GI cancer navigation, these patients often made multiple trips for diagnostic tests and consultations because of the lack of coordinated care and inefficient processes.

Multidisciplinary Care

Over the past decade, institutions have begun to apply the multidisciplinary team approach used with patients with breast cancer to patients with GI cancers. Fletcher Allen Health Care established the Upper GI (UGI) Multidisciplinary Care (MDC) Clinic in 2007 to streamline and improve the care of patients with esophageal, gastric, pancreatic, liver, and biliary tract cancers. Using a dedicated GI cancer nurse navigator, this program serves as "one-stop shopping" for patients and allows for more efficient and timely workups, evaluations, and treatment initiations within a well-coordinated program. The UGI MDC team provides an evaluation and develops a personalized treatment plan for patients, including all resources needed such as education, diagnosis, treatment, research, and support. The UGI MDC team comprises gastroenterologists; medical, radiation, and surgical oncologists; pathologists; radiologists; fellows, residents, and students; psychologists; primary nurses; research coordinators; and the GI cancer nurse navigator, American Cancer Society (ACS) patient navigator, dietitian, and social worker. The goals of the UGI MDC clinic are to

• Provide high-quality multidisciplinary care and increase efficiency of care

- Ensure that staging studies and clinical treatment are concordant with evidence-based practice guidelines from the National Comprehensive Cancer Network (NCCN)
- Increase the opportunity for physician-patient interaction, education, and research
- Increase patient satisfaction.

The UGI MDC clinic is held two or three times each month and is preceded by a one-hour multidisciplinary treatment planning conference. At this conference, the UGI MDC team reviews and discusses patient cases, including pathology slides and radiology films. Patients are then seen in the UGI MDC clinic by all necessary specialists, as well as the GI cancer nurse navigator, ACS patient navigator, dietitian, social worker, and psychologist. Patients meet with both the GI cancer nurse navigator and the ACS patient navigator, as each has a distinct role and scope of responsibility. The ACS patient navigator assists with psychosocial and logistical needs, whereas the GI cancer nurse navigator focuses on coordination of the patient's clinical and medical needs.

Nurse Navigator Roles and Responsibilities

Nurse navigators for patients with GI cancers serve as liaisons for referring providers and collaborate with all members of the multidisciplinary team. The GI cancer nurse navigator is often the first person a newly diagnosed patient with cancer will speak with upon referral for either a newly diagnosed cancer or a suspicious finding requiring further workup. Initial contact with the patient may be via telephone or in person. Referrals can come from both within and outside of the hospital and may be made by physicians, staff, or patients themselves. GI cancer nurse navigators regularly receive referrals from gastroenterologists and frequently visit the endoscopy suite to meet with patients just diagnosed with a GI cancer or those with a high suspicion for GI cancer.

The opportunity to meet with patients and caregivers following a biopsy is a crucial part of the GI cancer navigation process. In most cases, these patients have just been told of the cancer diagnosis and will need to meet with oncology specialists to determine a treatment plan. By connecting face-to-face with patients during this emotionally challenging and vulnerable time, the GI cancer nurse navigator becomes the single point of contact and guide throughout the cancer journey.

This initial meeting is a time to answer questions, discuss fears and concerns, and educate patients and families about diagnosis specifics. Nurse navigators may inquire about patients' medical histories and conduct assessments of physical needs and symptoms, as well as emotional, psychosocial, and financial concerns, thereby expediting referrals as appropriate. A review of the diagnostic testing performed should be completed, along with coordination of any additional studies needed to complete the diagnostic workup according to NCCN guidelines. The GI cancer nurse navigator discusses the need for and schedules consultations with the appropriate oncology specialists.

The National Coalition of Oncology Nurse Navigators refers to navigators as the "411 of cancer resources and community support services" (National Coalition of Oncology Nurse Navigators, n.d.). Nurse navigators spend ample time educating and answering questions for newly diagnosed patients with cancer and their families, providing both verbal and written education as well as links to community resources. The National Cancer Institute (NCI) and ACS provide information both online and in print for patients with GI cancers; in addition, for those with pancreatic cancer, the Pancreatic Cancer Action Network is a good source of information.

Whether the initial contact with newly diagnosed patients with GI cancer takes place in person or via telephone, the length of time required for that interaction can vary greatly, and the nurse navigators need to take cues from the patients and proceed accordingly. Some patients are straightforward and no-nonsense, preferring to know only the details that are of immediate relevance (i.e., those pertaining to the next test or appointment). Other patients want every possible detail that nurse navigators can provide and want to hear about each potential scenario. Average patients tend to fall somewhere in the middle of these two extremes, taking anywhere from 30–60 minutes for the initial contact depending on the specific needs identified. Additional follow-up is arranged based on patients' needs; as with the initial interaction, these telephone calls or face-to-face meetings can vary both in length of time and the extent of interactions and support needed. These additional and subsequent conservations often yield the most useful information for the GI cancer nurse navigator, including concerns regarding finances and insurance, marital issues, drug and alcohol abuse, and transportation. As relationships among GI cancer nurse navigators, patients, and families develop, much can be learned through active listening techniques.

GI cancer nurse navigators typically continue to work closely with patients and caregivers, serving as the primary contact at least until cancer treatment begins. Thereafter, if primary nurses of the treating physicians prefer to be the main contact for patients, nurse navigators may step back but remain available as a resource to patients, caregivers, and staff in the event that challenges or issues arise requiring additional assistance. Nurse navigators often stay in touch with patients by stopping by the infusion room or clinic departments to check in with patients and ensure that treatment is progressing as planned.

Palliative care is an important part of the GI cancer navigation program. In many institutions, palliative care programs support the physical and psychological needs of patients and caregivers facing the complex challenges associated with a GI cancer diagnosis (NCI, 2010). Patient referrals can be made at any time after diagnosis and can be related to a variety of issues including symptom management, goals of care, end-of-life discussions, and timing of the transition to palliative care or hospice.

Nurse Navigation Processes

Because nurse navigation for GI cancers is relatively new, evidence-based literature is particularly thin. To illustrate GI cancer navigation processes, Figure 6-1 provides a flow map that depicts each of the GI cancer nurse navigator's tasks for all new patients referred to the Fletcher Allen Health Care UGI MDC clinic. This process diagram serves as a guideline to help ensure patients move through the system in a timely and efficient manner.

Benefits of Nurse Navigation

Nurse navigation programs can have real-time and lasting effects for both patients and institutions, reducing time from a suspicious finding to diagnosis and treatment (Desimini et al., 2011). Since the initiation of the UGI MDC clinic at Fletcher Allen Health Care, the clinic has experienced more timely cancer staging in accordance with NCCN guidelines and a decrease in the number of unnecessary tests performed prior to treatment, resulting in decreased healthcare costs. The program has increased collaboration among multiple cancer specialists while decreasing the number of patient visits needed to complete cancer staging and initiate treatment. Increased satisfaction has been noted not only from patients and families but from the UGI MDC team as well. Overall, the success of the UGI MDC clinic can be attributed to open communication, participation, and buy-in of all key stakeholders—something that can be a challenge for many patient navigation programs to achieve (Varner & Murph, 2010).

According to Freeman and Rodriguez (2011), "the core function of patient navigation is the elimination of barriers to timely care across all segments of the healthcare continuum" (p. 3541). Nurse navigators have a common goal of identifying and removing barriers to timely and appropriate cancer care, but programs vary greatly based on patients' needs and institutional capabilities. What works for the GI cancer nurse navigator at Fletcher Allen Health Care, for example, may not necessarily work for a GI cancer nurse navigator working in a similar academic setting in another part of the country. Hence, navigation services must be tailored to meet the specific needs of the identified patient population and community served.

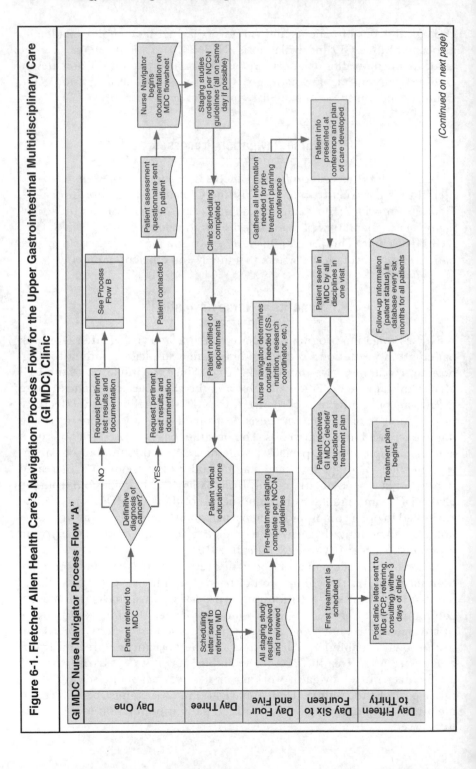

Figure 6-1. Fletcher Allen Health Care's Navigation Process Flow for the Upper Gastrointestinal Multidisciplinary Care (GI MDC) Clinic

(Continued on next page)

Figure 6-1. Fletcher Allen Health Care's Navigation Process Flow for the Upper Gastrointestinal Multidisciplinary Care (GI MDC) Clinic (Continued)

NCCN—National Comprehensive Cancer Network; PCP—primary care provider; SS—social services

Note. Figure courtesy of James M. Jeffords Institute for Quality and Operational Effectiveness at Fletcher Allen Health Care. Used with permission.

Today's healthcare system is complex, and patients with a newly diagnosed GI cancer can easily feel confused, overwhelmed, and alone. GI cancer nurse navigators have the opportunity to improve the healthcare experience by providing supportive, compassionate, and personalized care while educating and empowering patients and families to take an active role in treatment decisions.

Navigating Patients With Genitourinary Cancers

Benner's seminal work *From Novice to Expert* (1984) described how nursing practice develops and advances over time. Similarly, over the years, from assistance with access and logistics, to education, counseling, and transitioning into post-treatment care, the specialty of nurse navigation has evolved from a mere amenity to now a crucial component of cancer care, continuously assisting patients, families, and healthcare providers across the care continuum.

Most navigation programs initially focused on breast cancer navigation, but as program successes were demonstrated, attention turned to development of navigation services for other prevalent cancers as well. One such focus may be to establish a navigation program for genitourinary (GU) cancers, which might include prostate, bladder, kidney, and testicular cancers. Despite the wide range of diagnostics, treatment modalities, and possible side effects among GU cancers, one commonality is the potential impact upon intimate issues of sexuality and urinary elimination. GU cancer nurse navigators are well positioned to assist patients in dealing with these sensitive physical and psychosocial issues.

Prostate Cancer

Screening and Diagnosis

Referrals to GU cancer nurse navigators are often initiated by urologists upon disclosing biopsy results to newly diagnosed patients with prostate cancer. Although GU cancer nurse navigators could be used as key resources for increasing access to prostate cancer screening, most often the focus of GU cancer navigation services is based on the diagnosis and treatment phase of the cancer continuum.

Developing collaborative relationships with urologists serving a healthcare facility is crucial to building a successful GU cancer nurse navigator program. Urologists should understand that the navigator aims to support physicians' practice without causing significant overlap in responsibilities among those of physicians, urology nurses, and other healthcare providers. All healthcare providers involved with prostate cancer care should be familiar with the role of the GU cancer nurse navigator, as referrals can be generated from urology nurses, radiation oncologists, radiation oncology nurses, medical oncologists, other oncology nurses, case managers, and social workers. Taking awareness a step further, educating primary care providers (PCPs) and the community at large will optimize referrals such that the public perception views the GU cancer nurse navigator as one of the first healthcare professionals that newly diagnosed patients with prostate cancer should and will encounter.

Another method for ensuring that all newly diagnosed patients with prostate cancer are appropriately engaged with navigation services involves working with the organization's pathology department. A service agreement can be in place where pathology sends weekly lists of all positive prostate biopsies directly to the GU cancer nurse navigator, who then contacts patients to discuss the next steps and available services after the diagnosis has been shared by the physician.

Once prostate cancer navigation services are well established, the GU cancer nurse navigator is often engaged as a community resource for patients and providers when complex issues in screening arise. Because the potential number of patients with screening questions far outnumbers newly diagnosed patients, broader education methods such as lectures, written education materials, presence at health fairs and similar events, and the use of online tools, including websites and social media, allow the GU cancer nurse navigator to reach a wide audience and have a significant impact in addressing issues specific to prostate cancer screening.

Initial Visit and Treatment Shared Decision Making

Once patients are diagnosed with prostate cancer, attention soon turns to treatment decision making. Most GU cancer nurse navigators meet with patients and families for the first time at this point. The comprehensive navigator visit for newly diagnosed patients with prostate cancer should ideally include

- An explanation of clinical staging and review of the pathology report
- Pertinent treatment options based on national guidelines
- Possible side effects and appropriate management of each
- Nomograms and predictive tables
- A review of potential quality-of-life (QOL) issues
- Shared decision-making tools
- Referrals to support services as appropriate (e.g., social work, nutrition, genetics, psychiatry).

Key components of the clinical picture include tumor, node, metastasis (TNM) staging (American Joint Committee on Cancer, 2009), Gleason score, and prostate-specific antigen (PSA) levels. Using this data, the navigator can outline possible treatment options, which may include active surveillance or various forms of surgery, radiation, and hormonal therapy (NCCN, 2013d).

With localized prostate cancers, several options may be available to patients, even after analysis of the clinical picture and completion of risk assessment. Consideration of QOL issues can provide further insights regarding the best fit among treatment modality options. Structured shared decision-making tools can be used to help patients perform due diligence in order to consider all aspects and how each option compares with the others regarding QOL issues.

The term *due diligence* describes a systematic and thorough way of looking at the advantages and disadvantages of a situation. In an effort to help men to complete due diligence in prostate cancer treatment decision making, the Palo Alto Medical Foundation (2010) created a shared decision-making worksheet (see Figure 6-2) based upon a pilot study. Findings from the pilot revealed issues most important to men in deciding among prostate cancer treatment options, which included

- Avoiding side effects (urinary, erectile, bowel)
- Maintaining QOL
- Eliminating the cancer
- Being able to cover the cost of treatment
- Evaluating the operative risk
- Making treatment as convenient as possible.

During navigator visits, patients and families are asked to consider these issues with respect to each treatment option on the worksheet, taking into account everything learned about prostate cancer. Next, patients rank these issues or at least pick one or two high-priority issues. From there, one treatment option may stand out as most appropriate for patients. Using the shared decision-making worksheet within the navigator visits has demonstrated increased patient satisfaction with treatment decisions regardless of the clinical outcome, as opposed to patients who did not use such an approach prior to making a treatment decision (N. Brown, personal communication, March 13, 2013).

Treatment Navigation

Once treatment decisions are made, GU cancer nurse navigators strive to make processes as smooth as possible for patients. For patients on active surveillance, this includes ensuring that the schedule of PSA checks and urology follow-up visits are maintained. For patients undergoing surgery or radiation therapy, GU cancer nurse navigators work with the appropriate staff members from the treating physician's office to ensure scheduling of treatment dates and necessary planning appointments.

Although the GU cancer nurse navigators may not be directly involved in all steps necessary for coordinating or administering treatments, they serve as a constant resource for patients and families from treatment planning through completion of care. Collaborating with other healthcare providers is essential, as optimal navigation involves a team effort rather than reliance on the navigator's efforts alone. Developing trusting and collegial relationships with all staff and departments involved in the care of patients with prostate cancer will

Figure 6-2. Palo Alto Medical Foundation Research Institute's Prostate Cancer Shared Decision Making Worksheet*

Step 1: Where Do I Start?

A. My risk group is:
- ☐ **Low**—PSA < 10, Gleason score is ≤ 6, stage is T1 or T2a.
- ☐ **Intermediate**—PSA 10–20, Gleason score = 7, stage T2b or > 50% of their biopsies showing disease.
- ☐ **High**—PSA > 20, Gleason score is 8–10, or stage T3 or T4.

B. My doctor-recommended treatment options are:
- ☐ **Low Risk of Recurrence**
  - ☐ Watchful waiting
  - ☐ Surgery
  - ☐ Radiation
    - ☐ External beam
    - ☐ Brachytherapy

- ☐ **Intermediate Risk of Recurrence**
  - ☐ Watchful waiting
  - ☐ Radiation
    - ☐ External beam
    - ☐ Brachytherapy
  - ☐ Surgerý

- ☐ **High Risk of Recurrence**
  - ☐ Hormonal therapy plus radiation
  - ☐ Surgery and radiation

C. Other treatment options I want to explore are:
- ☐ _____
- ☐ _____
- ☐ _____
- ☐ _____

Step 2: Identifying My Goals (Rank your goals, "1" being the most important)

D. My Prostate Cancer Goals Are:
- ☐ **Avoiding Side Effects**
  Vignette 1: Age 73 (Low Risk; T2a, Gleason = 6) "The thought of being incontinent or needing a diaper depressed me … the options were surgery or radiation, and I thought proton therapy might reduce the possible side effects … and I have been extremely satisfied."

(Continued on next page)

Figure 6-2. Palo Alto Medical Foundation Research Institute's Prostate Cancer Shared Decision Making Worksheet* (Continued)

☐ **Maintaining Quality of Life**
Vignette 2: Age 55 (Low Risk; T1c, Gleason = 7) "I am a young, sexually active gay man ... I am unwilling to consider living the rest of my life without erections ... I chose to watch and wait."

Vignette 3: Age 83 (High Risk; T3b, Gleason = 9) "I wanted to stay active. I golf, ski, and work part time. I did hormones, then brachytherapy, then external beam radiation."

☐ **Getting the Cancer Out/Gone**
Vignette 4: Age 78 (Intermediate/High Risk; T1c, Gleason = 8) "I wanted to get rid of the cancer and live longer. Radiation was the best option. I did hormones while I was deciding what treatment to pursue."

Vignette 5: Age 58 (Low/Intermediate Risk; T2a, Gleason = 7) "I wanted to get rid of the cancer and know more about the disease. Surgery was the best option."

☐ **Cost of Treatment**

☐ **Operative Risk (fear of dying during surgery)**

☐ **Making Treatment as Convenient as Possible**
Vignette 6: Age 63 (Low Risk; T1c, Gleason = 6) "I wanted a short treatment phase, fewer complications, and a short recovery time. HDR brachytherapy was best for me."

Vignette 7: Age 63 (Low Risk; T2a, Gleason = 5) "I am the primary caretaker for ... and I have a job that requires my presence. I had to be able to miss zero days of work. I chose permanent seed brachytherapy."

Step 3: Setting Priorities (Rank your priorities, "1" being the most important, and "7" being the least important)

E. My priorities for treatment are:
☐ **Avoiding Immediate Side Effects of Treatment**
  ☐ Urine incontinence
  ☐ Bowel incontinence
  ☐ Impotency/erectile dysfunction
  ☐ Bowel problems
  ☐ Sexual potency

☐ **Avoiding Long-Term Side Effects of Treatment**
  ☐ Urine incontinence
  ☐ Bowel incontinence
  ☐ Impotency/erectile dysfunction
  ☐ Bowel problems
  ☐ Sexual potency

(Continued on next page)

Figure 6-2. Palo Alto Medical Foundation Research Institute's Prostate Cancer Shared Decision Making Worksheet* *(Continued)*

☐ **Maintaining Quality of Life**

☐ **Getting the Cancer Out/Gone/Controlled**

☐ **Cost of Treatment**

☐ **Operative Risk (fear of dying during surgery)**

☐ **Making Treatment as Convenient as Possible**
  ☐ Number of treatments
  ☐ Where treatment is administered

☐ **Other (please specify)** _____

_____

Step 4: Making a Decision

F. My realistic options for treatment are:

Priority	Treatment Option 1	Treatment Option 2	Treatment Option 3
1.			
2.			
3.			
4.			

G. The next steps I need to take are:

	Date I expect to accomplish this goal:	Support I need:
1. Find more information		
2. Talk to family members		

(Continued on next page)

Figure 6-2. Palo Alto Medical Foundation Research Institute's Prostate Cancer Shared Decision Making Worksheet* *(Continued)*

3. Make appointments		

Other comments:

Patient signature:	**Date:**
Navigator signature:	**Date:**

Instructions: Make a copy for the chart before patient leaves and give the original to the patient.

* With contributions from Nancy L. Brown, PhD, Palo Alto Medical Foundation Research Institute; Gordon Ray, MD, Palo Alto Medical Foundation; and D. Jeffrey Demanes, MD, California Endocurietherapy Cancer Center. Funded by Sutter Health Institute for Research and Education (SHIRE) and the National Cancer Institute (R21CA133340). The content is solely the responsibility of the authors and does not necessarily represent the official views of the National Cancer Institute or the National Institutes of Health.

Note. Figure courtesy of Palo Alto Medical Foundation. Used with permission.

ensure smooth transitions of care and minimal burden to patients in the process of obtaining well-coordinated, patient-centered care.

Post-Treatment Issues

Having already developed relationships with patients and families, GU cancer nurse navigators are in an ideal position to address survivorship issues concerning post-treatment care and management of any late and long-term side effects. Siegel et al. (2012) estimated that of the 13.7 million cancer survivors in the United States, about 2.8 million are prostate cancer survivors, potentially making survivorship a large component of GU cancer nurse navigator practice. Depending on the type of treatment, late effects may include incontinence; erectile dysfunction; bowel complications; loss of libido; menopausal-like symptoms including hot flashes, night sweats, and irritability; osteoporosis; and the risk of diabetes, cardiovascular disease, and obesity related to long-term hormone therapy (Siegel et al., 2012). GU cancer nurse navigators can arrange for follow-up visits after completion of treatment to address the issues of survivorship, coupled with an attention to wellness issues, such as diet, exercise, and sexual health. For issues beyond the navigators' scope of practice, navigators can initiate referrals to supportive services, such as nutrition, physical therapy, and counseling, while keeping PCPs informed of patients' post-treatment status.

In the event that follow-up care reveals progression of the prostate cancer, the GU cancer nurse navigator can assist with any necessary transitions to palliative care. Referrals to medical oncology or dedicated supportive care services may be necessary to pursue treatments with the primary goal being palliation, such as various forms of chemotherapy, hormone therapy, or immunotherapies and other emerging technologies and clinical trials. Several shared decision-making tools are available online (see Figure 6-3) to address issues in late-stage prostate cancer. Hospice referrals should be offered as appropriate to end-of-life care. Facing difficult issues in prostate cancer progression can be challenging for all involved, but GU cancer nurse navigators can serve to ensure smooth care transitions.

Bladder Cancer

As opposed to prostate cancer, where broad population-based screenings can identify hundreds of patients each year in need of GU cancer navigation services, newly diagnosed patients with bladder cancer are found much less frequently, often as an incidental finding of microscopic hematuria with a routine urinalysis. When developing GU cancer navigation programs, it is essential to identify services offered by the GU cancer nurse navigator and specific situations appropriate for patient referrals. For example, if a stage II (T2) muscle-invasive bladder cancer is found upon biopsy, the GU cancer nurse navigator can offer advice and decision-making strategies to help patients select among the available surgical options for treatment (J. Powers, personal communication, February 27, 2013).

Screening and Diagnosis

Currently, no recommended routine screening tests for bladder cancer exist (NCCN, 2013a). Smoking is associated with bladder cancer risk (Freedman, Silverman, Hollenbeck, Schatzkin, & Abnet, 2011); therefore, smoking cessation programs would be one diagnosis-specific task that GU cancer navigators could promote.

Figure 6-3. Web Resources for Shared Decision Making

- Informed Medical Decisions Foundation Decision Aids: www.informedmedicaldecisions
  .org/shared-decision-making-in-practice/decision-aids
- Ottawa Personal Decision Guide: http://decisionaid.ohri.ca/decguide.html
- Us Too International Prostate Cancer Education and Support Network Advanced Prostate Cancer Resource Kit: www.ustoo.org/Advanced_Disease.asp

Once pathology has confirmed a bladder cancer diagnosis, referral to the GU cancer nurse navigator can be offered. As with prostate cancer, possible sources of referral include urologists, urology nurses, case managers, and social workers. The initial visit with the GU cancer nurse navigator provides a great opportunity to review not only the clinical picture and treatment planning but also issues involving financial and insurance-related implications, as well as psychosocial and sexual issues.

Treatment Navigation

Medical care in urologic oncology is driven by national guidelines. Yet even with concrete treatment guidelines, situations may still arise when multiple options exist for a particular stage and grade of bladder cancer. Coordinating multidisciplinary GU tumor boards, involving urology, medical and radiation oncology, radiology, and pathology, allows all involved providers to discuss prospective cases as a group in an effort to present clear recommendations to patients. Individual meetings between the GU cancer nurse navigator and patients can include detailed discussions of the benefits and risks related to procedure choices, such as whether to use neoadjuvant chemotherapy or the surgical choice of a neobladder versus an ileal conduit. Guiding patients with bladder cancer and their families from diagnosis through treatment offers many opportunities for GU cancer nurse navigators to foster optimal care, particularly at critical points when assistance is needed with treatment decision making and identifying supportive services.

Post-Treatment Issues

Regardless of the treatment modality chosen, bladder cancer survivors often face side effects that directly affect urinary and sexual function. GU cancer nurse navigators can serve as a key resource to patients and significant others by offering assistance with symptom assessment and management and making referrals as needed to physical therapists who specialize in urologic issues or to specialists in sexual health. Patients and healthcare providers may be apprehensive in addressing sexual health (Albaugh, Kellogg-Spadt, Krebs, Lewis, & Kramer-Levien, 2009), so it is essential for GU cancer nurse navigators to create a trusting relationship and work to reduce these barriers. This can perhaps be accomplished through patient counseling and use of confidential online or printed self-reporting tools, as well as collaborating with fellow healthcare providers to identify available resources specific to sexual health.

Other Genitourinary Cancers

For GU cancers, such as testicular, kidney, and even rare cancers involving the penis or ureters, GU cancer nurse navigators should attempt to be involved with patients across the cancer care continuum, from screening and diagnosis through treatment and into survivorship or palliative care. Many care issues are similar to those found in prostate and bladder cancers, but unique diagnosis-specific needs and concerns can still be identified. During the process of setting up navigation services for these cancers, an essential first step would be to perform a needs assessment to identify potential disparities and barriers to optimal care. Some important baseline information, specific to each diagnosis, may include

- Number of cases diagnosed in the previous year
- Specialty departments involved in the care and how patients are referred
- Diagnosis-specific resources available
- Insurance-related issues and financial counseling
- Adherence to national treatment guidelines
- Availability of multidisciplinary tumor boards
- Patients' perceptions of care processes from diagnosis through treatment
- Physician needs, to help identify services and systems to best support the ongoing care of patients with GU cancers
- Nursing, administrative, and all frontline staff perspectives to identify areas for quality improvement and optimal patient-centered care and customer service.

Patient Counseling

With relatively rare cancers, GU cancer nurse navigators spend a majority of time coordinating logistics and ensuring that appointments, tests, and treatments are appropriately arranged. Treatment guidelines based on clinical diagnosis drive the care path forward, mainly under the guidance of the urologist or oncologist. Along this path, however, patients will encounter situations that require decisions or additional support, and again, the GU cancer nurse navigator can assist with questions that may arise, such as the following.

- When making treatment decisions, does the patient with kidney cancer choose partial nephrectomy, radical nephrectomy, ablative techniques, or active surveillance?
- When making treatment decisions, does the patient with testicular cancer choose surveillance or surgery?
- How does a patient with a GU cancer obtain information about insurance coverage?
- How does a patient with a GU cancer get connected with clinical trials or a second opinion?
- How does a patient with a GU cancer connect with other patients who have had a similar therapy?

Overarching Issues for Genitourinary Cancer Nurse Navigators

Sexuality

Sexual health is a vital and prevalent issue, but it is relatively overlooked and underassessed in GU cancer care. Sexual dysfunction and dissatisfaction is common among patients, and treatment often makes things worse. Ideally, counseling should be offered before treatment begins and after active treatment is completed. Elements of pretreatment counseling include sexual activity assessment and patient and partner education and inclusion in treatment decisions. Post-treatment counseling should include reassessment, as well as advice and referrals that offer psychological, pharmacologic, or mechanical aids to address sexual problems (Sadovsky et al., 2010). Interview techniques and assessment tools to assist cancer care providers in gathering information about patients' sexual health are readily available in the literature, and the NCI website contains a list of validated resources as well (NCI, 2013b).

Quality Improvement

Adherence to national treatment guidelines and multidisciplinary tumor board recommendations are fairly common methods used to address quality assurance in GU cancer care. Ideally, the core group involved should include urologists, medical and radiation oncologists, pathologists, radiologists, social workers or case managers, and the GU cancer nurse navigator. PCPs can add vital perspectives if able to participate.

Patient satisfaction surveys and symptom assessment tools are examples of conventional methods to gather quantitative feedback, but detailed qualitative feedback can be instrumental to quality improvement of GU cancer navigation programs and services. Conducting focus groups with patients who have completed therapy can reveal successes, as well as opportunities for improvement. Another group to assess, if available, includes patients who were diagnosed at the facility but then migrated out of the system to receive treatment elsewhere.

Future Implications for Genitourinary Cancer Navigation

The content in this section is by no means a comprehensive list of tasks for GU cancer nurse navigators. With a keen, progressive eye on logistics, education, counseling, and care transitions, GU cancer nurse navigators can develop focused programs and value-added services targeted at optimizing patient care while minimizing barriers and healthcare disparities. Starting with a comprehensive needs assessment will ensure that the GU cancer nurse navigation program is relevant and evolves into an integral component of GU cancer care for the patients and communities served.

Navigating Patients With Gynecologic Cancers

A paucity of evidence-based literature regarding gynecologic oncology (GYN/ONC) nurse navigation exists because this is a relatively new focus for formalized navigation programs. Rather, there seems to be universal acceptance of general oncology nurse navigation concepts and information, which have been further adapted in an ongoing "trial and error" fashion to this subspecialty of women's cancer care. Initial work in this area of navigation began by mapping the trajectory of gynecologic cancers and intuitively projecting the needs of
- Patients with newly diagnosed ovarian, cervical, or endometrial cancer, gestational trophoblastic neoplasm, and various sarcomas and neuroendocrine manifestations of malignancies
- Patients with recurrent disease
- Patients in need of palliative care or hospice services
- Patients completing treatment and engaging in survivorship activities along the continuum of care.

Patient Identification and Needs Assessment

For programs to establish optimal processes for GYN/ONC navigation, the juxtaposition with newly diagnosed patients with breast cancer is crucial to understand. Patients with breast cancer are often diagnosed after feeling a lump or having a dubious mammogram, which is then further evaluated with some type biopsy and a planning session regarding surgical modalities. By the time the breast cancer nurse navigator gets the patient's pathology report and makes initial contact with the patient, the patient not only has had some time to plan for the news of a potential cancer diagnosis but also now has the opportunity to participate in subsequent treatment-related surgical decisions. In stark contrast, GYN/ONC diagnoses usually are definitively established postoperatively unless prior scans and tumor markers were overwhelmingly indicative of disease. Some patients have come to the gynecologic oncologist for what is perceived to be extra testing or more extensive procedures to be done by a "specialist." Others may have been misdiagnosed for several months. Regardless, new patients can present with varying degrees of emotional reactions including hysteria, anger, fear, and a generalized inability to grasp much information. Additionally, as with a diagnosis of breast or GU cancers, the diagnosis of a GYN/ONC cancer can induce a profound perception of loss of oneself as a sexual being (Benigno, 2013), which can further perpetuate a sense of alienation.

Many entry points to navigation exist for GYN/ONC patients, with referrals coming from gynecologic oncologists, inpatient nursing staff, infusion nurses, and sometimes fellow patients. As GYN/ONC patients may be experiencing intense emotional responses to the cancer diagnosis, GYN/ONC nurse navigators must be flexible with the initial approach after the referral is received and use intuitive acceptance when working with patients and families. Furthermore, each GYN/ONC malignancy presents its own challenges, misconceptions, and anticipatory fears. Shame and embarrassment can be associated with human papillomavirus (HPV) in cervical cancer, as well as with treatment-related consequences such as surgical menopause and infertility.

The overall approach for the initial contact between GYN/ONC nurse navigators and patients and families is often contingent upon the setting in which the interaction occurs, as well as the unique and individual circumstances of the situation. The emotional response of patients and families in coming to terms with the cancer diagnosis often mirrors the grieving process. From the GYN/ONC nurse navigator's perspective, this is a time for simplicity rather than extensive education. Therapeutic communication is best limited to

- Introductions and a brief description of the GYN/ONC nurse navigator role
- Minimal educational materials, such as a simple brochure and business card with the nurse navigator's full contact information
- If appropriate, a notebook for patients to write down questions as they arise.

This is an opportune moment for the navigator to determine the support structure, if possible, and the knowledge level of patients and families. Yet, because of the shock and disbelief associated with a new diagnosis, patient comprehension is far from optimal, so the most productive approach is often an elementary one without the expectation of significant feedback from patients and families at this time.

Continuum of Care

As patients and families move into treatment, it is helpful for GYN/ONC nurse navigators to attend consultation visits and treatment appointments or to at least be available by telephone for questions that arise. If navigators are not able to meet with patients in person, it is helpful to instruct patients to write down any questions and then follow up with them by telephone as soon as possible to address concerns and thereby diminish the accumulation of fear, which can rapidly accelerate when there is a lack of understanding. For example, radiation procedures can seem overwhelmingly invasive, and chemotherapy often carries the stigma of poison, nausea, baldness, and whatever anecdotes patients might have heard from seemingly well-meaning commentators. The GYN/ONC nurse navigator can provide factual and objective information to help alleviate patients' fears and misconceptions and, thereafter, assist patients in moving forward with treatment-related decisions.

The time it takes for patients to advance from the initial stages of shock, disbelief, and fear into the ability for rational thought is unique to each patient situation. Thus, it is essential for GYN/ONC nurse navigators to continually assess cognitive abilities as patients progress into the active treatment phase.

It is important for patients to understand the GYN/ONC nurse navigator's availability for any ongoing questions or concerns. Sharing the GYN/ONC nurse navigator's contact information with the infusion and radiation nurses is helpful so that as patients express needs, the nurses can contact the GYN/ONC nurse navigator in a timely manner. Not only is this helpful to patients, but it also builds trust and confidence with staff and providers that the GYN/ONC nurse navigator is, indeed, available to guide patients through the cancer continuum.

The NCCN Distress Thermometer can be a very effective screening tool for both patients and staff to identify specific needs (Kendall, Hamann, & Clayton, 2012). At Northside Cancer Institute in Atlanta, Georgia, the implementation of the NCCN Distress Thermometer has had a secondary benefit of connecting many patients to services that might not otherwise have been identified. For example, a cervical cancer diagnosis can be a psychosocial and moral trauma for patients, so GYN/ONC nurse navigators must be alert for manifestations of this type of distress and encourage patients to express thoughts, feelings, and concerns. Additionally, navigators must be aware of the potential impact of cervical cancer on sexual function and intimate relationships (Hunter, 2011) and be ready to address these issues and appropriately refer patients to counseling services. GYN/ONC patients at Northside Hospital Cancer Institute have expressed feelings of relief and validation that distress is routinely assessed, recognized, and addressed.

As GYN/ONC patients equilibrate into treatment routines, GYN/ONC nurse navigators can introduce various educational modalities in a sequential manner as appropriate, relying upon the side effect profile observed at each encounter. Although such observations can preempt any planned learning opportunities, these may afford the nurse navigators the opportunity to assist patients in dealing with particular side effects. It may be helpful to review frequently asked questions and encourage patients to identify additional questions to discuss at the next appointment.

Genetic counseling and testing is particularly important for some GYN/ONC patients. Although this can be a very personal subject, it may ultimately have ramifications for the entire family and therefore must be handled in a deliberate and thoughtful manner. GYN/ONC nurse navigators must be knowledgeable of the various hereditary syndromes associated with GYN/ONC malignancies (i.e., hereditary breast and ovarian cancer, Lynch syndrome, Cowden syndrome, *PTEN* mutations, Sertoli-Leydig, *BRCA* mutations) to answer basic questions from patients and families (Babb & Parham, 2009). Identifying high-risk individuals and initiating genetic counseling referrals is a key responsibility of GYN/ONC nurse navigators (Matloff, 2013). Objective information can ameliorate guilt associated with this type of diagnosis. For example, patients of Ashkenazi descent are prone to multiple primaries of breast and ovarian cancer and need specific education on this risk. In communities with large Ashkenazi populations, GYN/ONC nurse navigators might consider approaching synagogues and offering to facilitate education programs in collaboration with genetic counselors to create an opportunity for increased community awareness, dialogue, and objectivity.

Survivorship Focus

Because women often seek the camaraderie of other women, a vibrant, productive, accessible support group is an important adjunct to navigating GYN/ONC patients through the cancer continuum. Groups can provide a vehicle for supportive care education including nutrition, sexuality and body image issues, integrative modalities, and ultimately a survivorship plan.

Support groups typically meet according to a defined frequency; this might be weekly, biweekly, or monthly. Groups may be restricted to patients only or open to patients, families, and caregivers. If a group is open to families and caregivers, at times facilitators may separate patients from families and caregivers to allow for therapeutic dialogue among each group without fear of burdening loved ones with sensitive information. Social media is another way to provide support to patients and can be an especially effective way to reach patients who either cannot travel to in-person groups or perhaps are not inclined to partake in social gatherings.

As patients near the completion of treatment, it is essential for GYN/ONC nurse navigators to discuss the availability of survivorship activities and encourage participation in order for patients to conceptualize themselves as survivors and feel a sense of forward motion. Finding survivorship support and helping patients to establish a sense of camaraderie with other survivors recently "cut loose" from the cocoon of care when treatment is completed can be extremely motivating.

Many cancer communities offer programs similar in structure to the Stress Therapy Empowering Prevention (STEP) program, which focuses on promoting health after cancer treatment through stress management, nutrition, exercise, and mind-body health (Burke, Ellsworth, & Vernalis, 2012). Patients who participate in these types of programs have been shown to develop a sense of personal empowerment in survivorship. Thus, nurse navigators should be aware of any locally available programs of this nature and encourage patients' participation as an integral component of survivorship (Burke et al., 2012).

Transition to Palliative Care

Sadly, in the GYN/ONC population, some patients progress relentlessly and are transitioned to palliative care. GYN/ONC nurse navigators can assist in alleviating patient and caregiver burden during this difficult time by ensuring that care transitions are as seamless as possible and facilitating open dialogue and communication. Usually at this juncture in care, an emotional bond forms between GYN/ONC nurse navigators and patients, which is predicated on reliability, trust, and availability; thus, the shift to palliative care must be graceful, keeping communication channels open but with refocusing to the new care team addressing the evolving goals of care. A gentle discussion regarding an advance directive can afford patients a sense of autonomy. Furthermore, having the support of an established patient-navigator bond can provide an ambience of comfort for patients and caregivers when considering difficult end-of-life decisions (Moore, 2008). These concepts also apply to GYN/ONC nurse navigators' role with hospice placement; each transition for GYN/ONC patients must be handled in the most delicate and thoughtful manner.

The role of the GYN/ONC nurse navigator can be extremely challenging. GYN/ONC nurse navigators have the unique opportunity to support patients in an intimate manner from diagnosis through the entire continuum of care. The resulting bond formed between patients and navigators can lead to profound professional satisfaction for nurse navigators who recognize the subtleties of this subspecialty by engaging in a sensitive and compassionate manner to guide patients through the cancer journey.

Navigating Patients With Head and Neck Cancers

The complexity of head and neck cancer (HNC) dictates that the majority of patients diagnosed will benefit from navigation services. HNCs comprise approximately 3% of cancers diagnosed in the United States (NCI, 2013a). Sites of HNCs vary and include tumors of the nasal cavity and paranasal sinuses, salivary glands, lip and oral cavity, pharynx, and larynx. Management of patients with HNC is highly individualized. NCCN guidelines provide clinical practice guidelines for sub-sites of HNC (NCCN, 2013b).

Squamous cell is the histologic cell type identified in more than 90% of HNC cases. The major risk factors for HNC are tobacco use (smoking and smokeless tobacco products), alcohol consumption, and HPV infections (Cabezón-Gutiérrez, Khosravi-Shahi, & Escobar-Álvarez, 2012). The combination of smoking and alcohol is known to have synergistic effects (Cabezón-Gutiérrez et al., 2012). During the 1980s, the number of HNC cases decreased, which many experts attributed to the decline in tobacco use. However, the incidence of HPV-associated HNC is on the rise, with HPV-positive oropharyngeal cancers increasing 225% between 1988 and 2004 (Splete, 2012). Experts are predicting a continued increase in HPV-associated HNC (Callaway, 2011; Splete, 2012). Splete (2012) indicated that "human papillomavirus-positive oropharyngeal tumors are increasing in incidence and exceed the number of tumors caused by the more traditional risk factors of tobacco and alcohol abuse" (p. 11).

According to NCCN (2013b) guidelines for HNCs, single-modality treatment of either surgery or radiation is recommended for the 30%–40% of patients presenting with stage I or II disease. The other 60% of the patients who present with locally or regionally advanced disease at diagnosis typically require multimodality treatment for optimal outcomes. Several studies have shown that treatment with chemotherapy and radiation (with or without organ-preservation surgery) can minimize morbidities, such as speech and swallowing deficits, with equivalent tumor control compared to organ removal surgery (Mouw et al., 2010).

The physical complexities of HNC are many and can include disfigurement; difficulty eating, swallowing, and speaking; xerostomia; pain; ageusia or hypogeusia; dental problems; trismus; fatigue; and voice changes (Devins et al., 2013). Psychosocial barriers include social stigma, depression, financial concerns, unemployment, difficulty communicating, difficulty maintaining intimate relationships, and fear of recurrence (Devins et al., 2013; Fang et al., 2012). Patients with HNC present with more complex and challenging psychological adjustments than patients with other cancers (Gil, Costa, Hilker, & Benito, 2012). Among the different cancer types, HNC, and more specifically oropharyngeal cancer, has the highest rates of major depressive disorder (Gold, 2012).

Referrals for Head and Neck Cancer Navigation

The journey to a definitive diagnosis of HNC often begins with a lump found in the neck or a persistent sore throat. Commonly, these complaints are first brought to the attention of a PCP, who prescribes one to two courses of antibiotics before referring the patient to an ear, nose, and throat specialist (ENT). At the time of consultation with an ENT, a rhinolaryngoscopy (a flexible endoscope or camera that is passed through the nose to visualize the aerodigestive tract) may be performed as part of the physical examination to potentially identify a visible lesion. If a patient presents with nodal involvement, a positron-emission tomography/computed tomography (PET/CT) scan may be considered (NCCN, 2013b). Further, a fine needle aspiration of a palpable or PET-identified neck node, which is usually the site of metastasis, may be recommended. The primary site is identified pathologically by tissue biopsy.

A positive pathology report may be the HNC nurse navigator's first notification of a newly diagnosed patient with HNC. Other methods of identifying patients include direct referrals from physicians, such as ENTs, medical oncologists, and radiation oncologists. Fostering positive working relationships with office staff can assist with the referral process. Additionally, some patients may self-refer to navigation services as a result of Internet research or community marketing. Referrals from previous patients, friends, or family members treated at a facility also drive newly diagnosed patients with HNC to the navigation program.

Initial Navigation Contact

Depending on the availability of services, geography, or barriers of each cancer center or disease site–specific program, the options for making initial patient contact may vary. Ideally, the first contact by an HNC nurse navigator is made when patients are given the diagnosis or at one of the consultation appointments immediately following diagnosis. Some healthcare facilities use a multidisciplinary clinic model in which patients are seen by a comprehensive team including oncologists (surgical, medical, and radiation), a dentist, the HNC nurse navigator, a dietitian, a speech pathologist, a social worker, and a health psychologist. Other institutions may require patients to attend a visual HNC conference, whereby the patient is examined via rhinolaryngoscopy while attendees watch the examination real-time on a video screen. Attendees typically include the treating ENT, medical oncologist, radiation oncologist, and other HNC specialists such as a dentist, dietitian, research staff, and HNC nurse navigator. Once the examination is completed, the patient is excused and the multidisciplinary team reviews the radiologic and pathologic findings to begin developing the patient's plan of care.

The convening of multidisciplinary tumor conferences and navigation programs for HNCs can decrease barriers regarding access to care and delays in treatment initiation. In a study by Patel and Brennan (2012), patients with early-stage disease experienced fewer treatment delays versus patients with advanced disease in which a multimodality treatment plan was needed. Other factors found to delay treatment are related to socioeconomic status, race, and preexisting comorbidities.

With the time constraints experienced by many physicians, HNC nurse navigators are ideally positioned to address patient concerns, needs, and healthcare system barriers. If present at the time treatment plans are discussed, HNC nurse navigators are available to provide education, clarify treatment plans, answer questions, and provide emotional support. HNC nurse navigators can serve as the linchpin to assist with referral processes and coordination of care for these very complex patient cases.

Coordination of care for patients with HNC can include scheduling imaging tests and arranging consults with a physical and occupational therapist, speech/swallow pathologist, dietitian, dentist, health psychologist, and social worker. Additionally, a gastroenterologist may be consulted if a percutaneous endoscopic gastrostomy (PEG) tube is indicated. Many of these referrals must be scheduled before the start of treatment. It is not unusual for HNC nurse navigators to spend 45 minutes or more with patients and families at the initial contact; this involves not only schedule coordination but also forming the basis for the therapeutic patient-navigator relationship.

Identification of Navigation Needs

The amount of information gathered by the HNC nurse navigator at the time of initial contact is extensive. A distress screening tool is useful to identify barriers and concerns with which the patient may present. Use of a distress screening tool ensures consistent assessment by the healthcare team and allows patients to identify physical, emotional, and practical stressors. Depending on the needs and concerns identified, referrals for smoking cessation, counseling for alcohol abuse, or referrals to a social worker, spiritual care provider, or health psychologist may be indicated. According to Patel and Brennan (2012), the underserved population is at increased risk for malnutrition, alcohol or substance abuse, and comorbidities. Socioeconomic factors such as lower education level, learning difficulties, limited access to transportation, lack of paid time off, and language barriers are additional obstacles that often require attention from HNC nurse navigators.

Patient Education

The quantity of information given to patients at the time of a consult can be overwhelming, and HNC nurse navigators can provide invaluable support during this time. Navigators provide and explain written information, as well as direct patients to electronic resources that can be reviewed at patients' convenience. Personalized calendars or checklists that include brief explanations for certain consultations or tests can be helpful organizational tools, alleviate anxiety, and promote compliance with scheduled services

(Robinson, Callister, Berry, & Dearing, 2008). An example of a brief explanation for a patient scheduled to start radiation therapy might be: A dental visit is necessary in order to have mouth stents fabricated and to ensure good dental health prior to starting radiation treatment.

NCI has multiple patient education publications that address general cancer topics such as chemotherapy, radiation, clinical trials, smoking cessation, and nutrition. Booklets specific to cancer of the oral cavity and larynx, which are written for newly diagnosed patients with cancer, are available as well. Organizations such as the National Institute of Dental and Craniofacial Research (www.nidcr.nih.gov) and CancerCare (www.cancercare.org) have pamphlets addressing oral cancer and oral care during radiation. Support for People With Oral and Head and Neck Cancer (www.spohnc.org) is a helpful resource for identifying local support groups, clinical trials, and educational materials.

Patient Contact

Depending on the individual needs of patients or corresponding treatment plans, continuing contact schedules may vary. Coordination of all of the pretreatment appointments is often labor intensive for HNC nurse navigators and requires multiple conversations with patients and caregivers. However, once treatment starts, contact may diminish, but it later increases again as side effects from treatment arise. If neoadjuvant chemotherapy is indicated, a key responsibility of HNC nurse navigators is the coordination and scheduling of concurrent chemoradiation. Coordination and communication with the treating medical oncologist and radiation oncologist will ensure a seamless transition of care. If any extensive dental work is required, a plan for adequate healing time is necessary prior to starting radiation therapy and may require additional coordination by the navigator to ensure the timeliness of the start of radiation or chemoradiation.

Supportive Care

Prior to or at the start of radiation therapy, a PEG tube may or may not be indicated. If one is placed, a visit from a home health nurse is important to meet patient and caregiver education needs including site care, tube flushing, and feedings. This can result in decreased fear, anxiety, and risk of post-procedure infection. It is beneficial for HNC nurse navigators to have a solid knowledge base on PEG tube management including site care, tube feeding options, tube maintenance, and medication administration. Engaging a registered dietitian in the care of patients with HNC is essential to closely follow patients' weight and body mass index, advise on nutrition and fluid needs, provide tips for easing swallowing and mouth pain, and make knowledgeable nutritional formula recommendations.

As patients progress through the course of treatment, their needs will change; thus, assessment is an ongoing responsibility for HNC nurse navigators. Management of side effects is a key component of navigation during multimodality treatment. Patients with HNC will experience a range of physical changes including fatigue, xerostomia, thick/ropy secretions, skin changes related to radiation or endothelial growth factor receptor inhibitors, dysgeusia, dysphagia, mucositis, and pain. Psychosocial issues may include anxiety, fear, difficulty coping, and depression. As side effects manifest, education and emotional support should be individualized for each patient. Fang et al. (2012) noted that patients who perceived having adequate information related to treatment, post-treatment, and psychological distress had better rehabilitation outcomes at two and six years after treatment.

Smoking cessation and alcohol counseling are key topics to address throughout the continuum of care. Approximately one-third to one-half of patients with HNC continue to use tobacco and/or alcohol after diagnosis and through treatment (Howren, Christensen, Karnell, & Funk, 2013). Continued tobacco and alcohol abuse has been shown to negatively affect treatment efficacy and survival (NCCN, 2013b).

Participation in a support group for patients with HNC can be empowering. Peer-to-peer education can be reassuring, encouraging, and provide a sense of normalcy for patients. One study of patients with HNC noted that the most common coping strategy was seeking social support (Howren, Christensen, Karnell, Van Liew, & Funk, 2013). A favorable QOL was reported one year after treatment in patients with greater perceived social support (Howren, Christensen, Karnell, Van Liew, et al., 2013).

A support group for caregivers of patients with HNC also can be beneficial. Spouses and other family members need support in dealing with the stresses of being a caregiver. Caregivers of patients with HNC experience high levels of distress and fear of recurrence and are at an increased risk for developing post-traumatic stress disorder. Caregivers' identified areas of concern included relationship conflicts, personal needs, the need for psychological care, and the desire for contact with self-help groups (Howren, Christensen, Karnell, Van Liew, et al., 2013). Family stressors often involve feelings of helplessness; fear of the cancer diagnosis and the possibility of a terminal illness; the effects of illness on employment, restriction of activities, and the ability to perform family functions; and concerns about the family's future (Gold, 2012).

The magnitude of side effects patients experience at the end of treatment may remain the same or even increase immediately following the completion of treatment and can be difficult to manage for several weeks. Studies have shown a decrease in QOL of patients with HNC at the time of diagnosis and in the first year after completion of treatment (Oskam et al., 2013).

Providing early palliative care interventions can improve QOL and reduce depressive symptoms (Peyrade et al., 2013). Late or long-term side effects are similar to those experienced during treatment, and unfortunately, some may not resolve (Tucker, 2012). For example, hypothyroidism may manifest after the thyroid gland is exposed to radiation, thus requiring the need for thyroid hormone management. Long-term xerostomia can place the patient at risk for dental caries and contribute to dysphagia. Deconditioning of the swallowing mechanism after use of a PEG tube or fibrosis from radiation also may contribute to dysphagia (Platteaux, Dirix, Dejaeger, & Nuyts, 2010). Direct interventions for late or long-term side effects can include continued assessment by a registered dietitian and rehabilitation and physical therapists. Therapies may include treatment for lymphedema and speech and swallow deficits. Gold (2012) identified the need for continued psychosocial support for both patients and caregivers after the completion of treatment.

As patients move into survivorship, concerns include physical changes related to speech, swallowing, eating, dry mouth, and appearance. Fingeret et al. (2013) identified the ability to speak as the most important indicator of health-related QOL, with swallowing being the second. Patients with oral cavity malignancies have impairments with eating related to pain, ageusia, trismus, and the ability to keep food in the mouth while chewing (Fingeret et al., 2013).

In a small study (99 patients enrolled; 16 evaluable), O'Brien, Roe, Low, Deyn, and Rogers (2012) identified barriers to intimacy for patients with HNC. These barriers were grouped into three categories: (a) personal identity, (b) reestablishing social networks, and (c) the ability to resume former intimate relations. Specific barriers related to personal identity included changes in appearance leading to a loss of confidence, the loss of independence, changes in a given role, and changes in speech. Obstacles for reestablishing social networks included the ability to resume work and to socialize while eating out. For resuming intimate relationships, the ability to communicate was essential. Restoring trust and being able to express feelings, needs, and desires along with fears are important to reestablishing closeness. Patients with HNC strongly desired the ability to embrace and kiss loved ones. Limited sensation, altered function of the lips and tongue, xerostomia, loss of teeth, and persistent fatigue were identified as barriers to resuming intimate relationships.

Patient education continues throughout the continuum of care and into survivorship. Fang et al. (2012) identified the following primary topics that patients desired more information on after treatment: strategies to stay healthy; adjusting to changes in swallowing and speaking; and ideas for making eating and speaking easier. Additional needs identified were communicating with family, coping with changes in appearance, reducing stress and anxiety, managing social situations, and obtaining information on intimacy and sexuality. Patients were interested in information that could be viewed at home, whether through books, pamphlets, DVDs, or Internet programs.

For long-term survivors, adaptation to a "new normal" takes place, which may include dietary or swallowing restrictions or an altered appearance. HNC survivors will return to normal life activities such as working, enjoying family and social events, and participating in physical activity or exercise. However, fear of recurrence is common at the slightest hint of symptoms or near the time of follow-up scans (Gold, 2012).

End-of-Life Considerations

Recurrence, metastasis, and end-of-life care bring about a unique set of stressors, anxiety, and fear for patients with HNCs (Gold, 2012). Locoregional failure at the end of life presents many complicated symptoms and side effects including dysphagia, aspiration, sleep disturbances, inability to communicate, secretion management, and pain (Peyrade et al., 2013; Shuman, Fins, & Prince, 2012). Wound concerns such as malodorous and disfiguring tumor growth, tumor bleeding, and fistulas may present, along with emergent airway obstruction and massive hemorrhagic events (Shuman et al., 2012). Nurse navigators should address advance directives, code status, medical power of attorney, and end-of-life wishes with patients prior to possible medical emergencies. Referral to a health psychologist or licensed social worker may improve outcomes related to end-of-life, legal, and medical decisions (Howren, Christensen, Karnell, & Funk, 2013). A health psychologist, palliative care team, and HNC nurse navigators can facilitate a sensitive discussion addressing choices about artificial nutrition and hydration, information on tracheostomy or laryngectomy management, and goals for communication if speech is compromised.

The complexities of HNC start at the time of diagnosis and extend well into survivorship. Long-term side effects, both physical and psychosocial, can persist for years after the completion of treatment. The HNC nurse navigator is an integral part of the healthcare team and an invaluable resource for this patient population.

Navigating Patients With Thoracic Cancers

The specialty of thoracic oncology manages cancers located within the chest. This includes primary tumors of the lung, esophagus, and trachea, chest wall tumors, mesothelioma, and thymomas, as well as any metastatic disease within the chest area. Similar to patients with other types of cancer previously discussed in this chapter, patients with thoracic cancers frequently require the services of multiple specialists (such as pulmonologists, thoracic surgeons, medical oncologists, and radiation oncologists), and thus, the role of thoracic cancer nurse navigators has begun to emerge as an essential component of comprehensive oncology programs.

Oncology nursing literature specific to the benefits of thoracic cancer nurse navigation is beginning to materialize. In particular, Seek and Hogle (2007) detailed the development of a multidisciplinary lung cancer clinic and the role of the thoracic cancer nurse navigator in the coordination of care for patients with lung cancer as a strategy to improve patient outcomes. Prior to establishing the multidisciplinary lung cancer clinic, delays of one to three months were noted between diagnosis and initiation of treatment, with the average being 29.3 days. After the first year, 92% of patients initiated treatment within 14 days of the multidisciplinary lung cancer clinic evaluation, with the average being 18.76 days. Patient satisfaction with the multidisciplinary lung cancer clinic process was extremely high, and the number of actual lung cancer cases evaluated and treated at the facility increased by 48%. Hunnibel et al. (2012) described navigation processes implemented at the Connecticut Veterans Affairs Healthcare System, whereby significant improvements in timeliness of care were identified, as well as a shift toward diagnosis at earlier stages. Chapter 8 provides further details of this case example.

Patient Identification and Referral

Patients with thoracic cancers present to the healthcare system in a variety of ways, which can contribute to multifactorial delays in definitive diagnosis and treatment initiation, as well as perceptions of fragmented care. Patients with lung cancer likely have the greatest variability in regard to entry into the healthcare system. For example, some patients may present to a PCP and be treated for several months for recurring pulmonary infections before a diagnosis of lung cancer is determined. Other patients may be referred to a pulmonologist for diagnostic evaluation after a suspicious chest x-ray. Additionally, patients may come in through the emergency department, perhaps after experiencing some sort of trauma, require a CT scan as part of that workup, and have an abnormality or incidental finding discovered on a chest CT scan. In other cases, patients with advanced lung cancer are admitted to the hospital in crisis with oncologic emergencies and are then definitively diagnosed. As results and implications of the National Lung Screening Trial have become more widely publicized (National Lung Screening Trial Research Team, 2011a, 2011b, 2013), high-risk patients are undergoing low-dose lung CT screening as a mechanism to identify early-stage lung cancers. These wide-reaching examples demonstrate the diversity with which patients with lung cancer enter the healthcare system and support the need for thoracic cancer nurse navigators to be engaged in proactive identification and orchestration of timely and efficient care processes.

As with any nurse navigation program, referrals are the lifeblood of thoracic navigation programs. At the Thomas Johns Cancer Hospital at Johnston Willis Hospital in Richmond, Virginia, for example, patients are typically referred to the thoracic cancer nurse navigator by PCPs, medical oncologists, radiation oncologists, pulmonologists, patients, and families; however, it has taken time, as well as thoughtful introspection, to engage referrals from the various members of the multidisciplinary team at the appropriate time. To illustrate this point, when the thoracic cancer navigation program was initially developed, navigation referrals were primarily identified through pathology reports faxed from the pathologist. The team soon realized, however, that this process was fraught with inefficiencies of wasted time and resources. In fact, many of those newly diagnosed patients underwent lung surgery and were already discharged before the thoracic cancer nurse navigator received and could act upon the referral from the pathologist.

After trying several different processes and approaches, the multidisciplinary team determined that the thoracic surgeon was most appropriate to initiate thoracic navigation referrals after the cancer diagnosis was determined. However, given the various entry points and pathways that patients with known or suspected thoracic cancer may take, it was important to empower all members of the multidisciplinary team to initiate navigation referrals so that patients could be connected with this valuable service at the earliest point possible. Currently, approximately 60% of patients with lung cancer at this facility are seen by the thoracic cancer nurse navigator through referrals from various members of the multidisciplinary healthcare team, including the thoracic surgeon, medical and radiation oncologists, the pulmonologist, nurses, and social workers, and self-referrals.

Patient Education

One of the primary roles of thoracic cancer nurse navigators is patient education regarding the disease, treatment modalities, and supportive care available. Often, navigators will create patient guidebooks or resource manuals to assist in the educational process. Content will likely vary depending on the thoracic navigation program's focus within the cancer continuum and may consist of materials produced by national organizations dedicated to cancer education, as well as pieces specific to organizational and local resources. While patient education materials might range in topics from diagnosis to survivorship, ultimately, the thoracic cancer nurse navigator must be thoughtful and selective in compiling materials and include only those items most pertinent to the situation at hand, because patients can become easily overwhelmed if bombarded with too much information. One strategy incorporated by the thoracic cancer nurse navigator at the Thomas Johns Cancer Hospital was to engage members of the local cancer support group as expert advisers on the educational manual being compiled for patients with thoracic cancer. This process was found to be extremely helpful in tailoring content to the cultural norms; the book contained enough information for patients to understand what they needed to do without being overly detailed. Another approach for obtaining feedback on a patient education manual might be to solicit the opinions of key providers and ancillary staff to ensure that content meets basic educational needs as viewed by the multidisciplinary team.

Navigation Processes and Referrals

Upon initial contact with patients, thoracic cancer nurse navigators collect information pertaining to past medical history, current condition, basic demographics, and current contact information. As part of the intake process, nurse navigators assess patients' understanding of the diagnosis, procedures, and proposed treatments. This is an opportune time to introduce educational materials and resource manuals to facilitate conversations and illustrate key constructs that might otherwise be difficult for patients to grasp. Educational topics commonly covered by thoracic cancer nurse navigators include an explanation of pathology results, staging and diagnostic procedures, rationale for additional specialty consultations, and what to expect as the next steps in the cancer journey.

After initial introduction, the thoracic cancer nurse navigator typically collaborates with the physician to determine additional diagnostics and staging evaluation studies needed and begins coordinating appointments for these procedures, as well as consultations with the appropriate oncology specialists. Such consultations may be arranged as part of a thoracic multidisciplinary clinic, if available, or may be arranged such that the appointments occur sequentially within a short period of time to facilitate collaborative dialogue among the providers to determine the most appropriate treatment. Based on the needs identified during the navigator's intake assessment, the navigator may initiate referrals to ancillary members and coordinate appointments. To ensure patient understanding of all that has been arranged, the thoracic cancer nurse navigator should consider preparing a calendar of scheduled appointments for the patient, as well as providing proper education on the necessary preparations for each appointment. Depending on the scope of thoracic navigation programs, the nurse navigators may attend oncology specialists' consultation visits, initiate referrals to the tumor board for case presentation, and assist with coordination of the recommended treatment.

Thoracic cancer nurse navigators must be thoroughly familiar with treatment guidelines to ensure that care is progressing according to nationally accepted best practices, such as NCCN guidelines. For example, patients diagnosed with stage IA non-small cell lung cancer (NSCLC) are typically recommended to undergo surgery; however, if patients are medically nonoperable because of comorbidities or other factors, radiation is an appropriate treatment modality (NCCN, 2013c). Thoracic cancer nurse navigators must understand the rationale and evidence behind the NCCN guidelines to be able to explain why one treatment option is being offered over another. A solid knowledge base with regard to chemotherapy regimens, specialized radiation therapy techniques, and the side effect profiles of various treatment modalities is essential in order to help guide patients in what to anticipate when treatment beyond surgery is needed.

It is not surprising that a high percentage of patients with thoracic cancer are active smokers, as tobacco exposure is a significant risk factor. Thoracic cancer nurse navigators should have a strong working knowledge of tobacco cessation strategies and available resources to assist patients in their efforts to kick the habit, including telephone quit lines and local tobacco cessation counseling services. Although many communities have tobacco cessation counselors and support groups available for thoracic cancer nurse navigators to refer to, navigators may want to consider becoming trained tobacco cessation specialists to be able to provide support and expertise to patients. Such training not only provides valuable information and approaches but also helps navigators to recognize the challenges associated with nicotine addiction and the need to support patients' efforts in a caring, compassionate, and encouraging manner.

A significant challenge for thoracic cancer nurse navigators working with patients with late-stage lung cancer is the need to have open and forthright conversations regarding goals of care and the importance of informed decision making when considering whether to pursue treatment. In a study regarding the effects of early palliative care with patients with stage IV NSCLC, Temel et al. (2010) found that patients had longer overall survival when they engaged with a palliative care team in addition to standard oncology care compared to those receiving standard oncology care alone. Furthermore, patients receiving the palliative care interventions reported improved QOL and less depression than the control group. As a result of this landmark study, thoracic navigation programs might consider building processes whereby patients with metastatic lung cancer are automatically referred to palliative care services. When looking at potential processes such as this, it is important to recognize and distinguish that palliative care does not equate to hospice. Palliative care aims to improve QOL without associated requirements such as limited life expectancy or termination of active treatment. For most palliative care services integrated within oncology practices, referrals to palliative care do not preclude patients from also seeking treatment.

Rather, integrated palliative care services provide additional support to patients with the intention of lessening the impact of cancer on patients and families.

Future Implications for Thoracic Cancer Navigation

Given the low five-year survival rates of many thoracic cancers, the role of thoracic cancer nurse navigators can be emotionally challenging. It can be especially difficult when working with late-stage patients to find the balance between advocating for aggressive treatment versus knowing when to talk with patients and families about quality rather than quantity of life.

Recognizing the potential for compassion fatigue, burnout, and moral distress is essential to the success of thoracic cancer nurse navigators. Acknowledging symptoms of these, along with grief, loss, and other stressors, and openly addressing these issues in a proactive manner are critical to nurse navigators' self-care. It is important for thoracic cancer nurse navigators to focus on the important role they play in helping patients and families navigate the healthcare system, establish realistic goals of care, and make the most of every day when time is limited.

Historically, nurse navigation has emerged as a mechanism to guide patients from diagnosis through multifaceted treatment and into survivorship or end-of-life care. Evidence has shown that thoracic cancer nurse navigators can have a positive impact on reducing diagnostic and treatment delays while providing positive patient experiences through coordination of services and additional psychosocial support. Future opportunity may evolve for thoracic navigation services in the screening phase of the cancer continuum as well. Given the drafted U.S. Preventive Services Task Force (2013) recommendation that current smokers ages 55–80 who have smoked the equivalent of a pack of cigarettes daily for 30 years undergo annual low-dose CT scans as a mechanism to screen for lung cancer, the adoption of CT screening for early-stage lung cancer presents potential for earlier engagement of thoracic cancer nurse navigators and optimism for earlier diagnosis with improved survival for this population.

Conclusion

The inception of oncology patient navigation, as conceived by Freeman, was primarily focused on expediting access to care. As oncology nurses and other professional disciplines stepped into the scenario, there has been an exponential evolution of the navigation paradigm to encompass therapeutic interventions across the trajectory of several site-specific cancers—each requiring multifaceted nuances of care.

Although several commonalities exist in all nurse navigation roles, this chapter has presented the various needs, procedures, and formats for several diagnoses, thereby creating an anthology of competencies for each.

References

Albaugh, J., Kellogg-Spadt, S., Krebs, L.U., Lewis, J.H., & Kramer-Levien, D. (2009). Sexual function and sexual rehabilitation with genitourinary cancer. In J. Held-Warmkessel (Ed.), *Site-specific cancer series: Genitourinary cancers* (pp. 121–148). Pittsburgh, PA: Oncology Nursing Society.

American Joint Committee on Cancer. (2009). *Prostate cancer staging* (7th ed.). Retrieved from http://cancerstaging.org/references-tools/quickreferences/Documents/ProstateSmall.pdf

Babb, S., & Parham, J.A. (2009). Cancer genetics. In S. Lockwood (Ed.), *Contemporary issues in women's cancers* (pp. 183–204). Burlington, MA: Jones and Bartlett.

Benigno, B.B. (2013). *The ultimate guide to ovarian cancer.* Atlanta, GA: Sherryben Publishing House.

Benner, P. (1984). *From novice to expert: Excellence and power in clinical nursing practice.* Upper Saddle River, NJ: Prentice Hall.

Burke, A.M., Ellsworth, D.L., & Vernalis, M.N. (2012). Stress Therapy Empowering Prevention (STEP): A healthy lifestyle program for breast cancer patients. *Journal of Oncology Navigation and Survivorship, 3*(1), 8–14. Retrieved from http://issuu.com/aonn/docs/jons-feb2012

Cabezón-Gutiérrez, L., Khosravi-Shahi, P., & Escobar-Álvarez, Y. (2012). Management of dermatitis in patients with locally advanced squamous cell carcinoma of the head and neck receiving cetuximab and radiotherapy. *Oral Oncology, 48,* 293–297. doi:10.1016/j.oraloncology.2011.10.019

Callaway, C. (2011). Rethinking the head and neck cancer population: The human papillomavirus association. *Clinical Journal of Oncology Nursing, 15,* 165–170. doi:10.1188/11.CJON.165-170

Desimini, E.M., Kennedy, J.A., Helsley, M.F., Shiner, K., Denton, C., Rice, T.T., ... Lewis, M.G. (2011). Making the case for nurse navigators: Benefits, outcomes, and return on investment. *Oncology Issues, 26*(5), 26–33. Retrieved from http://www.accc-cancer.org/oncology_issues/articles/SepOct2011/SO11-Desimini.pdf

Devins, G.M., Payne, A.Y., Lebel, S., Mah, K., Lee, R.N., Irish, J., ... Rodin, G.M. (2013). The burden of stress in head and neck cancer. *Psycho-Oncology, 22,* 668–676. doi:10.1002/pon.3050

Fang, C.Y., Longacre, M.L., Manne, S.L., Ridge, J.A., Lango, M.N., & Burness, B.A. (2012). Informational needs of head and neck cancer patients. *Health and Technology, 2,* 57–62. doi:10.1007/s12553-012-0020-9

Fingeret, M.C., Hutcheson, K.A., Jensen, K., Yuan, Y., Urbauer, D., & Lewin, J.S. (2013). Associations among speech, eating, and body image concerns for surgical patients with head and neck cancer. *Head and Neck, 35,* 354–360. doi:10.1002/hed.22980

Freedman, N.D., Silverman, D.T., Hollenbeck, A.R., Schatzkin, A., & Abnet, C.C. (2011). Association between smoking and risk of bladder cancer among men and women. *JAMA, 306,* 737–745. doi:10.1001/jama.2011.1142

Freeman, H.P., & Rodriguez, R.L. (2011). History and principles of patient navigation. *Cancer, 117*(Suppl. 15), 3539–3542. doi:10.1002/cncr.26262

Gil, F., Costa, G., Hilker, I., & Benito, L. (2012). First anxiety, afterwards depression: Psychological distress in cancer patients at diagnosis and after medical treatment. *Stress and Health, 28,* 362–367. doi:10.1002/smi.2445

Gold, D. (2012). The psychosocial care needs of patients with HPV-related head and neck cancer. *Otolaryngologic Clinics of North America, 45,* 879–897. doi:10.1016/j.otc.2012.05.001

Howren, M.B., Christensen, A.J., Karnell, L.H., Van Liew, J.R., & Funk, G.F. (2013). Influence of pretreatment social support on health-related quality of life in head and neck cancer survivors: Results from a prospective study. *Head and Neck, 35,* 779–787. doi:10.1002/hed.23029

Howren, M.B., Christensen, A.J., Karnell, L.H., & Funk, G.F. (2013). Psychological factors associated with head and neck cancer treatment and survivorship: Evidence and opportunities for behavioral medicine. *Journal of Consulting and Clinical Psychology, 81,* 299–317. doi:10.1037/a0029940

Hunnibell, L.S., Rose, M.G., Connery, D.M., Grens, C.E., Hampel, J.M., Rosa, M., & Vogel, D.C. (2012). Using nurse navigation to improve timeliness of lung cancer care at a veterans hospital. *Clinical Journal of Oncology Nursing, 16,* 29–36. doi:10.1188/12.CJON.29-36

Hunter, J. (2011). The impact of cervical cancer treatment on sexual function and intimate relationships: A crying shame. *Journal of Gynecologic Oncology Nursing, 21*(2), 10–17.

Kendall, J., Hamann, H., & Clayton, S. (2012). Oncology distress screening. *Oncology Issues, 27*(6), 22–24.

Matloff, E. (2013). Counseling BRCA, lynch carriers on prophylactic oophorectomy. *Oncology Nursing News. Retrieved from* http://nursing.onclive.com/publications/oncology-nurse/2013/march-april-2013/Counseling-BRCA-Lynch-Carriers-on-Prophylactic-Oophorectomy

Moore, C.D. (2008). Advance directives. In P. Esper & K.K. Kuebler (Eds.), *Palliative practices from A–Z for the bedside clinician* (2nd ed., pp. 3–9). Pittsburgh, PA: Oncology Nursing Society.

Mouw, K.W., Haraf, D.J., Stenson, K.M., Cohen, E.E., Xi, X., Witt, M.E., … Salama, J.K. (2010). Factors associated with long-term speech and swallowing outcomes after chemoradiotherapy for locoregionally advanced head and neck cancer. *Archives of Otolaryngology—Head and Neck Surgery, 136,* 1226–1234. doi:10.1001/archoto.2010.218

National Cancer Institute. (2010). Fact sheet: Palliative care in cancer. Retrieved from http://www.cancer.gov/cancertopics/factsheet/Support/palliative-care

National Cancer Institute. (2013a, February 1). National Cancer Institute fact sheet: Head and neck cancers. Retrieved from http://www.cancer.gov/cancertopics/factsheet/Sites-Types/head-and-neck

National Cancer Institute. (2013b, September 4). *Sexuality and reproductive issues (PDQ®)* [Health professional version]. Retrieved from http://www.cancer.gov/cancertopics/pdq/supportivecare/sexuality/HealthProfessional

National Coalition of Oncology Nurse Navigators. (n.d.). What is a navigator and how they help. Retrieved from http://www.nconn.org/patients

National Comprehensive Cancer Network. (2013a). *NCCN Clinical Practice Guidelines in Oncology: Bladder cancer* [v.1.2014]. Retrieved from http://www.nccn.org/professionals/physician_gls/pdf/bladder.pdf

National Comprehensive Cancer Network. (2013b). *NCCN Clinical Practice Guidelines in Oncology: Head and neck cancers* [v.2.2013]. Retrieved from www.nccn.org/professionals/physician_gls/pdf/head-and-neck.pdf

National Comprehensive Cancer Network. (2013c). *NCCN Clinical Practice Guidelines in Oncology: Non-small cell lung cancer* [v.2.2014]. Retrieved http://www.nccn.org/professionals/physician_gls/pdf/nscl.pdf

National Comprehensive Cancer Network. (2013d). *NCCN Clinical Practice Guidelines in Oncology: Prostate cancer* [v.1.2014]. Retrieved from http://www.nccn.org/professionals/physician_gls/pdf/prostate.pdf

National Lung Screening Trial Research Team. (2011a). Reduced lung-cancer mortality with low-dose computed tomographic screening. *New England Journal of Medicine, 365,* 395–409. doi:10.1056/NEJMoa1102873

National Lung Screening Trial Research Team. (2011b). The National Lung Screening Trial: Overview and study design. *Radiology, 258,* 243–253. doi:10.1148/radiol.10091808

National Lung Screening Trial Research Team. (2013). Results of initial low-dose computed tomographic screening for lung cancer. *New England Journal of Medicine, 368,* 1980–1991. doi:10.1056/NEJMoa1209120

O'Brien, K., Roe, B., Low, C., Deyn, L., & Rogers, S.N. (2012). An exploration of the perceived changes in intimacy of patients' relationships following head and neck cancer. *Journal of Clinical Nursing, 21,* 2499–2508. doi:10.1111/j.1365-2702.2012.04162.x

Oskam, I.M., Verdonck-de Leeuw, I.M., Aaronson, N.K., Witte, B.I., de Bree, R., Doornaert, P., … Leemans, C.R. (2013). Prospective evaluation of health-related quality of life in long-term oral and oropharyngeal cancer survivors and the perceived need for supportive care. *Oral Oncology, 49,* 443–448. doi:10.1016/j.oraloncology.2012.12.005

Palo Alto Medical Foundation. (2010). Shared decision making process: Prioritizing goals for treatment and outcomes. Retrieved from http://www.pamf.org/prostate/resources/binder/Chp4.pdf

Patel, U.A., & Brennan, T.E. (2012). Disparities in head and neck cancer: Assessing delay in treatment initiation. *Laryngoscope, 122,* 1756–1760. doi:10.1002/lary.23357

Peyrade, F., Cupissol, D., Geoffrois, L., Rolland, F., Borel, C., Ciais, C., … Guigay, J. (2013). Systemic treatment and medical management of metastatic squamous cell carcinoma of the head and neck: Review of the literature and proposal for management changes. *Oral Oncology, 49,* 482–491. doi:10.1016/j.oraloncology.2013.01.005

Platteaux, N., Dirix, P., Dejaeger, E., & Nuyts, S. (2010). Dysphagia in head and neck cancer patients treated with chemoradiotherapy. *Dysphagia, 25,* 139–152. doi:10.1007/s00455-009-9247-7

Robinson, J.H., Callister, L.C., Berry, J.A., & Dearing, K.A. (2008). Patient-centered care and adherence: Definitions and applications to improve outcomes. *Journal of the American Academy of Nurse Practitioners, 20,* 600–607. doi:10.1111/j.1745-7599.2008.00360.x

Sadovsky, R., Basson, R., Krychman, M., Morales, A.M., Schover, L., Wang, R., & Incrocci, L. (2010). Cancer and sexual problems. *Journal of Sexual Medicine, 7*(1, Pt. 2), 349–373. doi:10.1111/j.1743-6109.2009.01620.x

Seek, A.J., & Hogle, W.P. (2007). Modeling a better way: Navigating the healthcare system for patients with lung cancer. *Clinical Journal of Oncology Nursing, 11,* 81–85. doi:10.1188/07.CJON.81-85

Shockney, L.D. (2010). Evolution of patient navigation. *Clinical Journal of Oncology Nursing, 14,* 405–407. doi:10.1188/10.CJON.405-407

Shuman, A.G., Fins, J.J., & Prince, M.E. (2012). Improving end-of-life care for head and neck cancer patients. *Expert Review of Anticancer Therapy, 12,* 335–343. doi:10.1586/era.12.6

Siegel, R., DeSantis, C., Virgo, K., Stein, K., Mariotto, A., Smith, T., … Ward, E. (2012). Cancer treatment and survivorship statistics, 2012. *CA: A Cancer Journal for Clinicians, 62,* 220–241. doi:10.3322/caac.21149

Splete, H. (2012, January 25). Oral HPV infection more prevalent in men than women. Retrieved from http://www.oncologystat.com/news/Oral_HPV_Infection_More_Prevalent_In_Men_Than_Women

Temel, J.S., Greer, J.A., Muzikansky, A., Gallagher, E.R., Admane, S., Jackson, V.A., … Lynch, T.J. (2010). Early palliative care for patients with metastatic non-small-cell lung cancer. *New England Journal of Medicine, 363,* 733–742. doi:10.1056/NEJMoa1000678

Tucker, M.E. (2012, March 21). Oral complications after head/neck radiation 'underreported.' Retrieved from http://www.oncologystat.com/news/Oral_Complications_After_Head_Neck_Radiation_Underreported

U.S. Preventive Services Task Force. (2013). *Screening for lung cancer: Draft recommendation statement* (AHRQ Publication No. 13-05196-EF-3). Retrieved from http://www.uspreventiveservicestaskforce.org/uspstf13/lungcan/lungcandraftrec.htm

Varner, A., & Murph, P. (2010). Cancer patient navigation: Where do we go from here? *Oncology Issues, 25*(3), 50–53. Retrieved from http://accc-cancer.org/oncology_issues/articles/mayjune10/MJ10-VarnerMurph.pdf

CHAPTER 7

Setting-Specific Navigation

Marguerite A. Thomas, RN, MN, AOCN®, and Elissa A. Peters, RN, MS, OCN®

Introduction

Navigation, like nursing, is constantly changing and providing new opportunities to better support patients while eliminating barriers to optimal cancer care. One evolving area relates to patient navigation efforts focused on settings outside the acute diagnostic and treatment phases of the cancer continuum, including outreach (prevention education and early detection) and survivorship. Depending upon the needs of the institution, outreach and survivorship navigation may be stand-alone positions or included as part of the disease-specific navigators' responsibilities. However, for the purpose of this chapter, most of the discussion will be based upon models using stand-alone positions.

Outreach Navigation

Patient navigation started in 1990 in Harlem, New York City, when Harold P. Freeman, MD, noticed that African American women in the community experienced a higher incidence of breast cancer mortality (Freeman, 2012). He observed delays in follow-up after abnormal findings or cancer diagnoses and proposed that lay navigators from the community could help bridge the gap between the patient and the medical community. The role of lay navigators spanned a range of activities including providing education, engaging in advocacy, encouraging screening, and subsequently linking those with abnormal results to follow-up care, support, and guidance. Lay navigators assisted patients in overcoming barriers to care, thereby facilitating timely, quality care in a culturally sensitive manner (Mason et al., 2013). Freeman's approach of combining free or low-cost mammograms with lay navigation increased the number of women screened, reduced the time from abnormal finding to resolution of the finding, and decreased time between diagnosis and initiation of treatment, all of which resulted in an increased detection of early-stage cancers and increased five-year survival for women with breast cancer (Freeman, 2012).

Several studies have been published to support the value of navigation across the healthcare continuum, especially focusing on those patients at high risk for late diagnosis such as the poor, underinsured, and uninsured. Freeman was among the first to document this with African American patients with breast cancer (Freeman & Rodriguez, 2011). The Boston Patient Navigation Research Program also demonstrated that navigation addressed cancer health disparities by reducing time to diagnosis following an abnormal cancer screening event among a racially/ethnically diverse inner city population (Battaglia et al., 2012). In its 2012 standards, the American College of Surgeons (ACoS) Commission on Cancer (CoC) incorporated patient navigation as a standard of care for cancer programs seeking accreditation beginning in 2015 (ACoS CoC, 2012). To fulfill this standard, cancer programs must complete a community needs assessment to identify gaps in care, determine the type and settings for navigation, and develop a navigation plan to address these issues.

Types of Outreach Navigators and Settings

Outreach navigators frequently use a different skill set than disease-specific navigators. Essential knowledge for outreach navigators includes an awareness of early signs of cancer and current screening guidelines, as well as the available community and state resources for screening and diagnostics. Outreach navigators must be able to develop collaborative relationships with community partners and educate the community on the importance of cancer prevention and how early detection improves survival.

The outreach navigator may be a professional (nurse or social worker), a paraprofessional (community health worker), or a recognized community leader or peer (such as a cancer survivor) based in a clinic, health department, hospital, physician office, imaging center, or community setting (Braun et al., 2012). Because the outreach navigator's role may overlap with that of other community workers and healthcare professionals, it is essential to establish a clear scope of practice and defined responsibilities for the outreach navigator to avoid confusion.

Community leaders and peers are used in many communities as lay navigators to provide education, advocacy, and assistance in overcoming barriers to care in a culturally sensitive manner. These individuals usually understand the community served and the barriers involved. Depending upon the resources available in the community, lay navigators may be paid employees or volunteers. Some of the more well-known programs include Native American Cancer Research in Denver, Colorado; Hands of Hope in North Carolina (which provides rural navigation), PATH for Women in Orange

County, California (for the Asian and Pacific Islander community); Redes En Acción, the National Latino Cancer Research Network in Texas; and Kukui Ahi Patient Navigation Program at Molokai General Hospital in Kaunakakai, Hawaii (Braun et al., 2012). These programs studied the communities to be served and developed culturally sensitive training programs accordingly. In particular, the 'Imi Hale Native Hawaiian Cancer Network developed a training program for lay navigators by reviewing existing curriculums and conducting surveys and focus groups with patients and families with cancer within the community. Access to care and system barriers were identified and, from this, a training program was developed that focused on cancer knowledge, resources, patient advocacy, and communication. The outcomes of this program showed improvement in three categories: (a) access to care, (b) timeliness and completion of care, and (c) feelings of control and confidence (Domingo, Davis, Allison, & Braun, 2011).

A community health worker is often connected to public health departments and is considered a trusted member of the community. As a frontline worker with a primary focus on outreach, education, and early detection, the community health worker has a good understanding of the community, barriers to care, and services available to help decrease barriers. In a study done in New York City, the scope of practice for community health workers included outreach and community organizing, case management, home visits, health education, coaching, and navigation (Findley et al., 2012).

The outreach nurse navigator shares some of the basic roles of the lay navigator: education, advocacy, and formation of community partnerships. Nurses as outreach navigators typically have a better understanding of the diagnostic workup, disease process, treatment options, and symptom management for cancer. However, depending on the focus of the outreach and the work setting, the outreach nurse navigator is not always an oncology nurse. According to a study implemented at Group Health Cooperative, a nonprofit integrated healthcare delivery system based in Seattle, Washington, the role of the outreach nurse navigator is to provide proactive outreach to patients newly diagnosed with cancer by answering questions, providing emotional support to reduce distress, and addressing any early concerns about diagnosis or treatments (Horner et al., 2013). For the remainder of this chapter, unless otherwise indicated, the outreach navigator will be considered as a nurse.

Community Needs Assessment

For optimal success, outreach navigation programs must be tailored to meet the needs of the community, which are ideally identified through a comprehensive needs assessment. ACoS CoC recently adopted the following patient navigation standard:

A patient navigation process, driven by a community needs assessment, is established to address health care disparities and barriers to care for patients. Resources to address identified barriers may be provided either on-site or by referral to community-based or national organizations. The navigation process is evaluated, documented, and reported to the cancer committee annually. The patient navigation process is modified or enhanced each year to address additional barriers identified by the community needs assessment. (ACoS CoC, 2012, p. 75)

According to the ACoS CoC (2012) standard, the community needs assessment should include components such as (a) a description of the community served, (b) the assessment process used, (c) a list of the top priorities seen in the community, and (d) community partners. The assessment must be done every three years with subsequent programming changes implemented to address the identified health disparities and gaps. The results of the assessment, the improvements identified, and the new process for change are reported yearly to the cancer committee.

Community needs assessments can be homegrown, professionally devised, or a hybrid of both (Smith, 2013). Homegrown community needs assessments are developed by the cancer center to look at populations served by using patient satisfaction and tumor registry data. Patient and/or caregiver focus groups or surveys can address satisfaction with services, including access to care, timeliness of services, barriers or gaps in care, services used (as well as additional services needed), what worked well, and reasons for choosing the organization. Tumor registry data reflect the demographics and staging of patients with cancer treated at the organization, and this information is then compared to the county or state data to assess for gaps in service and local health disparities. According to Shockney (2010), cancer centers should analyze the delivery of care as seen through the eyes of patients, as this information reveals the true barriers to care within the system.

Hospitals could also obtain feedback from potential clients by surveying residences in one or two of the neighboring zip codes (Smith, 2013). Possible survey questions might include the following.

- What cancer screening has the individual completed in the past year?
- What is the individual's current health status and healthcare needs?
- Has the individual used the facility? (Why or why not?)
- What were the barriers to accessing health care?
- What were the advantages to utilizing the chosen healthcare system?

Questions could be related to the ease of scheduling, timeliness of care, services used, and accessibility, as well as basic demographic data such as insurance status, race and ethnicity, and socioeconomic status. Such a survey could be modified to include community partners such as physicians, imaging centers, faith communities, the American Cancer Society (ACS), insurance companies, and other referral sources. In addition to mailing of surveys, outreach staff can distribute them at community events with the goal of capturing basic demographics and screening patterns.

Many agencies conduct community needs assessments. Some assessments relate to the demographics and culture of the community, community resources, the community's education, economy, and environment, the social well-being of those living in the community, and general safety and health concerns. Other community assessments are more specific and focus on cancer. Examples include the United Way Quality of Life Indicators, public health department assessments, county health indicator reports, state cancer plans, Susan G. Komen community needs assessments, ACS facts and comparisons, state or hospital tumor registries, and local cancer screening program statistics.

When looking at existing community needs assessments and resources, the navigator can compare the institution's data to the previously described assessments by asking the following questions.

- Are the institution's demographics reflective of the community demographics?
- Are there opportunities for screening clinics?
- Does the institution meet the identified screening needs? If not, what steps need to be implemented to meet the needs?
- How does the institution's stage at time of diagnosis compare with county, state, and national data?
- What are the identified barriers to care, and what can be done to close gaps by utilizing either on-site services or referral to community resources?
- What programs are meeting the needs of the community, and what additional services are needed?
- How can the institution strengthen existing or establish community partners to better meet community needs?

Some organizations choose to use a hybrid model for community needs assessments. The following is an example of one cancer center's combined use of a homegrown survey along with data from existing resources to complete the community assessment. First, the program administrator evaluated the demographics of the community using existing community data and clients served at the cancer center, which confirmed that program demographics matched the community profile. Next, several gaps were identified in the community based on previously conducted community health surveys, including an increase in the use of tobacco among disparate populations, increase in skin cancer, rise in human papillomavirus–related head and neck cancers, breast and colorectal screening rates below the national average, and 25% of the community being either underinsured or uninsured. From these findings, the organization proposed several interventions to help address the gaps in care. The cancer committee and physician advisory board then approved this plan before implementation. Some of the specific interventions included the following.

- Develop a smoking cessation program for cancer, cardiac, and respiratory patients in the next two years to decrease tobacco use in disparate populations.
- Increase mammography rates in disparate populations by becoming a provider for the breast and cervical screening program. Provide funding for mammograms through grants for women not eligible for the breast and cervical screening program.
- Collaborate with nine local health fairs to provide fecal immunohistochemical testing (FIT) to increase colorectal cancer screening.
- Conduct an annual head and neck cancer screening event.
- Conduct an annual community skin screening event.
- Provide community education on the importance of early detection and screening for cancer.
- Further develop community partners, such as the safety-net clinics, to provide services for people with no medical home.

The community needs assessment requires the combined efforts of many talented individuals, not just the navigator, to compile data, identify areas of change, prioritize community needs, and implement necessary changes. Community assessments enable organizations to identify community partnerships to help fill identified gaps and minimize barriers to care. The outreach nurse navigator should be constantly evaluating the effectiveness of community programs and recommending necessary program adjustments as indicated.

Community Partnerships

Community partnerships can provide access to communities the outreach nurse navigator might not otherwise reach, facilitate better use of talents and resources, and possibly enable collaborative solutions to problems requiring expertise beyond that of a single organization (Ramanadhan et al., 2012). Community partnerships usually fall into one of three categories: (a) networking, (b) joint sponsorship of programs, or (c) formal relationships. Building partnerships takes time to develop levels of trust, commitment, and establish roles. Each level of partnership has its role in outreach, and it is essential for the outreach nurse navigator to know the level of commitment from each community partner. Most community partnerships reside at the networking level, with a few progressing to joint sponsorship and even fewer progressing to formal relationships.

The *networking* partnership centers around connecting with people and organizations to share resources, provide information, and create a broader referral base (Ramanadhan et al., 2012). These partnerships create an awareness of community resources, including what different agencies provide, changes that may affect the community, and upcoming community events. The role of networking participants is to learn and share information with the different agencies, as well as connect patients to community resources as appropriate. Examples of groups with which the outreach nurse navigator might establish networking partnerships include local nonprofit agencies, community educators, healthcare providers, health fair coordinators, and service organizations targeted toward specific populations.

As demonstrated by the following example, networking partnerships can occasionally evolve to *joint sponsorship*. In one community, several organizations were competing for the same audience on the same day for breast cancer awareness activities. A community grant provided funding to develop the Pikes Peak Breast Health Connection, which was composed of organizations involved in education, screening, diagnosis, treatment, and support services for breast cancer. The initial focus of the group involved education of other members about different community programs, sharing of community resources, and developing a community calendar of breast cancer–related events to decrease duplication of services. The group functioned in this capacity for several years. However, as new members joined the group, the focus evolved to creating an annual breast health awareness event held at a local community center. This fun and informational event targeted African American and Hispanic women. Educational information was available in both English and Spanish. Spanish-speaking lay navigators were available for the Hispanic population to teach breast health awareness and translate the program as needed. Participants were encouraged to visit the resource tables, meet with a bra fitter, listen to short presentations regarding breast health, and enjoy a fashion show and continental breakfast.

Joint sponsorship is more structured. Networking partnerships bring agencies together to share resources, whereas joint sponsorship involves a deeper level of commitment to the common goal or purpose and shared decision making. No written agreement is issued, but it is understood that each individual or agency will work toward the common goal using its specific skill set and available resources. Although each partner is expected to contribute equally, no formal process ensures this. Other examples of joint sponsorship include community screening task forces, disease-specific task forces, cancer coalitions, committees, and local chapters of the Oncology Nursing Society (ONS).

The Colorado Colorectal Cancer task force collaborated with a local Hispanic TV station and Hispanic community leaders to develop a telenovela program titled "Encrucijada" ("Crossroads"). The program is a local Hispanic soap opera that intertwines health messages into the story lines, including the importance of colorectal cancer screening, myths surrounding cancer screening, and available community resources. Task force members helped provide funding, staff a call center, evaluate program effectiveness, facilitate focus groups, and review the program's script for accuracy.

Many cancer centers have partnered with faith-based organizations to provide cancer education and outreach. This has been accomplished through collaborations with parish nurses and pastors. Health and wellness promotion has become increasingly common in many churches. In particular, African American churches have a long history of connecting members to community resources and providing culturally appropriate health education. Many churches recognize joint sponsorships with outreach nurse navigators and other community organizations as a natural expansion of promoting health and wellness within the parish (Rodriguez, Bowie, Frattaroli, & Gielen, 2009).

The third level is *formal partnerships*, which involve operating contracts between partners. Formal partnerships may include contracted providers for state and local cancer screening programs, nonprofit agencies (such as Avon, LIVESTRONG, and Susan G. Komen foundations) providing grants for screening and other community resources, and contracted language services. At this level, written program goals and objectives are established, and each partner is expected to fulfill designated obligations. Nguyen et al. (2006) developed a community-based program in Santa Clara County, California, that sought to increase Pap screening among Vietnamese Americans. A coalition composed of 15 partners, including Asian outreach groups, insurance companies, healthcare agencies, faith-based organizations, and two community members, developed an action plan with six major components. The plan included (a) a multimedia campaign, (b) a lay health outreach worker, (c) a Vietnamese Pap clinic with outreach navigation, (d) a registry and reminder system, (e) continuing medical education for Vietnamese physicians, and (f) restoration of the breast and cervical cancer control program. This program was highly successful because community members and agencies collaborated with healthcare agencies to provide services. The coalition secured the community's trust to pave the way for the medical community to increase screenings (Nguyen et al., 2006).

Avenues for Outreach

Once the community needs assessment is completed, target population identified, and community partners established, it is time to provide outreach navigation services. It is well established that certain cancers caused by tobacco use and sun exposure can be prevented. Pap screenings for cervical cancer and colonoscopy for colon cancer can prevent cancer if precancerous lesions are removed. Other screening tests, such as mammography and FIT stool tests, may detect cancer at earlier stages. Despite these mechanisms for cancer prevention and early detection, unfortunately, not everyone has equal access to care (Battaglia, Burhansstipanov, Murrell, Dwyer,

& Caron, 2011). Outreach nurse navigators help facilitate access to care by providing education on cancer, identifying barriers to care and linking patients to community resources to eliminate them, participating in screening activities, and facilitating resolution of abnormal screening findings.

Nurse navigators can accomplish community education regarding different types of cancer, screening guidelines, wellness, and community resources by participating in local health fairs and collaborating with community partners. Outreach nurse navigators can educate healthcare advocates or lay navigators to further provide education at churches, community centers, and service organizations. For example, the ANGEL Network (African American Women Nurturing and Giving Each Other Life) at Penrose Cancer Center in Colorado Springs, Colorado, is a hospital-based program initially funded by the local Susan G. Komen affiliate. The program used a lay navigator with a background in education. The initial focus for the ANGEL Network was education on breast health and screening, as well as the provision of free mammograms and clinical breast examinations. The highly successful program was the template for three sister groups in Ohio. Once Komen funding was no longer available, the hospital expanded the scope of the program. An extensive training program for healthcare advocates was developed so that members could bring information to local churches, health fairs, and groups on various cancers such as breast, ovarian, prostate, testicular, and colon cancer.

Community cancer screenings are a wonderful way to provide services for disparate populations. Screenings are commonly performed for early detection of breast, cervical, head and neck, colorectal, and skin cancers. Navigation is essential for participants with abnormal findings. Specifically, navigation has been shown to decrease the time to diagnosis and increase the number of people completing diagnostic procedures. The New York City Department of Health and Mental Hygiene studied the impact of patient navigation on colon screening and found a 61% increase in the monthly volume of colonoscopies with navigation (Elkin, Shapiro, Snow, Zauber, & Krauskopf, 2012). Markossian, Darnell, and Calhoun (2012) found a shorter time to diagnostic resolution for navigated breast patients in a Chicago-based program. The outreach nurse navigator also may need to work with community partners, such as health departments or safety-net clinics, to ensure that all screening participants have medical homes (Battaglia et al., 2012).

Cancer screenings may be done through a variety of settings and strategies. Services may be provided on-site at a local hospital or in mobile vans that travel to the communities. Screening may be the result of collaborations with local health departments, community centers, or local healthcare providers in rural communities. Regardless of the setting, when collaborating with community partners, all involved parties need to have a clear understanding of everyone's roles and responsibilities.

Funding

Budget and reimbursement changes have challenged every arena of health care, and outreach navigation is no exception. Depending upon the needs of the community, the scope of practice, and role of the outreach navigator, positions may be volunteer, grant funded, staff positions, or a combination of these.

Grant funding for outreach navigation programs might come from organizations such as Susan G. Komen, ACS, public health departments, state cancer programs, or the National Cancer Institute (NCI). Some organizations charge nominal fees for navigation, whereas some community partners contribute to programs by providing in-kind services or funding. Several cancer programs use grants to start navigation programs and then add additional hospital-funded positions as needed (Domingo et al., 2011).

Metrics

The impact of outreach navigation can be measured in four areas: (a) time to diagnosis, (b) time to initial cancer treatment, (c) patient satisfaction, and (d) cost-effectiveness (Campbell, Craig, Eggert, & Bailey-Dorton, 2010). Studies have shown that navigation increases screening rates in certain cancers (specifically, breast, cervical, prostate, and colorectal), decreases the time to diagnosis and start of treatment, and increases compliance with treatment (Whop et al., 2012). Cost-effectiveness of navigation has been demonstrated in colon cancer screening with an increased number of colonoscopies performed and decreased no-show rates (Elkin et al., 2012).

It may be difficult to measure the effectiveness of an outreach navigation program depending on the demographics of the community. If screening rates increase after outreach navigation efforts in a community with only one hospital, the increase could be attributed to the outreach program. However, in some areas with multiple settings where patients may receive care, it may be harder to measure and determine the effectiveness of outreach efforts. For example, an urban hospital could provide an educational event on the importance of colonoscopy for colon cancer. Participants at the event could receive services at that hospital, the community health department, or a local gastroenterology practice depending on insurance or personal preference. Unless all partners are sharing information, quantitatively measuring the effectiveness of the program is difficult.

Determining the most appropriate metrics for an outreach navigation program will depend upon community demographics, available resources, and the specific focus of the outreach program. Some possible outreach navigation metrics include

- Attendance at screening events
- Patient satisfaction
- Community partner satisfaction
- Number of referrals for breast, cervical, and colon screening from the targeted populations
- Number of new patients and returning patients
- Adherence to screening and recommended follow-up
- Access to care and identified barriers to care
- Downstream revenue from referrals
- Patient retention within the cancer program
- Time from screening to diagnosis
- Stage at time of diagnosis.

Case Example

Penrose Cancer Center is located in Colorado Springs, a metropolitan area 70 miles south of Denver. Penrose serves not only the metropolitan area, with an estimated population of nearly 600,000, but also approximately 300,000 individuals from the 2,000 square mile surrounding rural area. Penrose Cancer Center has been a member of the NCI Community Cancer Centers Program (NCCCP) since 2007. NCCCP is a public-private partnership with the NCI and consists of a network of community hospital-based cancer centers across the country working to improve access, quality of cancer care, and cancer research in the community. Through participation in the NCCCP, Penrose was able to support additional staff, such as nurse navigators and clinical trials coordinators. (This project was funded in whole or in part with Federal funds from the National Cancer Institute, National Institutes of Health, under Contract No. HHSN261200800001E. The content of this publication does not necessarily reflect the views or policies of the Department of Health and Human Services, nor does mention of trade names, commercial products, or organizations imply endorsement by the U.S. Government.)

The outreach department at Penrose was initially staffed by two lay navigators funded by a Susan G. Komen grant. When funding ceased, the hospital absorbed the program and expanded the focus beyond breast cancer to provide education and screening for several types of cancers.

The outreach nurse navigator position was developed in 2010. Primary responsibilities during the first year focused on developing and enhancing community partnerships, as well as participating in community screening events.

Before the outreach nurse navigator position was created, follow-up for outreach screening merely consisted of sending a letter with the screening results, as well as a telephone call to a limited subset of high-risk patients to ensure appropriate follow-up. One of the program enhancements with the implementation of the outreach nurse navigator included individual follow-up for all outreach screening participants with abnormal findings. This resulted in 145 individuals navigated during the first year, compared to 10 in the previous year. Primary responsibilities of the outreach nurse navigator involved assisting with referrals to safety-net clinics and specialists and following all patients until resolution of the abnormal findings. Through the collection and tracking of race and ethnicity data, the outreach nurse navigator was able to demonstrate a yearly increase in the number of Latino and African American participants in the outreach screening programs.

The outreach nurse navigator was invited by the community to serve as the chair for both the skin screening and prostate cancer task forces. In this role, the outreach nurse navigator collaborated with various community partners to plan the events, recruit staff (including professionals, lay volunteers, and Spanish interpreters), coordinate with the physician champion, market the events, develop workflow processes for the events, and conduct follow-up with all participants who had abnormal results until resolution of the problem.

The hospital began a cooperative agreement with a rural community medical center to provide breast surgery with immediate reconstruction. As part of this agreement, the outreach nurse navigator played a central role in assisting patients with the coordination of same-day appointments with breast team providers, including the breast surgeon, plastic surgeon, medical oncologist, and radiation oncologist, if indicated. Other key responsibilities included assessing for and eliminating barriers to care, such as transportation and lodging, and assisting with the transition of care to a community medical oncologist when desired.

In 2013, when the hospital secured a contract to provide screening services for the state breast and cervical program, navigation responsibilities for this program were aligned with the outreach nurse navigator. In this role, the outreach navigator screened participants for eligibility, coordinated the monthly clinic, navigated patients through the imaging process, and assisted with a smooth transition to the breast cancer navigator for patients who were diagnosed with cancer.

The outreach nurse navigator at Penrose Cancer Center has served in various capacities working with diverse underserved populations, such as racial and ethnic minorities, the under- and uninsured, and rural populations. Success has been demonstrated through increased screening participation and the provision of navigation services for patients with abnormal findings. Overall, the organization feels the role of the outreach nurse navigator has been extremely beneficial in continuing to build and strengthen community trust and partnerships, providing education within the community, and ensuring that the underserved have appropriate access to care.

Summary of Outreach Navigation

In summary, outreach navigation is constantly evolving depending on the needs of the community and the resources available. As with any navigation position, the role of the outreach navigator can be very rewarding. Key tasks in establishing an outreach navigation program include (a) developing a strategic plan by evaluating the needs of the community, (b) establishing strong community partnerships with organizations that share similar purposes in addressing healthcare disparities, and (c) defining meaningful program metrics that will clearly demonstrate program successes as well as opportunities for further program enhancements.

Survivorship Navigation

Freeman recognized the need for navigation after initial abnormal findings and cancer diagnosis. It has since morphed into navigation during the treatment phase, and more recently, there has been a focus on the importance of assisting patients with cancer in the post-treatment phase. A *survivorship nurse navigator* is a nurse whose focus and expertise are within the realm of post-treatment care of patients with cancer.

Cancer Survivorship

What exactly is a cancer survivor? NCI uses the following definition: "One who remains alive and continues to function during and after overcoming a serious hardship or life-threatening disease. In cancer, a person is considered to be a survivor from the time of diagnosis until the end of life" (NCI, n.d.). For the purposes of this chapter, the focus will be the cancer survivor after the acute phase of cancer treatment.

Fortunately, many more people are living longer with cancer. With an estimated 13.7 million Americans living with a history of cancer in 2012 (Siegel et al., 2012), the opportunity to focus on cancer survivors as they move beyond treatment into the future is one that will only be more prevalent as advances in cancer screening, diagnostics, treatment, and support continue to improve across many disease sites.

Cancer survivorship is a life-changing process of uncertainty beginning at the time of diagnosis and encompassing both positive and negative aspects (Doyle, 2008). This chapter focuses on cancer survivors who have completed the acute phase of cancer treatment and are celebrating remission or learning to face cancer as a chronic illness. This post-treatment phase is a "time of transition" (Grunfeld & Earle, 2010, p. 25). Some survivors have expressed feeling lost or abandoned and uncertain about how to cope with this part of the cancer journey (Landier, 2009). It is this uncertainty that lends itself to the need for survivorship navigation support.

In recent years, cancer care providers and community organizations have made a significant effort to develop programs and systems that support cancer survivors through the post-treatment period. The role of a survivorship navigator is one way to support the cancer survivor but has not been described in great detail in the literature. The ACS Patient Navigation Working Group published a report on the outcome measures for survivorship navigation (Pratt-Chapman, Simon, Patterson, Risendal, & Patierno, 2011). This report stated that the purpose of survivorship navigation is to diminish any barriers people may have as they complete treatment, access survivorship services, and accomplish high quality of life (Pratt-Chapman et al., 2011). Survivorship navigators are described as nurses, social workers, or other trained professionals. This chapter will focus on the role of a nurse as a survivorship navigator.

In 2005, the Institute of Medicine put out a call for increased attention to cancer survivors at the completion of treatment. The landmark publication *From Cancer Patient to Cancer Survivor: Lost in Transition* (Hewitt, Greenfield, & Stovall, 2006) identified needs that cancer survivors may have in the post-treatment phase. This report raised awareness of the issues that many cancer survivors face and demanded quality health care and improved quality of life for this population (Hewitt et al., 2006).

ACoS CoC has answered this call and in 2012 incorporated a new standard requiring all CoC-accredited cancer centers have survivorship support in place by 2015, with the goal that all patients undergoing cancer treatment receive a treatment summary and survivorship care plan as a standard of care at the end of cancer treatment (ACoS CoC, 2013).

The American Society of Clinical Oncology (ASCO) Quality Oncology Practice Initiative (QOPI®) (2013) recommends that a chemotherapy treatment summary be completed and provided to the patient and the primary care physician (PCP) within three months from the completion of chemotherapy. This was identified as one of 26 core measures abstracted from medical records for the biannual QOPI audits (ASCO, 2013). ASCO has also identified key initiatives through its Cancer Survivorship Committee that are meant to increase the quality of care for cancer survivors in post-treatment care (McCabe et al., 2013).

Post-Treatment Needs of Cancer Survivors

The period of time following completion of acute treatment is recognized as a distinct part of the cancer continuum. This often refers to the survivor's "new normal"—a key phrase many cancer survivors can relate to when attempting to redefine life after cancer treatment. Survivors may have unique needs, some of which are specific to the type of cancer, treatment, and other individual factors, whereas other needs (such as education, rehabilitation, etc.) are universal to all cancer survivors.

In 2006, the LIVESTRONG Foundation surveyed 2,307 post-treatment cancer survivors to identify specific survivor concerns and to determine whether these needs were being met by healthcare teams. The categories of concerns identified in the survey included physical, practical, and emotional. Results indicated that 99% experienced at least one concern after the completion of cancer treatment (LIVESTRONG, 2010).

While some physical concerns are unique to the disease, treatment, or cancer survivor because of preexisting comorbidities, other physical concerns are considered universal to all types of cancer. The 2010 LIVESTRONG report found that 91% of survivors had at least one physical concern, and the four areas that were most frequently cited were energy, concentration, sexual functioning, and neuropathy.

The LIVESTRONG (2010) survey also identified fear of recurrence as the top emotional concern. Other frequently reported concerns included grief and identity, personal appearance, family members' risk of cancer, sadness and depression, personal relationships, social relationships, and faith and spirituality (LIVESTRONG, 2010).

Ness et al. (2013) conducted a more recent survey of 337 cancer survivors and found similar post-treatment concerns. Fatigue was identified as the most prevalent physical concern, whereas fear of recurrence was the most common emotional concern. Other concerns identified through that survey included living with uncertainty, managing stress, and coping with sleep disturbances.

Practical concerns can include debt, insurance, employment, and school issues. The economic impact of cancer and its treatment and further surveillance cannot be ignored. One study of breast cancer survivors post-treatment reported the median annual cost of follow-up care to be $630 (Hensley et al., 2005). Returning to work can be an issue as well. Amir and Brocky (2009) identified factors reported in the literature that can impact return to work for cancer survivors after treatment, including the treatment received, cancer site, status of occupation, and others' roles in the workplace. A recent study of productivity among breast cancer survivors reported that "more than 40% of breast cancer survivors begin to or continue to experience productivity loss as long after surgery as 30 to 36 months" (Quinlan et al., 2011, p. 25). This productivity loss was mainly due to pain and range-of-motion disability in the affected arm (Quinlan et al., 2011).

Cancer survivors may have a knowledge deficit regarding post-treatment expectations. They may not know what to anticipate in relation to potential short- and long-term effects of cancer and its treatment or the follow-up plan for cancer surveillance; there may be a need for coordination of this follow-up care. Cancer survivors may want to start making healthier lifestyle choices but feel unsure about where to start. Needs during survivorship care may include health promotion education regarding increasing physical activity, healthy eating, stress management, or all of these.

Cancer survivors may also require coaching on how to communicate and be a central and active member of the healthcare team. Encouraging effective communication with the oncology physician and other providers of the multidisciplinary team can be helpful as survivors transition to less frequent provider visits. Needs may be specific to disease type and stage, treatment received, gender, and age. Some survivors are considered to be in remission, whereas others are living with cancer as a chronic illness. Some may still be receiving maintenance therapy but are finished with the acute stage of cancer treatment. Men and women may have different needs, especially in relation to body image and sexuality. The older adult (older than age 60) may have heightened needs after cancer treatment because of the normal changes that can come with aging, whether that may be physiologic, developmental, or life events (Schlairet, 2011).

Cancer survivors' needs may differ in relation to culture and heritage. Just as with other aspects of patient navigation, cultural and ethnic diversity requires individualized interventions (Shockney, 2010). Hamilton, Moore, Powe, Agarwal, and Martin (2010) explored how older African American cancer survivors perceived social support in a qualitative study and found that support from family, friends, and church members was important, but there were many remaining fears, negative beliefs, and misconceptions in regard to cultural beliefs that affected social support. Disparities exist in survivorship just as they do in other aspects of cancer care. Needs for the non–English speaking, underinsured, or uninsured are prevalent as well.

Models of Survivorship Care

Oncologists and PCPs attempt to meet the needs of cancer survivors in various ways, which may or may not include the role of a survivorship navigator. The variation in how care is delivered seems to depend on the awareness level of the institution, the demographics of the specific population served, and the resources available at the institution or in the community. Oeffinger and McCabe (2006) described multiple models for delivering survivorship care and noted that focus and flexibility were two keys to institutional success. Although survivorship care has evolved since 2005, focus and flexibility still remain pertinent concepts to keep in mind. No matter what model is used, the institution needs to be committed to the success of the survivorship program and make it an organizational priority (Campbell et al., 2011).

Survivorship care has not been found to be a one-size-fits-all model (Hahn & Ganz, 2011). Various methods and models have been created and tested at different institutions. For example, programs can be disease specific or include every disease type; visits may involve one-time consultations or encompass longitudinal follow-up. Survivorship clinics may be housed within a cancer center or exist as a separate entity, such as a nonprofit, grant-funded program. This type of program is often community focused and serves survivors from multiple settings (Pratt-Chapman et al., 2011).

The disease-specific model of survivorship care has evolved from survivorship clinics originally developed to address effects specific to breast cancer treatment, including lymphedema, body image, depression, weight issues, and long-term issues such as cardiac disease (Gilbert, Miller, Hollenbeck, Montie, & Wei, 2008). Another example is a survivorship program targeted toward survivors of Hodgkin lymphoma within an advanced practice multidisciplinary clinic (Gates, Seymour, & Krishnasamy, 2012). Specific interventions might include nurse-led consultations, individualized survivorship care plans, written educational materials individualized to each patient, and emotional distress screening.

Wheeler (2010) described a survivorship clinic specific to women with a history of gynecologic cancers that was multidisciplinary in nature. Although focusing on a specific type of cancer and post-treatment concerns for that population may have benefits, this model provides a mechanism to streamline education and anticipate needs of a specific survivorship population (Wheeler, 2010). The subspecialty of survivorship care for adults who had cancer as children or as young adults is more specific. These clinics are generally multidisciplinary in nature and serve adults who have survived different types of childhood cancers (McCabe & Jacobs, 2008).

An example of a treatment-specific model involves adult recipients of hematopoietic stem cell transplants (HSCTs). Beavers and Lester (2010) noted that many unique issues are faced by cancer survivors after HSCT, from the subacute survivorship period (first six months after acute treatment) to long-term care planning. These unique issues include risk for graft-versus-host disease, organ toxicity, and increased susceptibility to infections (Beavers & Lester, 2010).

When a survivor is seen in the consultative model, the one-time visit is comprehensive in nature and generally involves many different disciplines. The survivor's past treatment is reviewed, and a plan for follow-up is thoroughly explained and communicated to the PCP (Landier, 2009). Other disciplines such as nutrition, physical therapy, occupational therapy, social work, and spiritual care are often involved as well. These survivorship consultations are commonly performed by an oncology nurse practitioner, and the other disciplines are available the same day or by referral.

Longitudinal survivorship care is often provided by a nurse or oncology nurse practitioner and frequently is multidisciplinary in nature (Landier, 2009). The care is ongoing in this model and replaces the care that would otherwise be given by the oncologist.

The shared-care survivorship model is most prevalent in the literature. This model is a combination of care between the oncologist and the PCP. Mao et al. (2009) found that breast cancer survivors saw PCPs on an ongoing basis, and while the survivors were mostly satisfied with the general care received, there were concerns regarding care specific to breast cancer. Physicians working together across specialties to care for cancer survivors seem to enhance quality care (Gilbert et al., 2008). It is important to note that some survivors may continue to see other specialists (e.g., urology, surgery, dermatology) for a period of time based on the type of cancer and treatment received, with care eventually transitioned completely back to the PCP at a future point depending on individual factors, such as risk of recurrence and logistical factors.

The survivorship models described herein can be facilitated by an oncologist, a PCP, an advanced practice nurse, or an RN. Nurses (including oncology nurse practitioners, infusion nurses, and staff nurses) are in an ideal position to assist in coordination of care in survivorship (McCabe & Jacobs, 2012), and survivorship navigators could be great leaders of the endeavor. Even though follow-up care can be done by the oncology team, PCP, or shared among multiple specialties, a survivorship navigator can champion and coordinate the program. As a nurse, the survivorship navigator can focus on survivorship while the medical providers tend to specific aspects of treatment and follow-up care. When considering how to institute a survivorship program, it is vital to recognize that no one model will work in every setting (McCabe & Jacobs, 2008), but rather a thoughtful and deliberate approach must be taken to establish a model that best fits the needs of the community and overall objectives of the organization.

Components of a Survivorship Navigation Program

The essence of a survivorship navigation program is to meet the needs of the cancer survivor during this critical transition. Survivors' needs may be physical, emotional, or practical and may be disease specific or related to individual factors. Possible program components include (a) initiation of referrals and coordination of care, (b) compilation of treatment summaries and survivorship care plans, (d) the consultative visits, (c) PCP communication, (d) ongoing survivorship support and education, and (e) educating healthcare providers and the community at large about cancer survivorship.

Referrals and Coordination of Care

The referral process for the survivorship program can be unique to each setting. Cancer survivors may be referred to the program by an oncologist or oncology nurse practitioner, surgeon or other specialist, or PCP or through self-referral. Some programs may choose to have disease-specific nurse navigators continue to follow patients into survivorship, in which case a referral would not be necessary.

Once the referral has been made, the survivorship navigator reaches out to the survivor, either in person or by phone. Cancer survivors are often more open to meeting a survivorship navigator if previously informed about the survivorship program by other staff with whom trusting relationships have already been established. Ideally, the survivorship navigator will meet the survivor before the end of treatment and describe the post-treatment support offered. This introduction facilitates the beginning of a therapeutic relationship, after which a more comprehensive assessment can be conducted. Using open-ended questions and the National Comprehensive Cancer Network (2013) Distress Thermometer as a screening tool, the survivorship navigator can immediately begin addressing unmet needs and facilitating necessary referrals.

Treatment Summaries and Survivorship Care Plans

In addition to addressing unmet needs and providing support in the post-treatment phase, most survivorship programs incorporate the provision of patient-specific treatment summaries and survivorship care plans. The intent of the treatment summary and survivorship care plan is to provide information on past treatment and guidance for future follow-up care, health promotion, and wellness strategies. Faul et al. (2012) conducted a qualitative study with colorectal cancer survivors and PCPs regarding treatment summaries and survivorship care plans. They found that survivors felt peace of mind after receiving the documents, and most PCPs noted value in the treatment summaries and survivorship care plans. Another qualitative study using focus groups of cancer survivors found that patients may expect treatment summaries and survivorship plans, and nursing can play a key role in the supportive care processes for survivors (Marbach & Griffie, 2011).

Whereas the treatment summary can be thought of as what happened in the past, the survivorship care plan is the detailed future care plan for the survivor. Components of the treatment summary generally include date of diagnosis, type of cancer, stage, grade, dates and types of procedures done, and details of chemotherapy and targeted therapy (name of drugs, dates given, dosages, and site) and radiation details (type of radiation, dosages, and site) (Hewitt et al., 2006). Some treatment summaries include details of blood product transfusions, ejection fraction, banked sperm or eggs, menopausal status, and genetic test results.

The survivorship care plan is the written plan for the survivor's future health care in relation to the history of cancer. It may include contact information for all disciplines on the healthcare team, guidelines for cancer surveillance, signs and symptoms to watch for in case of cancer recurrence, risks of long-term or latent side effects, general health screening guidelines, and a list of available pertinent resources and education on general health promotion.

Currently, completion of the treatment summary and survivorship care plan falls to a variety of healthcare providers in a survivorship program. No foolproof, fully automated generation of these documents exists at this time, though many electronic medical record (EMR) systems are striving to meet the need. Survivorship navigators can be champions to drive the process and data-mine the medical record to complete the treatment summary and survivorship care plan. When completion of the documents does become an automated process within the EMR, a need for clinicians (such as survivorship navigators) to oversee the production and quality assurance of these documents will likely remain.

Consultative Visits

Delivering the treatment summary and survivorship care plan to the patient can be done by the survivorship navigator, oncologist, or oncology nurse practitioner. The best timing of this visit has not been established (Mayer, Gerstel, Leak, & Smith, 2011) but can be any time after the completion of acute treatment. Some cancer survivors may benefit from waiting a few weeks or months, as questions and concerns about the future and the "new normal" may arise as time passes.

Face-to-face delivery of the treatment summary and survivorship care plan is the optimal format because this facilitates explanation of the documents and time to answer questions and address post-treatment concerns. Some programs establish a one-time consultative survivorship visit with the oncology nurse practitioner to deliver and explain the documents (which is billable as a level 5 visit), whereas other programs have survivorship navigators conduct the visits despite the inability to bill for time (unless the survivorship navigators are advanced practice nurses).

Primary Care Provider Communication

The treatment summary and survivorship care plan can be a communication tool for the PCP as well. Survivorship navigators can facilitate the delivery of the documents to the survivor's PCP upon completion. Grunfeld and Earle (2010) asserted that

> survivorship care plans are viewed as the tool with the greatest potential to address the problems at the interface between primary care and specialist care during the transition period from active treatment to survivorship because of their focus on improving communication. (p. 28)

In a pilot study performed by Mayer et al. (2011), survivorship care plans were supported by all 29 survivors and 5 PCPs. Care coordination for cancer survivors during the survivorship phase is essential because of the continued complexity of care and the potential need for multiple providers (McCabe,

2007). Regular, effective communication and delineation of roles among providers is important for coordinated care during this phase (Mao et al., 2009). Although some cancer survivors may not have a PCP, part of the survivorship navigators' responsibilities may be to link survivors to a PCP and stress the importance of this connection.

Patient Support and Education

Education and ongoing support is a vital component of a survivorship navigation program. Survivorship navigators can be intensely involved with the facilitation and implementation of these programs. Many programs include a multidisciplinary approach to planning, incorporating social work, nutrition, physical and occupational therapy, and spiritual care. The time after treatment when a cancer survivor wants or needs support can vary from person to person. The individual may not be ready for support or may not need the same amount or type of support at the end of treatment versus a year or more out from treatment. Education and support needs may be more intense in the months to years after treatment rather than when treatment is initially completed. Some survivorship workshops and programs intermingle patients in treatment and out of treatment depending on the focus and topic of the discussion.

Education is focused on post-treatment topics, which were referenced earlier in this chapter. Cancer survivors may benefit from hearing about these topics in a group setting from a content expert with a chance to ask questions or discuss the topics with other cancer survivors. Topics may include how to effectively communicate with the healthcare team, side effects of treatment (e.g., lymphedema, fatigue, sexuality concerns, body image), stress management techniques, and how to manage fears of recurrence and insomnia.

Education and coaching about communication with the survivor's healthcare team can be an overlooked but very important topic. Survivorship navigators coordinate care among different members of the survivor's team but ultimately strive to empower the survivor to understand the follow-up plan and communicate his or her needs to the healthcare team. Survivors who assume a central role in the healthcare team may feel a renewed sense of control and hopefulness. This type of support can be done one-on-one or within a group setting.

Health promotion has an important role in survivorship care and is a great topic for educating survivors. This is especially true given the growing number of cancer survivors living longer after initial diagnosis, the majority of whom are older adults (Rowland, 2008). Health promotion can include topics such as increasing physical activity, healthy eating, and smoking cessation. The teachable moment during and after cancer treatment can be seen as an opportunity to help cancer survivors identify ways to improve one's health into the future (Rowland, 2008). A cancer diagnosis has long been considered a life-altering event, and providers can capitalize on the teaching moment that cancer can provide about the topic of health promotion (Demark-Wahnefried, Aziz, Rowland, & Pinto, 2005). The time when and if a cancer survivor is ready and willing to make healthy lifestyle changes varies from person to person. Some may already have a healthy lifestyle, and some may not have the motivation or interest in making these healthy changes. Survivorship navigators are there, when and if survivors are ready for more information and support regarding health promotion.

A fitness program can be one way to promote wellness in a cancer survivorship program. Survivorship navigators can be involved as the cancer center representative at the facility where the fitness program is held. From leading fitness classes (as skill set and time allows) to navigating, coaching, and educating cancer survivors involved in the specific fitness program, survivorship navigators play a vital role. Fitness programs can be as simple as a regularly scheduled yoga or exercise class to more complex programs held in hospital- or community-based fitness centers with personal training in place for cancer survivors.

Nutritional counseling is another facet of health promotion and can be done one-on-one and in a group setting. Survivorship navigators can facilitate nutrition specialists as guest speakers at survivorship workshops, as well as refer individuals for one-on-one nutrition counseling. Cooking classes, where practical day-to-day application of healthy eating can be demonstrated in front of the group, are another innovative idea for education related to nutrition's role in health promotion.

Smoking cessation is an important health promotion topic that cannot be ignored. Active smokers who have completed cancer treatment need to be referred to local resources for smoking cessation if they are ready to quit the tobacco habit.

Healthcare Provider and General Community Education

Educating other healthcare providers and the public about cancer survivorship is another role of survivorship navigators. The navigators are in an ideal position, as experts in post-treatment issues, to educate nurses, physicians, and other disciplines. Teaching opportunities within the community abound as survivorship concerns become more recognized and acknowledged.

Barriers to Survivorship Care

Unfortunately, many potential barriers to survivorship care exist. Multiple barriers have been identified as facilities have either launched survivorship programs or contemplated starting a program. First and foremost, the availability of survivorship services is not currently a universal standard of care (Pratt-Chapman et al., 2011). The potential complexity and unique nature of individual cancer survivor needs in this post-treatment phase can be a roadblock (Landier, 2009). Commonly identified challenges to survivorship program development include (a) resources, (b) logistics, (c) inadequate workforce, (d) physician buy-in, and (e) lack of evidence-based survivorship guidelines. According to Earle and Ganz (2012), the delivery of care to post-treatment survivors is a work in progress.

Resources, or the lack thereof, tend to be the universally identified barrier by most organizations (Campbell et al., 2011). The time it takes to datamine the medical record to compile a concise and accurate treatment summary and survivorship care plan can be very time consuming. Along with the time factor, challenges exist with identifying every survivor completing treatment and who is responsible for completing and delivering the treatment summary and survivorship care plan to the survivors. Survivorship navigators are one potential option for addressing these issues. Lack of reimbursement for time spent completing the treatment summary and survivorship care plan is another resource barrier commonly experienced by organizations (Campbell et al., 2011).

Referral logistics can be a challenge. For example, how does one capture every survivor at the end of treatment? Ideally, the oncologist, as the overall manager of care, would refer all patients completing cancer treatment to an existing survivorship program. However, in reality, survivorship navigators may be initially identifying survivors and seeking appropriate referrals from the managing oncologist, especially when launching a new survivorship program. This activity not only connects survivors to the valuable program resources but also is an effective marketing tool for survivorship navigators to educate team members regarding available services and to promote internal, external, and survivor self-referrals to the program.

Logistical barriers can include the EMR. Although the EMR is vitally important to the completion of the treatment summary and survivorship care plan, most do not have the functionality yet to concisely and accurately automate this task without intensive oversight from a clinical person. Yet, there is hope that in the future EMR systems will facilitate automated medical abstraction (Campbell et al., 2011). Survivorship navigators can complete treatment summaries and survivorship care plans. If and when EMR systems become fully automated and accurate in compiling the treatment summary and survivorship care plan, survivorship navigators could oversee and provide quality assurance to the process.

The oncology workforce is predicted to face a shortage in the years ahead. Numerous studies predict the number of physicians specializing in oncology will not be adequate to meet the needs of survivors in the future (Shulman et al., 2009). With this projected imbalance of supply and demand, having various healthcare professionals take part in survivorship care may be a necessity (Gerber, Stout, Schmitz, & Stricker, 2012). Utilizing mid-level practitioners, such as oncology nurse practitioners, physician extenders, and physician assistants, as well as RNs, may help resolve some of these workforce barriers (Shulman et al., 2009). Survivorship navigators can assist the oncologist or mid-level provider in facilitating a survivorship program or see survivors one-on-one and in group settings, as described earlier in the chapter. This does not replace the medical follow-up provided by the oncologist, oncology nurse practitioner, or PCP, but it could be part of the solution.

Getting physician buy-in for a survivorship navigator position, or even a survivorship program in general, can be a challenge. "Most providers have found it difficult to substantively change the way they care for cancer survivors" (Earle & Ganz, 2012, p. 3764). Physicians may not be convinced that the components of the survivorship program, namely the treatment summary and survivorship care plan, make a difference in patients' clinical outcomes.

The Children's Oncology Group (2008) long-term follow-up guidelines provide recommendations for cancer survivors who had cancer as a child, adolescent, or young adult. These guidelines are both evidence-based (when possible) and consensus-based recommendations. Lack of standardized guidelines to direct survivorship care for adult cancer survivors is an obstacle (Landier, 2009). ACS is in the process of developing survivorship guidelines to address the current gaps in survivorship care (Sharpe & Pratt-Chapman, 2012). The National Comprehensive Cancer Network provides follow-up guidelines for many cancer types based on cancer stage and the treatment received. These can be a helpful resource in putting together the survivorship care plan.

If logistically feasible at an institution, a multidisciplinary team can champion a process for each disease type, stage, and treatment modality to gather a general consensus of what follow-up will consist of at the institution. This may lessen confusion for the survivor and for the multiple providers who may be involved in follow-up care. For example, the team can decide the appropriate surveillance plan for a patient with breast cancer depending on the type of treatment(s) the patient received, agreeing that each patient in the same treatment scenario would have the same surveillance plan. The surgeon and radiation oncologist may agree to each see her six months after treatment, then alternate annual visits, and after five years, only see her on an as-needed basis. Effective communication of how the patient is doing after each visit could reduce confusion for the entire team and, most importantly, the patient.

Tools and Program Metrics

Marketing the role of the survivorship navigator is best done in the day-to-day support for the survivorship program. Having a presence at multidisciplinary conferences (known as "tumor boards" at some institutions), being visible in the waiting areas and infusion suites, checking in with the stakeholders of the program periodically, explaining the role and how the program is going, and providing formal education regarding cancer survivorship at staff meetings, cancer committee meetings, physician meetings, and conferences can help market the survivorship navigator role and the program. Having the survivorship program and the role of the survivorship navigator present, as applicable, on the institution's website can be an innovative way to increase awareness about the role. Ultimately, cancer survivors telling oncologists at follow-up appointments how they felt about the navigation services received may be the best way to substantiate the importance and impact of the survivorship navigator's role. This will only happen when survivorship navigators are able to make a difference in the post-treatment period for a cancer survivor and family.

The referral process is one that will evolve as survivorship navigators establish themselves. Referrals may come from oncologists, PCPs, or survivors themselves. Having a contact phone number and business cards to distribute are essential for survivorship navigators. As survivorship programs get started, navigators may find it necessary to proactively search out referrals and demonstrate the worth of the program.

The treatment summary and survivorship care plan are most conveniently abstracted when an established template is used. Side-by-side computer monitors for survivorship navigators facilitate ease of transcription of data from the EMR to the treatment summary template. Currently, many organizations have created treatment summary and survivorship care plan templates, which are available free of charge and very user friendly. These include the ASCO treatment plan and summary templates (www.asco.org/quality-guidelines/chemotherapy-treatment-plan-and-summaries), the Journey Forward Survivorship Care Plan Builder (www.journeyforward.org/professionals/survivorship-care-plan-builder), and NursingCenter.com's Prescription for Living Plan (www.nursingcenter.com/lnc/static?pageid=721732). In particular, ONS has partnered with Journey Forward regarding the survivorship care plan template (Belansky & Mahon, 2012). An institution also may create a custom template. Although the information included is roughly similar to publicly available templates, differences usually relate to the ease of completing and the institutional labeling of the completed document.

The LIVESTRONG Foundation provides an online care plan (www.livestrongcareplan.org), which can be compiled by either the survivor or healthcare provider. The person completing the care plan simply needs basic information about the type of cancer and treatment received. Once the care plan is completed, a brief summary with follow-up recommendations for the PCP and a more detailed, education-focused document for cancer survivors can be printed.

Pointing cancer survivors toward existing resources is a core component of the survivorship navigator's role. NCI provides a multitude of educational booklets on specific cancers, post-treatment concerns, and survivorship in general. ACS also provides educational resources for survivors during the post-treatment phase.

Communication with survivors' PCPs is a fundamental role to consider when developing a survivorship navigator position. Survivorship navigators can assume responsibility for communicating the treatment summary and survivorship care plan to PCPs. Including a cover letter that briefly explains the treatment summary and survivorship care plan can be helpful in establishing roles and expectations with regard to follow-up and also in marketing the survivorship navigator role and survivorship program. If time allows, survivorship navigators may consider meeting with PCPs up front to explain the documents as another innovative way to market the program as a whole.

Other program logistics include the gathering of multiple disciplines to support cancer survivors. Survivorship navigators cannot possibly be experts in everything, but through networking and awareness of resources, they can assemble the appropriate team and provide opportunities for survivors to gain important information and self-care skills. One way to accomplish this may be to co-facilitate survivorship workshops with oncology social workers, oncology nurse practitioners, or other nurse navigators. For optimal awareness of survivorship workshops, marketing personnel should be engaged to advertise the program within the community, as well as among oncology providers and staff to promote the program to current survivors.

Outcome measurements and the value of the survivorship navigator role can be difficult to directly measure. One citywide survivorship program reported tracking the number of individuals who received survivorship information, the number of care plans completed, and attendance at various educational sessions (Pratt-Chapman et al., 2011). Basic survivorship navigation metrics to track include the number of survivors referred to the program, referral sources and mechanisms, referrals initiated by the survivorship navigator, and attendance at survivorship support or education programs. Other considerations might include adherence to follow-up recommendations made in the survivorship visit, as well as satisfaction with the survivorship visit, survivorship navigator, and survivorship educational programs. Patient-reported outcomes might include quality of life, physical activity levels, changes in eating habits, and distress levels at different points in the post-treatment survivorship phase. Although it will be difficult to conclude with any certainty that positive or negative changes with patient-reported outcomes can be attributed to the survivorship navigator role, the information may be useful in establishing program development priorities to better support survivors' most challenging issues.

On another note, survivorship navigators may consider keeping a log of time spent on the telephone with cancer survivors. This does not replace documenting each encounter and outcome in the survivor's medical record, but it may provide ready access to quantifiable data to validate this aspect of the survivorship navigator role.

Case Example

Tanya is a 46-year-old cancer survivor who recently completed treatment for breast cancer. Because of the stage and risk features of her cancer, she underwent a lumpectomy, sentinel lymph node biopsy, chemotherapy, and radiation and is now considering five years of hormone therapy.

Tanya was referred to Mary, the survivorship navigator, by her oncologist. Mary initially met Tanya a few days before her last radiation treatment. This was a brief meeting to introduce the support available to Tanya as she finished treatment. Mary asked Tanya to complete a distress assessment and return it on her last day of radiation treatment.

When Mary received the distress assessment back, she noted that Tanya had self-reported a high level of distress during the last week. Issues identified as contributing to the distress included appearance, fatigue, pain, and insomnia. Mary called Tanya to assess the situation. She found that Tanya was struggling with her alopecia, discouraged that her hair has not grown back yet. Her fatigue was affecting her activities of daily living. The pain she was experiencing was related to neuropathy in her toes, and the insomnia was due to racing thoughts and fear of cancer recurrence. Mary provided support and encouragement over the telephone, facilitated referrals to physical therapy for fatigue and oncology social work for distress and insomnia, and invited Tanya to an upcoming survivorship workshop.

Eight weeks after Tanya's radiation was completed, she had a survivorship visit scheduled with her oncology nurse practitioner. Before this visit, Mary completed Tanya's treatment summary and survivorship care plan, abstracting the data from Tanya's medical record. This treatment summary and survivorship care plan was provided to the nurse practitioner to review with Tanya. At this survivorship visit, Tanya was given the chance to tell the story of her cancer experience from her perspective. The oncology nurse practitioner reviewed her treatment summary and answered all of Tanya's questions. Tanya felt grateful to go through the information because she had not asked many questions while on active treatment. The oncology nurse practitioner explained the follow-up plan for the next 5–10 years for Tanya. Tanya left feeling calm and more in control, knowing a plan was in place for her future. She made a telephone call to her PCP to schedule an annual physical, as she had not had this done since before her cancer diagnosis.

Participation at the survivorship workshop helped connect Tanya with others in similar situations. In a group setting, she was able to learn the benefits of exercise, practical healthy eating tips, stress management techniques, and how to effectively communicate with her healthcare team. She learned that it may be helpful to write down her symptoms and concerns in a journal to bring to her follow-up visits, and she made plans to do so.

Tanya is now a year out of treatment. She called Mary to register for an upcoming exercise class offered at the cancer center and thanked Mary for helping her through the difficult post-treatment transition. She felt she benefited greatly from meeting with the oncology social worker and physical therapist after treatment, as well as from the survivorship visit and workshop. She then asked Mary if any opportunities were available for her to give back to others who have been through similar situations. Mary encouraged Tanya to continue on her own cancer survivorship journey and congratulated her on her hard work. Mary urged her to continue attending the survivorship programs to connect with those just finishing treatment, as she may be able to inspire and spread hope to others just entering the post-treatment phase of cancer survivorship.

Summary of Survivorship Navigation

Although no consensus currently exists regarding the most effective way to provide care to survivors in the post-treatment phase, many models have been developed and are currently being used within the cancer community (Landier, 2009). Systems are needed to identify patients appropriate for survivorship care in a timely fashion (Campbell et al., 2011). The potential role of survivorship navigators in overseeing and facilitating the process for cancer survivors is immense. Although it is not the traditional form of navigation, it is an example of how the role has been expanded to creatively meet the needs of cancer survivors as they transition to life after cancer treatment.

Conclusion

Outreach navigation and survivorship navigation constitute the bookends of the cancer continuum. For both, the model used at any institution will vary depending on available resources, demographics of the patient population, and strengths of the nurse navigator. To create meaningful outreach and survivorship programs, institutions must invest time to identify the most prominent unmet needs within the community and then design systems that are focused on improving access to care and eliminating barriers. The importance of flexibility and continual evaluation of processes cannot be overemphasized. Navigation efforts spanning the cancer continuum provide much-needed support to the community and can be an incredibly enriching experience not only for nurse navigators coordinating these programs but also for underserved populations and the community at large.

References

American College of Surgeons Commission on Cancer. (2012). *Cancer program standards 2012: Ensuring patient-centered care* [v.1.2.1, released January 2014]. Retrieved from http://facs .org/cancer/coc/programstandards2012.html

American Society of Clinical Oncology. (2013). QOPI summary of measures, spring 2013. Retrieved from http://qopi.asco.org/Documents/QOPISpring13MeasuresSummary.pdf

Amir, Z., & Brocky, J. (2009). Cancer survivorship and employment: Epidemiology. *Occupational Medicine, 59*, 373–377. doi:10.1093/occmed/kqp086

Battaglia, T.A., Bak, S.M., Heeren, T., Chen, C.A., Kalish, R., Tringale, S., … Freund, K.M. (2012). Boston Patient Navigation Research Program: The impact of navigation on time to diagnostic resolution after abnormal screening. *Cancer Epidemiology, Biomarkers and Prevention, 21*, 1645–1654. doi:10.1158/1055-9965.EPI-12-0532

Battaglia, T.A., Burhansstipanov, L., Murrell, S.S., Dwyer, A.J., & Caron, S.E. (2011). Assessing the impact of patient navigation: Prevention and early detection metrics. *Cancer, 117*(Suppl. 15), 3553–3564. doi:10.1002/cncr.26267

Beavers, J., & Lester, J. (2010). Survivorship care for adult recipients of hematopoietic cell transplantations. *Clinical Journal of Oncology Nursing, 14*, 136–139. doi:10.1188/10.CJON.136-139

Belansky, H., & Mahon, S.M. (2012). Using care plans to enhance care throughout the cancer survivorship trajectory. *Clinical Journal of Oncology Nursing, 16*, 90–92. doi:10.1188/12. CJON.90-92

Braun, K.L., Kagawa-Singer, M., Holden, A.E.C., Burhansstipanov, L., Tran, J.H., Seals, B.F., … Ramirez, A.G. (2012). Cancer patient navigator tasks across the cancer continuum. *Journal of Health Care for the Poor and Underserved, 23*, 398–413. doi:10.1353/hpu.2012.0029

Campbell, C., Craig, J., Eggert, J., & Bailey-Dorton, C. (2010). Implementing and measuring the impact of patient navigation at a comprehensive community cancer center. *Oncology Nursing Forum, 37*, 61–68. doi:10.1188/10.ONF.61-68

Campbell, M.K., Tessaro, I., Gellin, M., Valle, C.G., Golden, S., Kaye, L., … Miller, K. (2011). Adult cancer survivorship care: Experiences from the LIVESTRONG centers of excellence network. *Journal of Cancer Survivorship, 5*, 271–282. doi:10.1007/s11764-011-0180-z

Children's Oncology Group. (2008). *Long-term follow-up guidelines.* Retrieved from http://www. survivorshipguidelines.org/pdf/ltfuguidelines.pdf

Demark-Wahnefried, W., Aziz, N.M., Rowland, J.H., & Pinto, B.M. (2005). Riding the crest of the teachable moment: Promoting long-term health after the diagnosis of cancer. *Journal of Clinical Oncology, 23*, 5814–5830. doi:10.1200/JCO.2005.01.230

Domingo, J.B., Davis, E.L., Allison, A.L., & Braun, K.L. (2011). Cancer patient navigation case studies in Hawai'i: The complimentary role of clinical and community navigators. *Hawai'i Medical Journal, 70*, 257–261. Retrieved from http://www.ncbi.nlm.nih.gov/pmc/articles/PMC3242420

Doyle, N. (2008). Cancer survivorship: Evolutionary concept analysis. *Journal of Advanced Nursing, 62*, 499–509. doi:10.1111/j.1365-2648.2008.04617.x

Earle, C.C., & Ganz, P.A. (2012). Cancer survivorship care: Don't let the perfect be the enemy of the good. *Journal of Clinical Oncology, 30*, 3764–3768. doi:10.1200/jco.2012.41.7667

Elkin, E.B., Shapiro, E., Snow, J.G., Zauber, A.G., & Krauskopf, M.S. (2012). The economic impact of a patient navigator program to increase screening colonoscopy. *Cancer, 118*, 5982–5988. doi:10.1002/cncr.27595

Faul, L.A., Rivers, B., Shibata, D., Townsend, I., Cabrera, P., Quinn, G.P., & Jacobsen, P.B. (2012). Survivorship care planning in colorectal cancer: Feedback from survivors and providers. *Journal of Psychosocial Oncology, 30*, 198–216. doi:10.1080/07347332.2011.651260

Findley, S.E., Matos, S., Hicks, A.L., Campbell, A., Moore, A., & Diaz, D. (2012). Building a consensus on community health workers' scope of practice: Lessons from New York. *American Journal of Public Health, 102*, 1981–1987. doi:10.2105/AJPH.2011.300566

Freeman, H.P. (2012). The origin, evolution, and principles of patient navigation. *Cancer Epidemiology, Biomarkers and Prevention, 21,* 1614–1617. doi:10.1158/1055-9965.EPI-12-0982

Freeman, H.P., & Rodriguez, R.L. (2011). History and principles of patient navigation. *Cancer, 117*(Suppl. 15), 3539–3542. doi:10.1002/cncr.26262

Gates, P., Seymour, J.F., & Krishnasamy, M. (2012). Insights into the development of a nurse-led survivorship care intervention for long-term survivors of Hodgkin lymphoma. *Australian Journal of Cancer Nursing, 13*(1), 4–10.

Gerber, L.H., Stout, N.L., Schmitz, K.H., & Stricker, C.T. (2012). Integrating a prospective surveillance model for rehabilitation into breast cancer survivorship care. *Cancer, 118*(Suppl. 8), 2201–2206. doi:10.1002/cncr.27472

Gilbert, S.M., Miller, D.C., Hollenbeck, B.K., Montie, J.E., & Wei, J.T. (2008). Cancer survivorship: Challenges and changing paradigms. *Journal of Urology, 179,* 431–438. doi:10.1016/j.juro.2007.09.029

Grunfeld, E., & Earle, C.C. (2010). The interface between primary and oncology specialty care: Treatment through survivorship. *Journal of the National Cancer Institute Monographs, 2010*(40), 25–30. doi:10.1093/jncimonographs/lgq002

Hahn, E.E., & Ganz, P.A. (2011). Survivorship programs and care plans in practice: Variations on a theme. *Journal of Oncology Practice, 7,* 70–75. doi:10.1200/JOP.2010.000115

Hamilton, J.B., Moore, C.E., Powe, B.D., Agarwal, M., & Martin, P. (2010). Perceptions of support among older African American cancer survivors. *Oncology Nursing Forum, 37,* 484–493. doi:10.1188/10.ONF.484-493

Hensley, M.L., Dowell, J., Herndon, J.E., II, Winer, E., Stark, N., Weeks, J.C., & Paskett, E. (2005). Economic outcomes of breast cancer survivorship: CALGB study 79804. *Breast Cancer Research and Treatment, 91,* 153–161. doi:10.1007/s10549-004-6497-9

Hewitt, M., Greenfield, S., & Stovall, E. (Eds.). (2006). *From cancer patient to cancer survivor: Lost in transition.* Washington, DC: National Academies Press.

Horner, K., Ludman, E.J., McCorkle R., Canfield, E., Flaherty, L., Min, J., ... Wagner, E.H. (2013). An oncology nurse navigator program designed to eliminate gaps in early cancer care. *Clinical Journal of Oncology Nursing, 17,* 43–48. doi:10.1188/13.CJON.43-48

Landier, W. (2009). Survivorship care: Essential components and models of delivery. *Oncology, 23*(Suppl. 4, Nurse Ed.), 46–53.

LIVESTRONG. (2010, June). *How cancer has affected post-treatment survivors: A LIVESTRONG report.* Retrieved from http://www.livestrong.org/What-We-Do/Our-Approach/ReportsFindings/LIVESTRONG-Survey-Report

Mao, J.J., Bowman, M.A., Stricker, C.T., DeMichele, A., Jacobs, L., Chan, D., & Armstrong, K. (2009). Delivery of survivorship care by primary care physicians: The perspective of breast cancer patients. *Journal of Clinical Oncology, 27,* 933–938. doi:10.1200/JCO.2008.18.0679

Marbach, T.J., & Griffie, J. (2011). Patient preferences concerning treatment plans, survivorship care plans, education, and support services. *Oncology Nursing Forum, 38,* 335–342. doi:10.1188/11.ONF.335-342

Markossian, T.W., Darnell, J.S., & Calhoun, E.A. (2012). Follow-up and timeliness after an abnormal cancer screening among underserved, urban women in a patient navigation program. *Cancer Epidemiology, Biomarkers and Prevention, 21,* 1691–1700. doi:10.1158/1055-9965.EPI-12-0535

Mason, T.A., Thompson, W.W., Allen, D., Rogers, D., Garbram-Mendola, S., & Arriola, K.R.J. (2013). Evaluation of the Avon Foundation community education and outreach initiative community patient navigation program. *Health Promotion Practice, 14,* 105–112. doi:10.1177/1524839911404229

Mayer, D.K., Gerstel, A., Leak, A.N., & Smith, S.K. (2011). Patient and provider preferences for survivorship care plans. *Journal of Oncology Practice, 8*(4), e80–e86. doi:10.1200/JOP.2011.000401

McCabe, M.S. (2007). Living beyond cancer: Survivorship is more than surviving. *Nature Clinical Practice Urology, 4,* 575. doi:10.1038/ncpuro0947

McCabe, M.S., Bhatia, S., Oeffinger, K.C., Reaman, G.H., Tyne, C., Wollins, D.S., & Hudson, M.M. (2013). American Society of Clinical Oncology statement: Achieving high-quality cancer survivorship care. *Journal of Clinical Oncology, 31,* 631–640. doi:10.1200/JCO.2012.46.6854

McCabe, M.S., & Jacobs, L. (2008). Survivorship care: Models and programs. *Seminars in Oncology Nursing, 24,* 202–207. doi:10.1016/j.soncn.2008.05.008

McCabe, M.S., & Jacobs, L.A. (2012). Clinical update: Survivorship care—Models and programs. *Seminars in Oncology Nursing, 28*(3), e1–e8. doi:10.1016/j.soncn.2012.05.001

National Cancer Institute. (n.d.). Survivor. In *NCI dictionary of cancer terms.* Retrieved from http://www.cancer.gov/dictionary?cdrid=450125

National Comprehensive Cancer Network. (2013). NCCN Distress Thermometer for patients. Retrieved from http://www.nccn.org/patients/resources/life_with_cancer/pdf/nccn_distress_thermometer.pdf

Ness, S., Kokal, J., Fee-Schroeder, K., Novotny, P., Satele, D., & Barton, D. (2013). Concerns across the survivorship trajectory: Results from a survey of cancer survivors. *Oncology Nursing Forum, 40,* 35–42. doi:10.1188/13.ONF.35-42

Nguyen, T.T., McPhee, S.J., Bui-Tong, N., Luong, T.-N., Ha-Iaconis, T., Nguyen, T., ... Lam, H. (2006). Community-based participatory research increases cervical cancer screening among Vietnamese-Americans. *Journal of Health Care for the Poor and Underserved, 17*(Suppl. 2), 31–54. doi:10.1353/hpu.2006.0078

Oeffinger, K.C., & McCabe, M.S. (2006). Models for delivering survivorship care. *Journal of Clinical Oncology, 24,* 5117–5124. doi:10.1200/JCO.2006.07.0474

Pratt-Chapman, M., Simon, M.A., Patterson, A.K., Risendal, B.C., & Patierno, S. (2011). Survivorship navigation outcome measures: A report from the ACS patient navigation working group on survivorship navigation. *Cancer, 117*(Suppl. 15), 3575–3584. doi:10.1002/cncr.26261

Quinlan, E., Maclean, R., Hack, T., Tatemichi, S., Towers, A., Kwan, W., ... Tilley, A. (2011). Breast cancer survivorship and work disability. *Journal of Disability Policy Studies, 22,* 18–27. doi:10.1177/1044207310394439

Ramanadhan, S., Salhi, C., Achille, E., Baril, N., D'Entremont, K., Grullon, M., ... Viswanath, K. (2012). Addressing cancer disparities via community networking mobilization and intersectoral partnerships: A social network analysis. *PLOS ONE, 7,* 32130. doi:10.1371/journal.pone.0032130

Rodriguez, E.M., Bowie, J.V., Frattaroli, S., & Gielen, A. (2009). A qualitative exploration of the community partner experience in a faith-based breast cancer educational intervention. *Health Education Research, 24,* 760–771. doi:10.1093/her/cyp010

Rowland, J.H. (2008). Cancer survivorship: Rethinking the cancer control continuum. *Seminars in Oncology Nursing, 24,* 145–152. doi:10.1016/j.soncn.2008.05.002

Schlairet, M.C. (2011). Needs of older cancer survivors in a community cancer care setting. *Journal of Gerontological Nursing, 37,* 36–41. doi:10.3928/00989134-20100730-05

Sharpe, K., & Pratt-Chapman, M. (2012). Clinical survivorship guidelines: What navigators need to know. *Journal of Oncology Navigation and Survivorship, 3*(6), 28. Retrieved from http://issuu.com/theoncologynurse/docs/jons_december_2012_web

Shockney, L.D. (2010). Evolution of patient navigation. *Clinical Journal of Oncology Nursing, 14,* 405–407. doi:10.1188/10.CJON.405-407

Shulman, L.N., Jacobs, L.A., Greenfield, S., Jones, B., McCabe, M.S., Syrjala, K., ... Ganz, P.A. (2009). Cancer care and cancer survivorship care in the United States: Will we be able to care for these patients in the future? *Journal of Oncology Practice, 5,* 119–123. doi:10.1200/JOP.0932001

Siegel, R., DeSantis, C., Virgo, K., Stein, K., Mariotto, A., Smith, T., ... Ward, E. (2012). Cancer treatment and survivorship statistics, 2012. *CA: A Cancer Journal for Clinicians, 62,* 220–241. doi:10.3322/caac.21149

Smith, W. (2013). Community health needs assessments: Everything community cancer centers need to know today. *Oncology Issues, 28*(1), 32–34.

Wheeler, T. (2010). Gynecologic oncology survivorship care. *Journal of Gynecologic Oncology Nursing, 20*(1), 14–16.

Whop, L.J., Valery, P.C., Beesley, V.L., Moore, S.P., Lokuge, K., Jacka, C., & Garvey, G. (2012). Navigating the cancer journey: A review of patient navigator programs for Indigenous cancer patients. *Asia-Pacific Journal of Clinical Oncology, 8*(4), e89–e96. doi:10.1111/j.1743 -7563.2012.01532.x

CHAPTER 8

Example of a Successful Nurse Navigation Program

LaTonya E. Mann, FNP-BC, MSN, OCN®, CRNI, and Patricia M. Strusowski, RN, MS

Introduction

Many Americans are unable to gain access to high-quality care, with nearly half reporting a breakdown in the coordination of health care (Collins, Wender, & Altshuler, 2010). Nowhere is this breakdown more evident than in cancer care, where effective delivery and quality of care have suffered as costs have risen exponentially, creating a "perfect storm" for patients with cancer and survivors (Collins et al., 2010). Nurse navigators can minimize the effects of this storm. This chapter will discuss the development of a nurse navigation program at Christiana Care Health System in Delaware. In particular, the role and responsibilities of the head and neck cancer (HNC) nurse navigator will be highlighted with a case example.

Christiana Care Health System

Christiana Care Health System (2013), headquartered in Wilmington, Delaware, is one of the country's largest healthcare providers, ranking 22nd in the nation for hospital admissions. Christiana Care is a major teaching hospital with two campuses and more than 270 medical and dental residents and fellows. Christiana Care is recognized as a regional center for excellence in cardiology, cancer, and women's health services. As a not-for-profit, nonsectarian health system, Christiana Care includes two hospitals with more than 1,100 patient beds, a home health service, preventive medicine, rehabilitation services, a network of primary care physicians (PCPs), and an extensive range of outpatient services. With more than 10,500 employees, Christiana Care is the largest private employer in Delaware and the 10th largest employer in the Philadelphia region. In fiscal year 2013, Christiana Care had more than $2.51 billion in total patient revenue and provided the community with approximately $27 million in charity care (Christiana Care Health System, 2013). Figure 8-1 depicts a few statistics to demonstrate Christiana Care's national and regional rankings for various healthcare services provided.

Development and Implementation of the Nurse Navigation Program

Before Christiana Care opened the Helen F. Graham Cancer Center and Research Institute, patients with cancer were treated in a variety of settings, including physician offices, hospital departments, and outpatient clinics scattered throughout the system with no coordination among departments. As a result of this fragmented approach to cancer care, patients often had to wait as long as three weeks to undergo diagnostic procedures and consultative visits with appropriate specialists.

In 1997, Christiana Care hosted a retreat with the goal of forming a planning team for cancer program development. Participants included board members, medical staff leaders, administrative personnel, and community members. A consulting group was also engaged to assist with creating the cancer program's strategic model (see Figure 8-2). The model identified necessary key components driving the vision to become an academic community cancer center. Early priorities centered on the development of a multidisciplinary cancer care management structure to navigate patients and families across the continuum of care with the primary purpose of increasing communication among the healthcare team and decreasing duplication for patients. Subsequently, health improvement teams (HITs) were created to focus on the continuum of care for patients with cancer and their families.

Members of the HITs included surgeons, medical oncologists, radiation oncologists, radiologists, pathologists, PCPs, social workers, cancer outreach staff, and clinical trial nurses. Additional support staff members were hired,

---

Figure 8-1. Christiana Care Health System Rankings by Volume for Healthcare Services Provided, 2013	
Among hospitals in the United States, Christiana Care ranks:	**Among hospitals on the East Coast, Christiana Care ranks:**
• 22nd in admissions	• 12th in admissions
• 30th in births	• 14th in births
• 22nd in emergency visits	• 12th in emergency visits
• 24th in total surgeries	• 12th in total surgeries

Note. Figure courtesy of Christiana Care Health System. Used with permission.

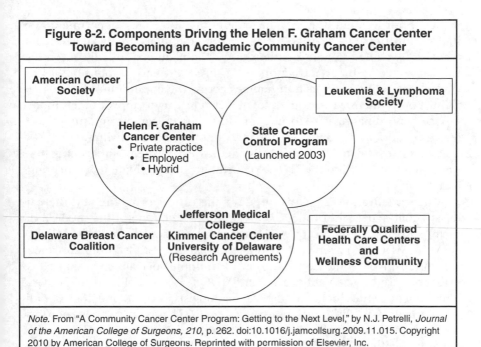

Figure 8-2. Components Driving the Helen F. Graham Cancer Center Toward Becoming an Academic Community Cancer Center

American Cancer Society

Leukemia & Lymphoma Society

Helen F. Graham Cancer Center
• Private practice
• Employed
• Hybrid

State Cancer Control Program (Launched 2003)

Delaware Breast Cancer Coalition

Jefferson Medical College Kimmel Cancer Center University of Delaware (Research Agreements)

Federally Qualified Health Care Centers and Wellness Community

Note. From "A Community Cancer Center Program: Getting to the Next Level," by N.J. Petrelli, *Journal of the American College of Surgeons, 210*, p. 262. doi:10.1016/j.jamcollsurg.2009.11.015. Copyright 2010 by American College of Surgeons. Reprinted with permission of Elsevier, Inc.

including nurse navigators, dietitians, a health psychologist, and genetic counselors. Initial activities for which the HITs assumed responsibility included a complete review of national guidelines for prevention, screening, early detection, diagnosis, treatment, supportive and palliative care, and surveillance. The teams reviewed patient educational materials, initiated site-specific prospective tumor conferences, provided guidance for cancer outreach, reviewed clinical trial portfolios and promoted enrollment, identified gaps in support services, defined clinical outcomes for the cancer program, and monitored outcome metrics and trends.

The following year, focus groups were conducted with patients with cancer and their families. The common theme from participants was the desire for a healthcare team that is willing to communicate and welcome patient and family involvement with the treatment plan. Participants also requested improvements whereby history information would not need to be repeatedly provided to each new physician or department across the continuum. Bottom line, patients and families wanted to increase communication and decrease duplication in care.

As a result of the focus group findings, the Christiana Care board of directors designated a $25 million endowment from unrestricted funds to support enhancements to the cancer program. First, a new multidisciplinary department, Cancer Care Management, was created as part of the Performance Improvement/Care Management division. This department was staffed with nurse navigators, social workers, dietitians, financial assistants, a health psychologist, and inpatient discharge planners. Initially, seven disease site–specific nurse navigators were hired. Primary responsibilities included navigating patients and families across the continuum of care, providing comprehensive assessment of needs, referring to appropriate support services, coordinating care for the multidisciplinary centers and tumor conferences, and facilitating performance improvement activities. After the Cancer Care Management department was established, nurse navigators were incorporated into the HITs to coordinate and facilitate team meetings and activities.

A new medical director was hired for the cancer program, and thereafter a 72,000-square-foot cancer center was opened. One of the medical director's first priorities was to establish cancer site–specific multidisciplinary centers (MDCs) coordinated by nurse navigators because optimal cancer care often involves the collaboration of multiple specialists committed to evidence-based and quality care. The MDC teams established at the Graham Cancer Center included medical oncologists, surgical oncologists, radiation oncologists, clinical trial nurses, nurse navigators, and other appropriate support staff. Initially, three MDCs were created: thoracic, HNC, and a general oncology MDC for all other cancers. The program has since expanded to 19 MDCs (see Figure 8-3).

A physician champion, someone passionate about quality cancer care and timely evaluation of findings suspicious for cancer, is essential to the successful launch and enduring sustainability of MDCs. For example, the HNC MDC was one of the first MDCs initiated at the Graham Cancer Center because of the efforts of an extremely dedicated HNC surgeon who understood the multidisciplinary process and advocated the benefits of coordinated care for patients and families. Annually, the Graham Cancer Center sees only about 90 new analytical HNC cases; although this is a lower volume than other types of cancer, the complexity and coordination of care necessary for this high-risk population were key drivers in the creation of the HNC MDC.

According to Petrelli (2010), several key elements are part of the multidisciplinary care process. The process begins with a referral to the MDC scheduler; such referral can be from a physician, patient, or family member. The referral source is notified of the need for the patient's current contact information, as well as pertinent medical records related to the cancer diagnosis (e.g., pathology report[s] confirming the cancer diagnosis, diagnostic studies, physician progress notes). Once medical records are received, the MDC scheduler and nurse navigator review them. The patient is then contacted with the date, time, and location of the appointment, as well as educated on the MDC process and team members who will be present at the visit. If diagnostic studies were completed at an outside facility, the patient

Figure 8-3. The Helen F. Graham Cancer Center Multidisciplinary Centers Weekly Schedule

Time	Monday	Tuesday	Wednesday	Thursday	Friday
7:00					
8:00	Spinal Tumor/Metastatic Lesion -(2nd & 4th)		General/Melanoma/Soft Tissue Sarcoma/Upper GI	Head & Neck	Dupuytren -(1st & 3rd)
9:00		Pulmonary			Skin -Last Friday of the month
10:00			Interventional Pain Management		Young Adult F/U -(2nd) / Lymphoma (Heme) -(1st, 3rd, & 4th)
11:00				Breast	
12:00					
1:00		Thoracic/Esophageal	Ostomy - every other Wednesday		Gynecology
2:00		Bone Lesion -(2nd & 4th)	Neuro CyberKnife		Bone Lesion -(1st & 3rd)
3:00	Genito-Urinary/Prostate Center	Hepatobiliary Pancreatic	Head & Neck		
4:00					
5:00		Rectal/Anus	Thyroid		
6:00					

Revised 7/2013

Note. Figure courtesy of Christiana Care Health System. Used with permission.

is asked to bring the disk with images to the MDC appointment. The nurse navigator introduces the role of the navigator and addresses any needs or concerns the patient may have before the MDC visit. Centralized registration is essential for one point of patient entry and to use information technology as a systemwide communication tool. Coordinated supportive care services must be present, such as nutrition, social services, palliative care, and pastoral care. Steward (2006) emphasized "one stop shopping" as a major advantage of the MDC structure and asserted that six to eight weeks of time can be saved by using such a model instead of patients traveling to various physician offices for consultations.

Early gaps in care that nurse navigators at Graham Cancer Center focused on eliminating included (a) inappropriate referrals to the MDC if the patient only needed to meet with one team member, (b) ensuring that all necessary records and documentation needed were available for the MDC consultations, (c) transportation concerns, and (d) not having all appropriate team members available at the time of the MDC visit. For example, at times, a genetic counselor, endocrinologist, or nuclear medicine physician may be indicated, and the nurse navigator then makes arrangements as needed to ensure that all necessary team members are scheduled for the MDC consultation.

Nurse Navigators' Role and Responsibilities

The role of the nurse navigators at the Graham Cancer Center was designed to predominantly focus on personalized care coordination to help overcome healthcare system barriers and expedite timely access to quality health care from diagnosis throughout cancer survivorship. According to Wilkes (2011), "nurses have much power to help patients and their families value and participate in adherence and persistence of cancer treatment" (p. 309). The nurse can act as a catalyst to minimize many of the institutional or health system barriers and provide effective communication to establish a trusting relationship with patients and families and reinforce teaching (Wilkes, 2011).

Nurse navigators can identify patients through many routes, of which the most common at the Graham Cancer Center is physician referral to the MDC. Nurse navigators may receive direct referrals from other team members; for example, the inpatient discharge planner may coordinate patient's discharge but refer the patient to the nurse navigator for coordination of follow-up needs. Patients also may self-refer to the nurse navigation program.

A primary role of nurse navigators at the Graham Cancer Center is to serve as the main contact person for patients and the healthcare team. The nurse navigators use a holistic approach for assessing and supporting the needs of patients and families. This is accomplished through introducing appropriate support services, linking patients with community agencies, performing follow-up calls to patients at home, providing information about support groups and educational programs for patients and families, and reinforcing education regarding disease, treatments, side effects, and adverse reactions. While serving as the single point of contact to help resolve problems that patients, families, and physicians encounter, nurse navigators monitor patients' progress through the cancer continuum and assist with communication among the patient, family, and healthcare team members. Other responsibilities include performance improvement projects, HIT participation and facilitation, program planning, and health promotion and disease prevention education for patients, caregivers, and the community. The nurse navigators work closely with agencies in the community, such as the American Cancer Society, the Cancer Support Community, the Leukemia & Lymphoma Society, and the Ovarian Cancer Coalition, to offer support groups and educational programs.

The responsibilities of the nurse navigators at the Graham Cancer Center at times overlapped with those of other team members, which enabled early learning opportunities and assisted with defining the unique role for nurse navigators as compared to other support staff (see Figure 8-4). Although each member of the Cancer Care Management team plays a distinct part in the shared goal of improving or maintaining patients' health, extensive interdisciplinary collaboration exists among departmental staff (see Figure 8-5). For example, the nurse navigator may discuss services available through Cancer Care Management, support groups, and symptom management. The social worker and dietitian may reinforce the same information, yet each team member advances the patient's knowledge with the overall objective of improving health and self-care abilities.

Program Metrics

The Graham Cancer Center identified several program metrics to measure navigation outcomes, including inpatient length of stay, clinical trial accrual, patient satisfaction, patient-reported quality of life, and referrals to outside agencies for coordination of services. Specific initiatives that nurse navigators have focused on related to these metrics include
- Decreasing wait time from diagnosis to first treatment modality
- Increasing referrals to registered dietitians for high-risk cancer diagnosis
- Decreasing wait time for dental clearance for patients with HNC and patients started on bisphosphonate therapy
- Partnering with the inpatient oncology department to decrease length of stay by initiating daily multidisciplinary rounds
- Auditing tumor conference recommendations to ensure discussion and follow-through of National Comprehensive Cancer Network (NCCN) guidelines with compliance rates presented quarterly to the cancer committee

Figure 8-4. Major Responsibilities for Core Members of the Helen F. Graham Cancer Center Cancer Care Management Department

Nurse Navigators
- Assess patient and family needs, introduce appropriate support services
- Link patients with community agencies
- Conduct follow-up calls to patients and families at home
- Provide information on support groups and educational programs to patients and families
- Facilitate and coordinate care in the multidisciplinary centers
- Reinforce education regarding disease, treatments, side effects and adverse reactions, and reportable signs and symptoms
- Assess for discharge planning needs and coordinate with inpatient staff; follow up after discharge to ensure services are set up as planned
- Complete tumor conference documentation and audits

Social Workers
- Perform psychosocial assessments
- Identify community resources
- Address insurance questions and provide financial counseling assistance
- Coordinate hospice referrals and placement at skilled nursing facilities
- Arrange transportation for treatment
- Assist with skilled nursing facility placement
- Counsel patient and families
- Facilitate support groups
- Assist with end-of-life decision making
- Provide bereavement support
- Participate in performance improvement projects and facilitate health improvement teams

Financial Assistants
- Verify insurance benefits and obtain authorization for treatment
- Complete charitable care and medication assistance applications
- Evaluate patients for Medicaid/Medicare eligibility
- Assess patients for Special Needs fund
- Assist patients with application for Health Care Center
- Coordinate Community Assistance Program
- Assist in connecting patients with community resources

Registered Dietitians
- Provide individual and group nutrition counseling

Health Psychologist
- Provide individual and group counseling to patients, families, or those with a cancer history
- Conduct psychological assessments, including cognitive screening
- Provide bereavement support

Note. Figure courtesy of Christiana Care Health System. Used with permission.

Figure 8-5. Interdisciplinary Collaboration Within the Helen F. Graham Cancer Center Cancer Care Management Department

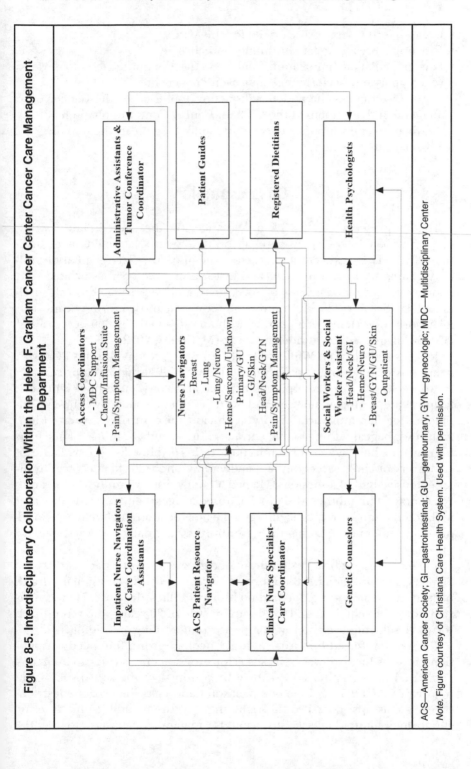

ACS—American Cancer Society; GI—gastrointestinal; GU—genitourinary; GYN—gynecologic; MDC—Multidisciplinary Center

Note. Figure courtesy of Christiana Care Health System. Used with permission.

- Creating order sets by disease site for the MDCs
- Creating a breast cancer continuum spreadsheet
- Forming a Patient- and Family-Centered Care Committee to help develop yearly goals and performance improvement activities.

Figure 8-6 depicts the patient satisfaction tool used by the Cancer Care Management department at the Graham Cancer Center to obtain feedback on navigation and support services, and Figure 8-7 reflects the tool used for feedback from providers.

Case Example

HNC represents roughly 3% of all cancers in the United States, with a staggering $3.6 billion spent annually on treatment (National Cancer Institute, 2013). These cancers are limited to the oral cavity, larynx, pharynx, salivary glands, and nasal passages and historically have been associated with poor treatment outcomes. As of 2008, head and neck squamous cell carcinoma (HNSCC) was the 10th most commonly diagnosed form of cancer in men worldwide (Jemal et al., 2011), with an estimated 650,000 new cases of HNSCC diagnosed worldwide each year (McCreery, 2012).

Joe was a 68-year-old White male who initially presented to his PCP with symptoms of hoarseness, pain, and difficulty swallowing for approximately two weeks prior to developing a palpable and slowly enlarging right neck lymph node. Unfortunately, he had no relief after a seven-day course of antibiotic. Joe had a medical history significant for controlled hypertension, gastroesophageal reflux disease, chronic rhinitis, and chronic left knee pain for which he had had multiple injections by his orthopedist. Joe had a surgical history of cholecystectomy, appendectomy, and right hemicolectomy after extensive lysis of adhesions. He had a family history significant for stomach cancer in his mother who was diagnosed at age 64 and remains alive and well. Joe had no known drug allergies. His medications included aspirin 81 mg daily, omeprazole 20 mg daily, lisinopril 20 mg daily, and carvedilol 25 mg daily.

Joe had a distant history significant of cigarette use (one pack per day for 35 years, a habit which he discontinued 15 years ago). He occasionally drank beer in the social setting. Joe had no history of illicit drug use. He was married with adult children and lived with his wife of 30 years, who was retired. Joe was a self-employed contractor, performing roofing and siding.

Joe's PCP referred him to a surgical oncologist for a fine needle aspiration biopsy, which showed cells suspicious for squamous cell carcinoma. A computed tomography (CT) scan (with contrast) of the soft tissue of the neck revealed a 2.5 × 3.1 cm complex solid and cystic heterogeneously enhancing mass just dorsal to the right angle of the mandible and anterior sternocleidomastoid muscle, suspicious for malignant metastasis to level IIA

Figure 8-6. Patient Satisfaction Survey Used at the Helen F. Graham Cancer Center for Navigation and Support Services Feedback

HELEN F. GRAHAM
CANCER CENTER

CHRISTIANA CARE ⊕ HEALTH SYSTEM

NCI COMMUNITY
CANCER CENTERS
P R O G R A M

Dear Madam/Sir,

In an effort to improve the services provided by the Cancer Care Management program, we are asking for your help. Please complete the following survey and return in the postage paid envelope provided.

Age: ____

Gender:
M ____   F ____

Type of Cancer: _____

Ethnicity: ____
N = Non-Hispanic
H = Hispanic
U = Unknown

Race: ____
1. WHT = White
2. BL = Black or African American
3. ASN = Asian
4. HW = Native Hawaiian or Pacific Islander
5. AI = American Indian/Alaskan Native
6. MUL = More than one race
7. UNK = Unknown or other
8. Do not wish to provide information

Directions: Please rate each statement with a number indicating your agreement	Agree				Disagree
	1	2	3	4	5
Was friendly and courteous	O	O	O	O	O
Answered questions in a manner easily understood	O	O	O	O	O
Showed sensitivity/concern about your cultural beliefs/practices	O	O	O	O	O
Provided explanation of services available through the Cancer Center	O	O	O	O	O
Provided assistance with your appointments and referrals	O	O	O	O	O
Provided helpful educational materials and/or community resources	O	O	O	O	O
Helpfulness of understanding your treatment plan	O	O	O	O	O

Comments

(Continued on next page)

Figure 8-6. Patient Satisfaction Survey Used at the Helen F. Graham Cancer Center for Navigation and Support Services Feedback *(Continued)*

If you were seen by a support service below please circle which one and answer the questions related to your satisfaction with that service.
1. Social Worker
2. Dietitian
3. Financial/Transportation Coordinator
4. Health Psychology
5. Mind, Body, and Spirit Wellness Program
6. Survivorship Program
7. Pain/Palliative Care Team

	Agree				Disagree
	1	2	3	4	5
Was friendly and courteous	O	O	O	O	O
Answered questions in a manner easily understood	O	O	O	O	O
Showed sensitivity/concern about my cultural beliefs/practices	O	O	O	O	O
Provided helpful educational materials and/or community resources	O	O	O	O	O

Comments

If you were seen by a second support service below please circle which one and answer the questions related to your satisfaction with that service.
1. Social Worker
2. Dietitian
3. Financial/Transportation Coordinator
4. Health Psychology
5. Mind, Body, and Spirit Wellness Program
6. Survivorship Program
7. Pain/Palliative Care Team

	Agree				Disagree
	1	2	3	4	5
Was friendly and courteous	O	O	O	O	O
Answered questions in a manner easily understood	O	O	O	O	O
Showed sensitivity/concern about my cultural beliefs/practices	O	O	O	O	O
Provided helpful educational materials and/or community resources	O	O	O	O	O

(Continued on next page)

Figure 8-6. Patient Satisfaction Survey Used at the Helen F. Graham Cancer Center for Navigation and Support Services Feedback _(Continued)_
Comments:
Additional comments and/or suggestions for improvement:
Name (optional):
Thank you for taking the time to respond to this survey. Your input is very important and will enable us to offer the best possible care.
Note. Figure courtesy of Christiana Care Health System. Used with permission.

lymph nodes. In addition, there was asymmetric prominence and enhancement of the mucosa in the right vallecula and lingual tonsil, suspicious for squamous cell carcinoma. A chest x-ray revealed no active disease in the chest. No clear-cut primary site was identified on radiographic scans.

The surgical oncologist performed an evaluation under anesthesia where biopsies were obtained from the nasopharynx, oral cavity, and base of the tongue. He performed a tonsillectomy and right neck dissection at that time. Pathologic review of the neck contents revealed that one of the 24 lymph nodes contained metastatic squamous cell carcinoma. There was a suggestion of extranodal extension. Pathologic review of biopsies from the base of the tongue confirmed the presence of moderately to poorly differentiated squamous cell carcinoma and human papillomavirus (HPV).

The surgical oncologist then referred Joe to the navigation program at the Graham Cancer Center for an MDC evaluation regarding treatment options for his locally/regionally advanced base of the tongue squamous cell carcinoma. Management of HNC brings unique physiologic and psychosocial issues, which often are amplified by the complexities of multimodality treatment. The initial evaluation and treatment plan for patients with HNC requires a team approach with expertise in caring for these complex cases. Figure 8-8 identifies specific roles of the various HNC MDC team members.

Team members reviewed Joe's records and diagnostic studies. During the MDC consultations, Joe acknowledged a 30-pound weight loss over the past three months along with persistent dysphagia. He had several teeth that appeared decayed, and he admitted to not seeing a dentist in more than five years. A neck examination revealed that the neck dissection scar was healing well. The surgical oncologist performed a fiber-optic nasopharyngeal laryngoscopy, which showed no visible residual disease. Treatment options were discussed with Joe and his wife.

Figure 8-7. Provider Satisfaction Survey Used at the Helen F. Graham Cancer Center for Navigation and Support Services Feedback

HELEN F. GRAHAM
CANCER CENTER

CHRISTIANA CARE ⦿ HEALTH SYSTEM

NCI COMMUNITY
CANCER CENTERS
P R O G R A M

Dear Physician,

Please rate these support services in terms of their consistency in meeting your expectations (1 being the lowest and 5 being the highest).

	Poor				Excellent
	1	2	3	4	5
Nurse Navigator	O	O	O	O	O
Social Work	O	O	O	O	O
Registered Dietitian	O	O	O	O	O
Financial/Transportation Coordinator	O	O	O	O	O
Health Psychology	O	O	O	O	O
Mind, Body, and Spirit Wellness Program	O	O	O	O	O
Survivorship Program	O	O	O	O	O
Pain/Palliative Care Team	O	O	O	O	O

I was aware these services existed.
Yes ___ No ___

Additional comments regarding the Cancer Care Management program:

Name (optional):

Thank you for taking the time to respond to this survey. Your input is very important and will enable us to offer the best possible care.

Note. Figure courtesy of Christiana Care Health System. Used with permission.

Most patients with HPV-associated HNSCC are diagnosed with stage III or IV disease. These patients should receive multimodality treatment including surgery, chemotherapy, and radiation in accordance with NCCN (2013) guidelines. NCCN (2013) suggests all patients with HNC are best managed with clinical trials. After the MDC team assessed Joe, they determined he was ineligible for treatment on clinical trial due to the extranodal extension of the disease. Of interest, HPV-associated HNSCC is receiving special consideration in clinical trials because of its unique char-

---

Figure 8-8. Team Member Roles Within the Head and Neck Cancer Multidisciplinary Center at the Helen F. Graham Cancer Center

Surgical oncologist—Lead the team with input and treatment planning; evaluate for removal of tumor

Medical oncologist—Input with treatment planning; evaluate for chemotherapy or biologic therapy

Radiation oncologist—Input with treatment planning; evaluate for radiation therapy

Dentist or prosthodontics—Assess dental status and need for extractions; prevention of dental problems

Nurse navigator—Coordinate scheduling of multidisciplinary center evaluations, provide education and guidance to the patient through the cancer continuum

Research nurse—Assess for clinical trial candidacy and coordinate trial elements

Social worker/health psychologist—Assess psychosocial needs and help address the emotional concerns of cancer diagnosis

Speech pathologist—Evaluate for ability to improve speech and swallow

Dietitian—Evaluate and assist in maintaining nutrition status

Rehabilitation specialist—Evaluate for ability to improve physical functioning

Note. Figure courtesy of Christiana Care Health System. Used with permission.

---

acteristics, and future clinical trials are expected to assess and analyze HPV status.

Joe was, however, an excellent candidate for biologic therapy in conjunction with radiation therapy. Survival and quality of life for people with HNC has progressed over the past few years because of new treatments. Preservation of form and function is a key element in the overall care of patients with HNC (Sivesind & Pairé, 2009). Patients with HNC are greatly affected physically, socially, and mentally by facial disfigurement and dysfunction of speech and swallow as a result of disease and treatment. Targeting the epidermal growth factor receptor with monoclonal antibodies such as cetuximab has resulted in clinical gains (Sivesind & Pairé, 2009).

Current standards of care include radiation therapy alone or surgery alone for stage I–II oropharyngeal cancer. Available options established through prospective trials for more locally advanced cancers include radiation with concurrent cisplatin or cetuximab, induction chemotherapy followed by radiation with or without concurrent systemic therapy, and surgery with postoperative radiation with or without concurrent cisplatin (Sturgis & Ang, 2011). A newer technique, intensity-modulated radiation therapy (IMRT), has significantly improved the efficacy of radiation therapy while minimizing side effects. IMRT uses three-dimensional computer planning to more accurately target malignant tissue and adjusts the radiation dose intensity across the treatment field to spare more unaffected tissue.

Managing and preventing sequelae of radical surgery, radiation therapy, and chemotherapy (e.g., pain, xerostomia, speech and swallow problems, depression) require professionals who are familiar with the disease (Pfister et al., 2011). To ensure prompt referral to these supportive services, the HNC nurse navigator developed a set of standing orders to assist with the coordination of appointments (see Figure 8-9). To facilitate patient understanding of the many MDC consultations, the HNC navigator developed a multipurpose tool (see Figure 8-10) to provide patient and family education, empowerment, and an organized method to manage multiple appointments. The three-page checklist is sectioned for appointments likely to be scheduled (such as dental, positron-emission tomography, CT, magnetic resonance imaging, dietary consultation, feeding tube placement, speech and swallowing evaluation, home care, chemotherapy, radiation therapy, and surgery). This "at-a-glance" document has resulted in more efficient scheduling, ease in communication and patient education, and decreased likelihood of scheduling conflicts or missed appointments causing stress and additional coordination. This checklist was provided to Joe and lessened some of the anxiety of what appointments to expect.

It is essential for people with HNC to be evaluated by a dentist before, during, and after cancer treatment, especially when treatment involves radiation therapy. Radiation can cause dry mouth, mouth sores, taste changes, and jaw stiffness. Because of this, a dental appointment is usually the first appointment to be coordinated by the nurse navigator. Good oral health decreases complications during and after cancer treatment. Because only a few weeks are typically available in which to complete the dental evaluation and treatment, it is critical for the nurse navigator to forward information to the dentist as soon as possible. Figure 8-11 depicts the dental clearance letter developed by the HNC navigator at the Graham Cancer Center as a result of a project focused on identifying and removing barriers to treatment initiation. Any delay in dental care can cause a subsequent postponement of cancer treatment, which may put the patient at risk for cancer relapse.

Early results of this process improvement project revealed a 65.8% decrease in time from MDC consultation to initial dental visit and a 10% decrease in time from MDC consultation to dental clearance. In Joe's case, the nurse navigator arranged an appointment for Joe with a local dentist who prescribed topical fluoride trays prior to radiation therapy to reduce the risk of infection of the teeth and gums.

At the time of the MDC visit, the nurse navigator obtained an order to coordinate a dietitian consultation. Patients with HNC often are malnourished at diagnosis because of the tumor and the tumor-associated symptoms of dysphagia and odynophagia. Poor dietary habits result from a history of alcohol and tobacco abuse and can lead to changes in metabolism and vitamin and mineral deficiencies, which further contribute to malnutrition. The outcome of chemotherapy and radiation treatment is not as favorable when there is an interruption of treatment; therefore, it is essential to address and incorporate nutritional interventions into the care plan for every patient with HNC before initiating definitive treatment.

The nurse navigator obtained an order to coordinate a speech and swallow evaluation. HNC often results in significant functional changes including alterations in or loss of voice, disruptions in speech production, and deterioration of swallowing ability (Lewin & Hutcheson, 2009). The pa-

Figure 8-9. Standing Orders for the Head and Neck Cancer Multidisciplinary Center at the Helen F. Graham Cancer Center

CHRISTIANA CARE
HEALTH SERVICES

DOCORD

DOCTOR'S ORDER SHEET
Instructions:
Do not return charts with new or changed orders to rack.
No conditional (dependent on the approval of another physician) medication orders will be honored

HELEN F. GRAHAM CANCER CENTER
HEAD AND NECK CANCER PATIENTS ORDERS
MD5412 (03/11)

MARK REQUESTED ORDERS AND/ OR BOXES IF INDICATED.
PRE-MARKED BOX ORDERS WILL BE PERFORMED UNLESS OTHERWISE NOTED.

DOCTOR'S ORDER	REQUISTIONED	NOTED
Patient: _____ Date of birth (DOB):_____		
Allergies (include reaction):_____		
Diagnosis:_____Date:_____ICD-9 Code:_____		
Mark below all orders which are to be implemented in accordance with Cancer Care Management Head and Neck Program Protocols		
❑ Test tissue biopsy for HPV, P-16 and EGFR		
❑ Dental evaluation Dentist:_____		
❑ Positron Emission Tomography (PET)		
❑ CAT Scan Type: with IV contrast. Is patient diabetic? ❑ yes ❑ no		
❑ Magnetic resonance imaging (MRI)Type:_____		
❑ Feeding Tube consult: Dr:_____Agency:_____		
❑ Nutritional Consult – Registered Dietitian		
❑ Speech/swallowing evaluation with speech pathologist ❑ Pre-op ❑ Post-op ❑ Pre-radiation therapy		
❑ Radiation Oncology Dr:_____		
❑ Medical Oncology Dr:_____		
❑ Surgical Follow up Dr:_____		
❑ Return to Multidisciplinary Center Date:_____		
❑ Rehabilitation: Dr:_____ ❑ Pre-op ❑ Post-op ❑ Inpatient ❑ Outpatient		
❑ Health Psychologist consult		
❑ Cancer Care Management Team		
❑ Discharge Planner Consult		
❑ Smoking Cessation Referral		
❑ Alcohol Cessation Referral		

_____
Signature/Title

Cell phone number
__/__/__
_____
Print Name or ID#   Date   Time

16758 S (49140) (0510)C   DOCTOR'S ORDERS-Order

Note. Figure courtesy of Christiana Care Health System. Used with permission.

Figure 8-10. Patient Appointment Checklist for the Helen F. Graham Cancer Center's Head and Neck Cancer Multidisciplinary Center

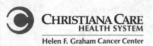

CHRISTIANA CARE
HEALTH SYSTEM
Helen F. Graham Cancer Center

Head and Neck Multidisciplinary Center Patient Appointment Checklist

Appointment	Why this appointment is important
Dental Date _____ Time _____ Robert N. Arm, D.M.D. Location: Wilmington Hospital Floor _____ Room _____ 302-428-6468 **Or:** **Your dentist** Dentist _____ Date _____ Time _____	■ **Priority Appointment** – You must have dental work done prior to radiation treatment or planning. ■ You may need teeth cleaning. ■ You may need fillings checked. ■ You may need teeth extracted. ■ You may need a fluoride treatment. ■ If seeing your own dentist, please have your dentist call Dr. Arm at 302-428-6468.

PET Scan
Date _____ Time _____
Location: Christiana Hospital, First Floor
Outpatient Way Station 7, Room 1520
302-733-1528
Or:
Agency: _____
Date _____ Time _____
Location: _____
Phone Number _____
	■ This scan allows physicians to see if tumor cells are located in parts of the body other than the head and neck area.
	■ **This test must be done before having any teeth extracted.**
	■ Please let your Cancer Care Coordinator know if you are claustrophobic.
	■ **Required preparation:**
	  ● Do not eat or drink anything for four (4) hours prior to the test.
	  ● Limit carbohydrate intake for 24 hours before test.
	  ● Test may take up to two (2) hours.

CT Scan of _____
Date _____ Time _____
Location: Christiana Care
Helen F. Graham Cancer Center
Or:
Agency _____
Date _____
Time _____
Location _____
Phone _____
	■ This scan provides physicians with a clear picture of tumor size and location.
	■ Please let your Cancer Care Coordinator know if you take oral medications for diabetes.
	■ **Required preparation:**
	  ● You may not be able to eat or drink anything for four (4) hours prior to the test. Ask your Cancer Care Coordinator for specific instructions.
	  ● You may be asked to drink a contrast material two (2) hours prior to the test. Ask your Cancer Care Coordinator if you need to do so.

(Continued on next page)

Figure 8-10. Patient Appointment Checklist for the Helen F. Graham Cancer Center's Head and Neck Cancer Multidisciplinary Center (Continued)

Appointment	Why this appointment is important
MRI of_____ Date_____Time _____ Location: Christiana Hospital (Christiana Care Imaging Services located on the walkway between the hospital and Medical Arts Pavilion I) Or: Agency _____ Date_____ Time _____ Location_____ Phone	■ An MRI gives physicians a three-dimensional view of your internal organs. ■ Please let your Cancer Care Coordinator know if you are claustrophobic. ■ **Required preparation:** ● Do not wear any metal objects (jewelry, hairpins, watches, etc.).
Dietary Consultation Date_____Time _____ Dietitian: _____ Location: Christiana Care Helen F. Graham Cancer Center 302-623-4500	■ The dietitian will help you maintain your normal body weight and proper nutrition throughout treatment. ■ The dietician will make recommendations for tube feedings, if needed.
Feeding Tube Consultation Physician _____ Date_____ Time _____ Location _____ **Feeding Tube Insertion** Date_____Time _____ Location _____	■ This type of tube is inserted into your stomach for feedings when it is hard to swallow. ■ You will get more detailed information on how the tube works and what it will do for you during your consultation.
Speech/Swallowing Evaluation Date_____Time _____ Speech Language Pathologist: Phone _____ Location: Christiana Hospital (not at the Cancer Center) Or: _____ _____	■ The speech language pathologist will check your speech and swallowing ability and provide exercises to help you maintain your speech and swallowing function throughout your treatment.
Home Care Agency _____ Phone Number _____ Date of 1st visit _____	■ Your home care provider will help educate you about your feeding tube.

(Continued on next page)

Figure 8-10. Patient Appointment Checklist for the Helen F. Graham Cancer Center's Head and Neck Cancer Multidisciplinary Center *(Continued)*

Head and Neck Multidisciplinary Center
Patient Appointment Checklist (continued)

Physicians	Roles in your Treatment
Chemotherapy Charles Schneider, M.D., FACP Date_____Time _____ Location: Christiana Care Helen F. Graham Cancer Center, Suite 2200 302-366-1200 **Or:** Dr: _____ Location: _____ Date_____Time _____ Phone: _____	▪ This physician will recommend the most appropriate chemotherapy medications and dosages for your treatment. ▪ He/she will help you manage any chemotherapy and cancer-related side effects such as pain or nausea.
Radiation Therapy Adam Raben, M.D. Date _____Time _____ Location: Christiana Care Helen F. Graham Cancer Center, Suite 1100 302-623-4800 **Or:** Radiation Oncologist _____ Location:_____ Date_____Time _____ Phone:_____	▪ This physician will determine the appropriate type and extent of radiation therapy you will receive. ▪ He/she will help you manage the side effects of radiation therapy such as skin irritation and trouble swallowing.
Surgeon Name _____ Location: _____ Date_____Time _____ Phone: _____	▪ For recommended surgery.

Note. Figure courtesy of Christiana Care Health System. Used with permission.

tient may be at risk for choking on solid food, liquids, or even saliva. These problems can occur as a result of not only the disease but also treatment. During the evaluation, the speech pathologist assessed Joe for xerostomia and reduced trismus. Specialized exercises and swallowing techniques were taught to Joe to reduce the risk of speech, voice, or swallowing complications. Although not necessary for Joe, other tests, such as a video fluoroscopic swallowing study (an x-ray) or a fiber-optic endoscopic evaluation of swallowing (known as FEES) study, may be done to better evaluate swallowing function.

Because of Joe's self-employment and insurance needs, the nurse navigator arranged a meeting for him with the outpatient social worker. Patients with HNC often need assistance in sorting through the complex emotions and issues that arise. Social workers are able to educate patients and families

---

Figure 8-11. Dental Clearance Form for the Helen F. Graham Cancer Center's Head and Neck Cancer Multidisciplinary Center

HELEN F. GRAHAM
CANCER CENTER
CHRISTIANA CARE ⊕ HEALTH SYSTEM

NCI COMMUNITY
CANCER CENTERS
PROGRAM

DENTAL CLEARANCE FOR HEAD AND NECK CANCER PATIENTS:

Your patient is presenting to you for a dental evaluation in preparation for cancer treatment. Good oral health may minimize complications during and after his/her cancer treatment. Elimination of all potential sources of oral infection is an important aspect of preparation of head and neck cancer treatment and we ask for your assistance in achieving this.

Please give your patient priority for an appointment to expedite dental care as limitations on time available for dental care may exist due to your patient's cancer treatment. You probably have only a few weeks in which to complete your evaluation and treatment. Keep in mind treatment decisions will not only affect your patient's dental health now and during treatment but for the rest of your patient's life.

Please read the following instructions carefully:
1) Perform a complete dental evaluation with full mouth periodontal charting. If the patient is edentulous, a panoramic film should be taken.
2) Fill in completely the attached dental evaluation report, including your treatment plan. Fax the evaluation to LaTonya Mann at XXX-XXX-XXXX.

Thank you for helping to prepare your patient for his/her cancer treatment. Your expeditious care of your patient will hopefully improve the course and outcome of his/her cancer treatment. If you have any questions, please do not hesitate to contact me or your patient's radiation oncologist.

LaTonya E. Mann, RN, MSN, OCN, CRNI
Head and Neck Oncology Nurse Navigator
Helen F. Graham Cancer Center
Phone:
Fax:
E-mail:

(Continued on next page)

Figure 8-11. Dental Clearance Form for the Helen F. Graham Cancer Center's Head and Neck Cancer Multidisciplinary Center *(Continued)*

CHRISTIANA CARE
HEALTH SERVICES
Helen F. Graham Cancer Center

HFGCC

PRE CANCER TREATMENT
DENTAL CLEARANCE/EVALUATION

Patient name:

Date of birth:

SECTION 1: DENTAL CLEARANCE/REFERRAL
Sections 1 and 2 to be completed by Oncologist or Nurse Navigator and faxed to Dental Office prior to patient appointment.

Diagnosis: _____

Treatment plan: _____

Anticipated dose to oral cavity and mandible: _____

Referring physician: _____

Comments: _____

_____

Signature/Title   Print Name or ID#   ___/___/___   _____
                                                  Date   Time

SECTION 2

Faxed to: Dentist (print name): _____ at: (___) ____ – ____

Signature/Title   Print Name or ID#   ___/___/___   _____
                                                  Date   Time

SECTION 3: DENTAL CLEARANCE/EVALUATION
Section 3 to be completed by Dentist and faxed back to Oncology Office.

Panorex/full mouth x-ray (FMX) performed: ☐ No   ☐ Yes

Further dental work required: ☐ No   ☐ Yes

Does patient require extractions: ☐ No   ☐ Yes, scheduled date: ___/___/___ How many: ____
                                                       Post extraction follow-up date: ___/___/___

Fluoride trays made: ☐ No   ☐ Yes

Patient cleared to start radiation therapy: ☐ No   ☐ Yes

Further treatment plan and expected dates: _____

_____

_____

_____

_____

Dentist Signature/Title   Print Name or ID#   ___/___/___   _____
                                                  Date   Time

23158 S(84655)(0112)C

Note. Figure courtesy of Christiana Care Health System. Used with permission.

about support groups, psychosocial assistance, and other practical resources that are available.

Joe's navigator was aware that anxiety is a very common response in patients who are coping with a cancer diagnosis. During the post-team visit, Joe and his wife expressed candid concerns about the diagnosis and treatment plan. During this critical time, the nurse navigator provided education and further information about various resources within the cancer center as well as within the community. The nurse navigator reassured Joe that all initial appointments would be coordinated and he would be notified of specific date, time, and location of appointments. The nurse navigator provided Joe with a patient treatment journal containing contact information of all team members and National Cancer Institute education materials. Joe confirmed that he understood the treatment plan and said he would contact the nurse navigator with further needs or concerns. The nurse navigator further reassessed Joe's needs at each telephone and face-to-face encounter. The nurse navigator not only followed up with Joe but also the radiation oncology nurse, medical oncology nurse, and other members of the multidisciplinary team to obtain information regarding the patient's status and any changes in the treatment plan.

According to Ridge, Mehra, Lango, and Feigenberg (2013), surveillance after treatment of HNC is mandatory because early detection of second primary cancers or locoregional recurrence yields the best chance for disease control. Nearly two-thirds of patients whose HNC recurs develop a tumor at or near the primary site or in the neck nodes, with locoregional relapse accounting for approximately 80% of primary treatment failures. The majority (80%) of HNC recurrences occur within two years (Ridge et al., 2013). Joe's radiation oncology nurse asked the survivorship nurse navigator to meet with Joe and his wife during the final week of treatment. The focus of this visit was to educate Joe regarding the potential late and long-term physical and psychosocial effects of treatment. The survivorship nurse navigator arranged to meet with Joe at his first follow-up appointment to assess for any unmet mental and physical needs using an abbreviated quality-of-life scale.

At the first follow-up appointment, the survivorship navigator made referrals to the dietitian and surgical oncologist based on Joe's nutrition concerns and limited range of motion in his right arm. The survivorship nurse navigator also assessed Joe's need for other services, such as speech therapy, health psychology, social work, and genetic counseling, and determined he did not require further referral. The navigator obtained consent for release of Joe's medical information to compile the survivor treatment summary and care plan and then used the Journey Forward treatment summary template to prepare these documents. After completion of the treatment summary and care plan documents, the survivorship nurse navigator scheduled an appointment to meet with Joe and his wife to review these and ensure understanding of the follow-up and surveillance schedule.

Conclusion

The nurse navigation program at Christiana Care reflects the philosophy of providing patients with cancer and their families with the best possible multidisciplinary care. A multidisciplinary team approach provides optimal care for the challenging population of patients with cancer. Communication and collaboration among healthcare professionals will increase the quality of care provided while acknowledging and respecting each team member's talents and expertise.

When professionals within the healthcare team have mutual goals and work in a cooperative and collaborative manner, efficiency of the specialty consultations and coordination of care is maximized. Lack of communication among members of the healthcare teams can lead to confusion about the diagnosis, prognosis, and treatment plan. This is not only stressful for patients but frustrating for healthcare professionals as well. Initial barriers experienced by the HNC nurse navigator at the Graham Cancer Center included missed appointments, lack of efficiency in obtaining orders for necessary diagnostics prior to MDC consultations, lack of dental guidelines, transportation concerns, and insurance issues. Most of these were eased with tools developed by the nurse navigator and referrals to available organizational and community resources.

References

Christiana Care Health System. (2013). Christiana Care Health System 2013 year in review. Retrieved from http://www.christianacare.org/yearinreview

Collins, L.G., Wender, R., & Altshuler, M. (2010). An opportunity for coordinated cancer care: Intersection of health care reform, primary care providers, and cancer patients. *Cancer Journal, 16*, 593–599. doi:10.1097/PPO.0b013e3181feee9a

Jemal, A., Bray, F., Center, M.M., Ferlay, J., Ward, E., & Forman, D. (2011). Global cancer statistics. *CA: A Cancer Journal for Clinicians, 61*, 69–90. doi:10.3322/caac.20107

Lewin, J.S., & Hutcheson, K.A. (2009). General principles of rehabilitation of speech, voice, and swallowing function after treatment of head and neck cancer. In L.B. Harrison, R.B. Sessions, & W.K. Hong (Eds.), *Head and neck cancer: A multidisciplinary approach* (3rd ed., pp. 168–177). Philadelphia, PA: Lippincott Williams and Wilkins.

McCreery, H. (2012). Advancements in head and neck cancer: Better treatment options offer more promise. *ONS Connect, 27*(3), 10–14. Retrieved from http://connect.ons.org/issue/march-2012/up-front/advancements-in-head-and-neck-cancer

National Cancer Institute. (2013, October). A snapshot of head and neck cancer. Retrieved from http://www.cancer.gov/researchandfunding/snapshots/pdf/headandneck-snapshot.pdf

National Comprehensive Cancer Network. (2013). *NCCN Clinical Practice Guidelines in Oncology: Head and neck cancers* [v.2.2013]. Retrieved from http://www.nccn.org/professionals/physician_gls/pdf/head-and-neck.pdf

Petrelli, N.J. (2010). A community cancer center program: Getting to the next level. *Journal of the American College of Surgeons, 210,* 261–270. doi:10.1016/j.jamcollsurg.2009.11.015

Pfister, D.G., Ang, K.K., Brizel, D.M., Burtness, B.A., Cmelak, A.J., Colevas, A.D., … Worden, F. (2011). Head and neck cancers. *Journal of the National Comprehensive Cancer Network, 9,* 596–650.

Ridge, J.A., Mehra, R., Lango, M.N., & Feigenberg, S. (2013). Head and neck tumors. In D.G. Haller, L.D. Wagman, K.A. Camphausen, & W.J. Hoskins (Eds.), *Cancer management: A multidisciplinary approach; Medical, surgical, and radiation oncology.* Retrieved from http://www.cancernetwork.com/cancer-management/head-and-neck-tumors

Sivesind, D.M., & Pairé, S. (2009). Coping with cancer: Patient and family issues. In C.C. Burke (Ed.), *Psychosocial dimensions of oncology nursing care* (2nd ed., pp. 1–28). Pittsburgh, PA: Oncology Nursing Society.

Steward, N. (2006). Implementing and operating a thoracic multi-disciplinary center: The Helen F. Graham Cancer Center experience. *Association of Cancer Executives Update, 7*(4), pp. 1, 3, 5.

Sturgis, E.M., & Ang, K.K. (2011). The epidemic of HPV-associated oropharyngeal cancer is here: Is it time to change our treatment paradigms? *Journal of the National Comprehensive Cancer Network, 9,* 665–673.

Wilkes, G.M. (2011). *Targeted cancer therapy: A handbook for nurses.* Burlington, MA: Jones and Bartlett.

CHAPTER 9

Program Assessment and Outcome Metrics

Jay R. Swanson, APRN, MSN, Laura S. Hunnibell, APRN, DNP, AOCN®, and Sharon Bartelt, RN, MSN, MBA, CPHQ, CSSBB, OCN®

Introduction

Patients with cancer increasingly express a desire for navigation services at cancer centers. Through increased public awareness, patients have learned the benefits of navigation, either firsthand or from friends and family. Healthcare organizations focus marketing campaigns on navigation programs to promote the optimal patient experience. In addition, national organizations are working to concisely define the role of the oncology navigator (Brown et al., 2012). From a systems perspective, navigation is a mandatory component of any cancer center accredited by the American College of Surgeons (ACoS) Commission on Cancer (CoC) program (ACoS CoC, 2012). Therefore, the desire for cancer centers to quickly and efficiently build navigation programs is gaining focus.

The endeavor to create an effective navigation program begins early in the development process. A review of the literature shows that navigation programs are extremely diverse; this can be attributed to successful navigation programs being built on the needs of the populations served (Braun et al., 2012). For example, a navigator working with a population of predominantly urban African Americans will likely identify different needs and use distinct strategies to facilitate those needs than a navigator working with a population of rural individuals. Therefore, each navigation program must determine specific operational methods to implement.

Most research done on navigation programs has focused on program outcomes (Campbell, Craig, Eggert, & Bailey-Dorton, 2010; Koh, Nelson, & Cook, 2011; Pedersen & Hack, 2010). Although one cannot assume that all navigation programs provide the same level of care, research has begun to more accurately define navigation and the value it provides (Case, 2011). Even with these efforts moving the practice of oncology navigation forward, once a program is developed, no standardized framework exists for evaluating the navigation program.

Current evidence focuses mostly on patient and programmatic outcomes of navigation. These outcome measures provide the initial framework that begin to illustrate the importance of patient navigation (Fillion et al., 2012; Pedersen & Hack, 2011). Although programs differ, the evidence points to a few consistencies in program evaluation: (a) patient satisfaction, (b) barrier reduction, (c) provider satisfaction, (d) diagnostics, (e) completion of therapy, (f) length of stay, (g) patients' perceived quality of life (QOL), (h) cost analysis, (i) cancer surveillance, and (j) appointment attendance (Jean-Pierre, Hendren, et al., 2011; Korber, Padula, Gray, & Powell, 2011; Thygesen, Pedersen, Kragstrup, Wagner, & Mogensen, 2011; Whitley et al., 2011).

Given the information that can be gathered on the value of navigation programs, navigators and program administrators must ascertain those elements that are vital in demonstrating the achievement of program goals and objectives. It is practical to assemble a broad range of data points to monitor past trends and extrapolate meaning from this analysis. Early in the establishment of a navigation program, the navigator is often responsible for gathering the data. Without advanced electronic methods, it can be challenging for the navigator to amass large amounts of data and have the time to provide the level of navigation services patients need. Therefore, careful tailoring of data collection toward specific outcomes will create an easier workflow for the navigator and be more helpful to the program's continued development, maturity, and prosperity.

Today, the healthcare industry is more focused on the effect of an intervention rather than the mere availability of such; thus, to provide navigation services without justification of merit will likely prove unsuccessful in program sustainability. The national movement to standardize the roles and benefits of navigation will assist in the overall development of stronger navigation programs (Brown et al., 2012). For individual programs, outcome evaluation provides a mechanism for resource allocation to the most needed and potentially beneficial programmatic pieces. Monitoring outcomes can provide valuable information on community needs and guide future discussion of program offerings. This identification of pressing needs encourages the navigation program to adapt and be able to meet this gap in care (Thygesen, Pedersen, Kragstrup, Wagner, & Mogensen, 2012). Without outcomes assessment, this process is difficult and unpredictable. It is unacceptable to believe that a program may exist within the same context of its genesis; rather, the program will need to adapt to the changing needs of the cancer population, the community, and the resources around which the program is located (Fiscella et al., 2011).

A program should be built, advanced, and evaluated through thoughtful and deliberate planning. It is no longer sufficient to simply have navigators available, but rather navigation programs must strive to improve program elements to continue to meet patients' needs (Yosha et al., 2011). Navigation provides essential psychosocial, financial, and physical benefits for patients with cancer (Hendren et al., 2011; Hook, Ware, Siler, & Packard, 2012; Robinson-White, Conroy, Slavish, & Rosenzweig, 2010; Swanson & Koch, 2010). Quality improvement and program evaluation enable navigators to provide the highest quality of care and support. Navigation involves anticipating and mobilizing available resources that patients may require throughout their cancer journey.

Navigation programs are developed within the boundaries of the system, focused on meeting the needs and expectations of the patients, communities, and healthcare organizations served. These needs and expectations assist in the development of overall program goals, objectives, and measurable outcomes, which typically are unique to each navigation program. Therefore, an adaptive approach to program development that meets the needs of the populations served allows programs to grow stronger and become more sustainable. Navigator programs that focus on meeting patients' evidence-based needs will perform better on national quality indicators (Chen et al., 2010; Weber, Mascarenhas, Bellin, Raab, & Wong, 2012). As programs improve their quality indicator scores, patient care is improved and disease morbidity and mortality, as well as hospital readmissions, are potentially reduced (Gilbert et al., 2011). Furthermore, initial efforts to cost-define navigation have shown programs with particularly well-defined outcomes to be more cost-effective (Markossian & Calhoun, 2011), which, in the end, results in more sustainable navigation programs.

In this chapter, an assessment tool related to the development and advancement of navigation programs will be presented. This tool was created in response to the lack of standardization in navigation program development. Following this, information will be covered regarding how to establish and measure program outcomes. Through the development of meaningful program metrics and targeted outcomes, navigation programs are able to best meet community needs and substantiate the crucial role of navigation in the delivery of superior cancer care. A case example of one facility's efforts to establish meaningful metrics and improve patient outcomes through navigation services will also be shared.

The Navigation Assessment Tool

Development

Navigation programs exist to bridge gaps in care within the communities served and connect patients to available resources. Often, it is the navigator's responsibility to assess the community to identify barriers to and gaps in care and then build a system that facilitates an efficient and seamless patient experience. However, navigators quickly learn that many challenges exist in this process, such as (a) attempts to distinguish navigation services from those of other team members without replicating services, (b) resistant physicians and staff, (c) lack of understanding (from patients, staff, providers, and even navigators) regarding navigator roles and responsibilities, (d) identification of resources and how to efficiently access them, (e) high turnover rates in local community resource offices, (f) complex or inefficient screening processes, (g) creation of navigation forms and documentation processes, and (h) promotion of navigation services, to name a few.

Navigation programs, as a whole, need to establish relevance within the healthcare system. As the programs become more common, this will become less of an issue. However, even established programs struggle to precisely define program merits and return on investment (ROI) to administration and other key stakeholders. As more patients express an expectation for navigation assistance, additional personnel and interventions may be necessary to deliver optimal program outcomes. Unless navigation programs are able to meet the needs of the community and demonstrate value to key stakeholders, program sustainability may be in jeopardy.

The National Cancer Institute (NCI) Community Cancer Centers Program (NCCCP) is a network of community hospitals throughout the United States focused on improving the quality of care delivered in the community setting (NCI, n.d.-a). One of the NCCCP's quality focus areas is patient navigation. Despite varied programmatic structures and populations served, collaboration among diverse navigation programs led to the development of a Navigation Assessment Tool (NAT) (see Figure 9-1). (This project was funded in whole or in part with Federal funds from the National Cancer Institute, National Institutes of Health, under Contract No. HHSN261200800001E. The content of this publication does not necessarily reflect the views or policies of the Department of Health and Human Services, nor does mention of trade names, commercial products, or organizations imply endorsement of the U.S. Government.)

Consistencies of program development and maturation were identified and characterized to create an evaluation tool that any program, from inception to maturity, could use to assess current program status and establish priorities for further enhancements.

Use of the Navigation Assessment Tool

The NAT is a mechanism for navigation programs to assess program maturity and establish a means for growth. Swanson, Strusowski, Mack, and Degroot (2012) provided an analysis of the tool's development and purpose,

Figure 9-1. National Cancer Institute Community Cancer Centers Program's Navigation Assessment Tool

As all navigation programs are built uniquely, we encourage you to rate your program as you feel appropriate. The purpose of this form is not to gauge one program against another, but to assist you in building a stronger navigation program. The form can be used to assess an individual tumor site or the entire program.

Definitions:

Key stakeholders: Those people that you feel are essential to making a program work, including Administration, Navigators, Staff, Physicians (both employed and those in private practice). Specialty areas include medical, surgical and radiation oncology, rehab, palliative care, and hospice.

Community partnerships: Those entities that exist within and outside of your program that you need the support of or are a referral source for patient use and contribute to the support of patients along the continuum of their care.

Acuity system: Ability to determine appropriate level of care/intervention based on patient need and disease process.

Risk factors: Variable associations with increased risk of complications with disease and treatment of cancer.

Metrics/reporting measures: Measuring activities and performance.

Percentage of patients navigated: Patients with cancer inclusive of analytic cases, new diagnosed primaries, reoccurrences, advanced diseases, metastatic of defined cancer site(s) within your program setting.

Continuum of navigation: Navigation functional areas include: Outreach/Screening, Abnormal Finding to Diagnosis, Treatment, Outpatient and/or Inpatient, Survivorship and End-of-Life Care. Navigation can occur along any or all of these. One single person may do all of these or you may have one person designated to cover one area of the continuum. They may be disease-specific navigators or cover all diseases within that category. The sign of a level 5 site is that navigation is continuous across the cancer care continuum.

Disparity: Is any underrepresented group that your program is able to focus on. Providing outreach and effort in this population is a hallmark of navigation according to its original conception and should be continued as part of a navigation program.

Tools for reporting navigator statistics: Documents to help evaluate and measure a navigation program.

MDC involvement: Multidisciplinary team approach to care including physicians (med onc, rad onc, and surgeon) and other healthcare providers to create a plan of care for patient; patient may not always be present to be considered an MDC.

(Continued on next page)

Figure 9-1. National Cancer Institute Community Cancer Centers Program's Navigation Assessment Tool (Continued)

	Level 1	Level 2	Level 3	Level 4	Level 5
*Key stakeholders	Administrative support	At least one physician champion referring to navigation program	Two physicians involved and referring to navigation program; one is not an oncologist.	Most specialty physicians support the navigation program.	The navigation program receives referrals from employed and non-employed MDs, PCPs, or community partners.
*Community partnerships	Navigator works with departments outside of cancer but within own facility	**Plus,** works with at least one national group such as NCI, ACS, LLS, Wellness Community, Susan G. Komen for the Cure, or LIVESTRONG	**Plus,** supports state cancer control goals and objectives.	**Plus,** connects with other local community partners such as churches, community centers, other community organizations	Includes a formal connection to national/state/local organizations as an active committee or board member
Acuity system/patient *risk factor	No risk factor or acuity system available.	Some patients are assessed but no formal tool is used. Acuity based on dependence of patient vs. actual patient risk factors.	Use of a formal tool, which may be disease specific.	Utilizing formal assessment tool, has a well-defined referral process for identified issues.	Provides periodic reevaluation as a proactive approach to intervene or prevent issues and ensure quality of care during specific treatment points.
*Quality improvement measures	None in place.	Brainstorming and discussion regarding metrics and reporting within the multidisciplinary team or cancer committee.	One QI initiative in place measured and reported to all stakeholders on hardcopy file annually.	QI initiatives developed in collaboration with patient feedback or patient satisfaction surveys reported to administration.	Multiple QI initiatives in place monitored to demonstrate program improvement and financial contribution and cost savings services of navigation (i.e., compliance to POC).

(Continued on next page)

Figure 9-1. National Cancer Institute Community Cancer Centers Program's Navigation Assessment Tool (Continued)

	Level 1	Level 2	Level 3	Level 4	Level 5
Marketing of the navigator program	Occurs by word of mouth	Includes level 1 as well as some basic written material (i.e., pamphlet)	**Plus,** navigator participation at health fairs, cancer screening events as a means of marketing cancer program	**Plus,** effort made to promote navigation in some media form	**Plus,** multiple sources of media used to support navigation (video, print, audio, web, etc.)
Percentage of patients offered navigation	0%–20%	21%–40%	41%–60%	61%–80%	> 80%
*Continuum of navigation	One functional area within the cancer continuum	Two functional areas within the continuum	Three functional areas within the continuum	Four functional areas within the continuum	Navigation across all functional levels of the continuum.
Support services available and used by navigation team	No resources available	Hospital resources (social worker and/or case manager) are available to assist with cases	Outpatient social services available within cancer program	Level 3 plus a minimum of two additional outpatient oncology-specific services available	All services available or can be accessed within the community or organization (dietitian, social worker, psychologist, clinical trials, speech therapy, physical/occupational therapy, pastoral care, oncology rehab, financial counselors, palliative care, volunteer dept., genetic counselor, or survivorship).

(Continued on next page)

Figure 9-1. National Cancer Institute Community Cancer Centers Program's Navigation Assessment Tool *(Continued)*

	Level 1	Level 2	Level 3	Level 4	Level 5
*Tools for reporting navigator statistics	No reports or tools, paper records, paper record (patient chart) narrative of services provided for patients and their family	Basic homegrown Access file/Word, Excel. Basic info tracked (i.e., number of patients, disease site, supportive services provided)	High level homegrown Access database created by hospital information technology dept. Collects stats and support services provided for patient/family.	Formal hospital system EMR database used to collect support services and stats. Not a database specific for navigation.	Reporting of all support services provided to the patient via EMR specific for navigation including outcome information. Documents all support services.
Financial assessment	No financial assessment performed	Financial assessment and assistance only available in the inpatient setting.	**Plus,** financial assessment and assistance available for outpatients within cancer program	**Plus,** proactive financial assessment completed for all oncology patients	**Plus,** data collection completed on types of services provided and number of patients assisted on a regular basis.
*Focus on disparities	None defined.	Underserved population defined.	At least one culturally sensitive activity devoted to reaching underserved population provided annually	Patient service mechanism defined to integrate underserved patients into the program.	Cultural sensitivity assessment completed on cancer center staff with cultural objective created on at least an annual basis.

(Continued on next page)

Figure 9-1. National Cancer Institute Community Cancer Centers Program's Navigation Assessment Tool (Continued)

	Level 1	Level 2	Level 3	Level 4	Level 5
Navigator responsibilities	Navigator is unaligned with any physician and responsible only for support of the patient	**Plus,** navigator coordinates care between multiple disciplines within the cancer program	**Plus,** navigator participation in support groups, family/patient center programs	**Plus,** navigator maintains an active role in disease-specific MDC/tumor conference	**Plus,** navigator is an integral part of quality improvement audits, and strategic planning
Patient identification process	No formal patient identification. Path reports, daily schedule, radiology reports used to identify patients.	N/A	Patients self-refer or are referred by oncology provider	N/A	Primary care provider and/or specialist (GI, pulmonary, interventional radiology) refers at the time of abnormal finding
Navigator training	No formal training in place	Core competencies of navigation defined	Local/in-house training curriculum developed specific to navigator core competency and development of navigator role	Local/in-house training program completed by all navigators, or navigators are certified in oncology in their respective disciplines	Navigators formally trained by nationally recognized training program and certified.

(Continued on next page)

Figure 9-1. National Cancer Institute Community Cancer Centers Program's Navigation Assessment Tool *(Continued)*

	Level 1	Level 2	Level 3	Level 4	Level 5
Engagement with clinical trials	Navigator shares basic understanding of clinical trials in cancer	Navigator has greater depth understanding of clinical trials, has completed specific training (NCI, ONS, etc.)	Navigator shares information regarding the availability of clinical trials in their community cancer center with patients	Navigator engages with research team in providing general referrals	Navigator engages with research team, assists with specific trial referrals, for underserved populations
*Multidisciplinary care/conference involvement	Basic Commission on Cancer requirements met, including discussion of NCCN guidelines or other national oncology standards	Navigator attends tumor conference but does not participate, documents physician discussion of plan of care in narrative note but not formal part of patient record	Navigator assists with case finding for MDC presentations. No treatment plan documented. Dictation completed by MD regarding plan of care.	Navigator provides formal review of discussions of MDC with patient after care presentation.	Patient informed of presentation at MDC with full formal report on treatment planned; discussion shared with patient referring MD and primary care, formal audits completed.

ACS—American Cancer Society; EMR—electronic medical record; GI—gastrointestinal; LLS—Leukemia & Lymphoma Society; MDC—multidisciplinary conference; NCI—National Cancer Institute; NCCN—National Comprehensive Cancer Network; ONS—Oncology Nursing Society; PCP—primary care physician; POC—plan of care; QI—quality improvement

Note. Items with an asterisk (*) are further explained under the definition section at the beginning of the Assessment Tool. Navigation Assessment Tool Version 1.0 was created by the National Cancer Institute Community Cancer Centers Program (NCCCP) and approved by the NCCCP Executive Subcommittee on 7/14/2011. This tool has not been validated. Retrieved from http://ncccp.cancer.gov/files/NavAssessTool_508Comp_20130318-2.pdf.

suggesting that programmatic growth is twofold: (a) systematic relevance and (b) patient focused. Within the systematic relevance arm, categories are designed to create a lattice of importance of the navigation program to the larger system as a whole. For example, breast-imaging nurses may call patients with negative biopsies, whereas primary care physicians (PCPs) call patients with positive findings. Breast nurse navigators could instead perform this service for patients with both positive and negative findings, while providing anticipatory guidance and coordination of further care for patients who require additional intervention for positive findings.

Swanson et al. (2012) suggested that the NAT guides programs in establishing resources and other infrastructure to improve patient outcomes. Using the previous example, waiting for a call with biopsy results from either the PCP or breast-imaging nurse can be stressful for patients; however, some of this stress can be alleviated when the news is delivered by a navigator with whom the patient has already met and discussed concerns. In fact, the navigator can arrange a specific time to call the patient or even allow the patient to initiate the call to the navigator at a decided time when the results would be available so that the patient has as much control of the situation as desired.

In this example, establishing the process for results notification may evolve over time through patient feedback and adaptation based on patient needs and systematic requirements. Through the use of the NAT, programs are encouraged to continue identifying system gaps and establishing process improvements that prevent patients from being subjected to healthcare inadequacies.

As of yet, little research is available regarding the financial benefits of navigation programs to healthcare administrators or cost savings associated with implementing disease-reducing interventions for patients. At a time when navigation programs struggle to quantitatively demonstrate relevance and success, the NAT provides a systematic tool for framing navigation program assessment so that stakeholders can see system benefits and continued program development and process improvements.

Early Program Development

When establishing a new navigation program, there is usually much excitement about the program. It is not uncommon for a navigator to be hired and simply instructed to begin a program; yet, this is often a time when many questions arise without easy answers. Using the NAT, Swanson et al. (2012) suggested a path to identify program elements already in place and those in need of further development. New program administrators and navigators need not feel inadequate; rather, they can leverage the excitement and enthusiasm associated with the program inception to focus on initial priorities for building upon early successes. Swanson et al. (2012) cautioned not to expect rapid growth and asserted that it is impossible to evaluate program effectiveness after a mere six months. Rather, an annual evaluation is more feasible, as program advancement takes time and continued focus.

In using the NAT, Swanson et al. (2012) suggested bringing together a multidisciplinary team representing all cancer program stakeholders. This team should thoroughly discuss and accurately self-assess the navigation program's level in each of the different categories. Considering that the levels build upon one another, a program usually will not be at a level four without first achieving the three lower levels. An honest assessment about the current status of a navigation program will allow more appropriate placement of resources for programmatic growth. Resources and finances should be directed toward strategic areas prioritized for growth rather than areas already established and functional.

Furthermore, Swanson et al. (2012) suggested the establishment of a target level for each category to promote program growth. Because programs are tailored to the needs and resources of a community, not every navigation program needs to aspire to a level five in each of the categories. Rather, in most cases, a level three or four may be sufficient in meeting the needs of the patient population. Swanson et al. (2012) also advised that if a specific level is working for the patient population without concern, continuing to focus on system enhancements in this area may lead to frustration and wasted efforts, as well as resource diversion from other categories in need of attention.

Established Programs

Navigation programs with established structures and resources have likely assessed the program and implemented strategies for ongoing improvements. However, an initial evaluation using the NAT may provide answers to systematic failures and sources of patient dissatisfaction. After the assessment process is completed, the NAT functions as a quality improvement tool in which program elements scoring below goal levels can receive additional focus and development.

Established programs require growth and innovation to continue to meet the needs of the populations served as new resources become available, other resources lose funding, and systems change to meet other disease-site needs. For the program to be relevant, Swanson et al. (2012) recommended periodic reassessment with the NAT to assist in keeping a focus on continued development and resource allocation toward the program's greatest needs, which are ultimately patient driven. Although navigation programs should stretch when establishing goal levels for each of the NAT elements, the key to success is to avoid overreaching and instead prioritize the focus on one category until it is as close to goal level as possible before moving to the next identified area in need of advancement.

Categories of the Navigation Assessment Tool

Each of the 16 NAT categories will be described. Within each category, criteria are defined for each of the five levels, incrementally moving from basic program components to more advanced components. Remember, although a level five intuitively seems to be the most desirable level, this may not be achievable or even necessary for the specific category being evaluated. Rather, each program reflects its own best practice, and through use of the NAT, defining that best practice is perhaps more visible (Swanson et al., 2012).

Category 1. Key Stakeholders

Key stakeholders are individuals whose support is considered essential to the success of the navigation program. As the different levels indicate, administrative engagement is imperative. To further the program's strength and sustainability, provider loyalty is essential.

Category 2. Community Partnerships

Navigation programs must identify and establish community partnerships for optimal patient support. First, a navigation program must look internally for resources that could provide patient benefit. Stronger navigation programs establish collaborative relationships with other community entities to provide additional assistance for patients, screening opportunities, and survivorship support on a local, state, or national level.

Category 3. Acuity System and Risk Factor Identification

An acuity system provides a method to assess the degree of complexity of patient cases and, based on the disease, the level of support that patients require. Early identification of disease-modifying needs is critical and should be done as close to diagnosis as possible to increase the potential for successful treatment completion (Gilbert et al., 2011). For example, at the Gibbs Cancer Center and Research Institute in Spartanburg, South Carolina, the navigation team created a simple acuity system consisting of a score of either 1 or 2: a score of 1 indicates that a patient needs education on the diagnosis but does not require intensive interventions, whereas a score of 2 means the patient is complex and requires multiple navigator interventions. For example, patients with head and neck cancer have a multitude of physical and psychosocial issues that navigators may need time to resolve. As a result, head and neck cancer navigators are not able to work with as large a volume of patients as another disease-specific navigator. In this example, the patient with head and neck cancer would be scored as a 2. These data, taken in context, can provide basic information to support the productivity of each navigator.

Given the overwhelming workload potential for navigators, a concise and standard process for assessing patients should be developed for each program. In this process, a stratification of patients may begin to materialize. Navigators may identify certain patient characteristics that require more attention. As navigators notice these characteristics, they can incorporate referral patterns to resources and educational information into the care for those particular patients. In this way, navigators understand the needs of their patient populations and provide comprehensive support as concerns arise. Simultaneously, navigators are developing a risk-factor system based on patient needs and the time required for patients. For example, navigators may notice that patients with head and neck cancer require one hour of counseling regarding the side effects of treatment before starting therapy, and thus, they can better allocate this time in their schedule.

Navigators begin to preemptively provide information and support before patient concerns arise as a result of their prior experience and expertise in working with similar patients. For example, a head and neck navigator is likely to recognize that patients with head and neck cancer undergoing radiation treatment experience oral mucositis and esophagitis and thus provides preventive oral hygiene teaching before radiation begins, as well as frequent reinforcement of this education.

Although the previous examples seem intuitive, the NAT urges navigation programs to be systematic in the process of patient need stratification in order for navigators to budget time and resources more effectively.

Category 4. Quality Improvement

Navigation programs cannot grow and improve without analyzing gaps in the system and navigation delivery process. Therefore, periodic quality improvement efforts seek to improve overall program function. Furthermore, quality improvement should not be undertaken in a clandestine manner. Periodic sharing of efforts strengthens program function and physician loyalty.

Category 5. Marketing

Navigation programs should seek to be visible and use as many sources of media as possible to exhibit the benefits of navigation to the community. Initially, these efforts should begin within the institution, informing all employees about the navigation program and its benefits. From there, employees will share the information with family and friends. However, word-of-mouth advertisement may not be as effective as other measures. Navigation programs must consider other opportunities to advertise services, such as signs, billboards, commercials, and web content.

Category 6. Percentage of Patients Offered Navigation

This category was purposefully left vague (Swanson et al., 2012). Each navigation program must determine the denominator of this category based on the specific population the program intends to navigate. For example, a breast navigation program would not want to consider the total number of cancer diagnoses accessioned by the institution's cancer registry; this would yield a low percentage, and it would seem to administrators as though the navigator is ineffective. Rather, a breast navigator would want to compare the number of patients with breast cancer navigated with the total number of breast cancer cases diagnosed at the facility. Other considerations for appropriate denominators might include disease-specific percentages (e.g., breast, colon, head and neck, hematologic), total treatment visits, or cancer registry totals. The intended purpose of this category is to assist programs in navigating as many patients and as close to diagnosis as is feasible. For example, in reviewing this information, a lung cancer navigator may identify that percentages are lower than expected. This may prompt a discussion with the pathologist, where it is discovered that lung biopsies performed in outpatient centers do not reach the navigator's desk. This subsequently could result in a system enhancement opportunity to establish a better referral pattern so that patients are connected in a timely manner with the navigator. The purpose of this category is not to attempt to reach 100% of all patients diagnosed at the facility but rather to identify areas of improvement to facilitate earlier navigation of all appropriate patients.

Category 7. Continuum of Care

Freeman's model of navigation suggested that navigation is appropriate at any time during the continuum of cancer (Freeman, 2012). Therefore, it is appropriate for navigation programs to provide tailored resources to patients during all phases of the cancer care continuum: screening, abnormal findings, diagnosis, treatment, survivorship, palliative care, and the end of life.

Category 8. Support Services

Navigators cannot possibly possess the expertise to provide direct services for all the potential resources and support needed for every patient. Rather, connections with institutional and community resources to assist patients with potential concerns (e.g., nutrition, social services, finance, insurance, mental health, pharmacology) can provide the optimal resolution of those concerns.

Category 9. Reporting Tools

Navigation programs must establish specific outcome metrics to coincide with overall program goals and objectives. These metrics are then monitored and periodically reported to stakeholders as a mechanism to demonstrate program successes. Navigators must understand the specific metrics and operational definitions of each and then implement a process to gather and present the data in a succinct and understandable manner. This process can be as simple as a monthly tally kept up to date in a navigator-developed database or by using more sophisticated computer software integrated with the institution's electronic health record. Clearly, the latter seems to offer a more efficient and intuitive approach to data management and monitoring of program outcomes, thus providing for more patient navigation time. However, a navigation program must work within existing systems and may not be able to justify the purchase of such software or successfully interface the selected software with the electronic health record.

Category 10. Financial Assessment

Many patients' needs are unique; however, one need seems to be ubiquitous: financial support (Hendren et al., 2011). Therefore, providing financial counseling and assessment before treatment and periodically thereafter allows a program to anticipate patients' financial concerns. Patients may experience difficulty not just with the cost of treatment but also with other bills such as the mortgage, groceries, and medications for side effect management. Identifying financial concerns early in the cancer continuum will allow navigators to better connect patients with appropriate resources and handle additional concerns as they arise (Korber et al., 2011).

Category 11. Focus on Disparate Populations

Underserved and disparate populations have higher disease morbidity and mortality from all cancer diagnoses (Centers for Disease Control and Prevention, 2013). This concern has continued to be a focus of navigation programs. Programs that seek to understand underserved populations accessing (or not accessing) navigation services will have a better connection with that population and perhaps, in time, will be able to reduce disease burden in these populations. Of course, racial and ethnic minorities are seen as underserved populations, but so are rural, older adult, and uninsured patients. Navigation programs will most likely have more than one underserved population requiring resources and assistance.

The focus on disparities has gained national attention as an expectation in oncology (Center to Reduce Cancer Health Disparities, 2013). Information is available concerning the ability of navigators to obtain resources, as well as remove barriers to care throughout the patients' continuum of care (Yosha et al., 2011). Navigators at the Gibbs Cancer Center and Research Institute focus on African American and Hispanic populations. Figure 9-2 depicts an increase in the navigation of African Americans with breast, lung, colorectal, and prostate cancer from 2010 to 2011; this was due, in part, to hiring an additional navigator and focusing outreach to those populations.

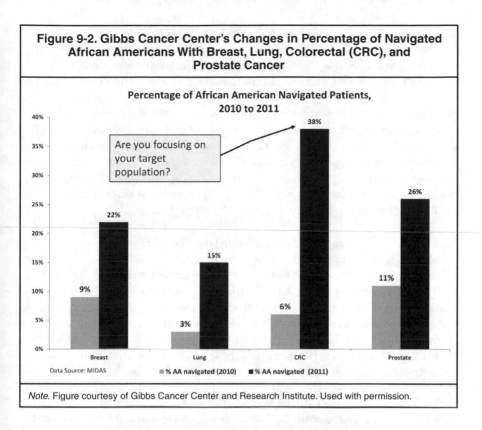

Figure 9-2. Gibbs Cancer Center's Changes in Percentage of Navigated African Americans With Breast, Lung, Colorectal (CRC), and Prostate Cancer

Percentage of African American Navigated Patients, 2010 to 2011

Are you focusing on your target population?

Data Source: MIDAS   ▨ % AA navigated (2010)   ■ % AA navigated (2011)

Note. Figure courtesy of Gibbs Cancer Center and Research Institute. Used with permission.

Category 12. Navigator Responsibilities

Beyond coordinating care and providing patients with necessary resources and information, navigators are key to program development. In general, the more visible navigators are, the more a part of the system framework they become. Therefore, navigator involvement with multidisciplinary rounds, support groups, cancer conferences, the clinical research team, and quality improvement initiatives integrates navigators directly into cancer programs and strengthens their position within the system.

Category 13. Patient Identification

Although physician champions are a great resource for patient referrals, other sources for patient identification exist and, in some cases, are more feasible for a beginning program. These sources include (a) the cancer registry, (b) daily pathology reports, (c) daily treatment schedules, and (d) patient self-referral. The efforts of navigation programs should be to identify patients as close to the time of diagnosis as possible. This not only provides patients with navigation resources at this most stressful time but also potentially builds patient loyalty with the cancer program.

Category 14. Navigator Training

Although formal navigator training programs are beginning to form, most navigators receive little education regarding navigation duties and responsibilities. Some institutions have sought to define the roles of navigation; however, navigators must work within the confines of the individual program and patient population (Francz & Simpson, 2013). Minimally, programs should establish standards of navigation that can serve as a framework for basic orientation to the role. Perhaps consideration can be given to a national training program or conference for navigators to establish network connections and gain a broader understanding of the specialty. Regardless, the strength of navigation programs lies with successful orientation and cultural assimilation for new navigators.

Category 15. Engagement With Clinical Trials

Although most navigators do not enroll patients into clinical trials, they should be knowledgeable about the research studies available. Patients will likely have questions about clinical trials and look to navigators for information. Furthermore, a well-integrated system could engage navigators' assistance with the prescreening process. For example, a navigator could inform the clinical trials staff of a new patient with lung cancer so that a review of available lung trials and eligibility criteria could be completed prior to the physician consultation. Should a clinical trial be available, the navigator could coordinate a discussion among the provider, patient, and clinical trial staff. The intent of this category is to provide more patients with the opportunity to be educated about, and possibly enroll in, clinical trials, particularly minority and underserved patients, who generally are underrepresented in clinical trials (Center to Reduce Cancer Health Disparities, 2013). From a navigation perspective, clinical trials are potential revenue generators and could assist in establishing the financial merit of navigation programs.

Category 16. Multidisciplinary Conference Involvement

All cancer centers accredited by ACoS CoC must have a tumor board or multidisciplinary conference (MDC) (ACoS CoC, 2012). This category of the NAT encourages navigation programs to define the multidisciplinary conference—whether it is a face-to-face conference where patients are able to meet with all members of the multidisciplinary team or a virtual conference where patients receive information about the recommendations after the conference has taken place. Regardless of how the MDC is defined, navigators are well positioned to not only provide information but also coordinate appointments and facilitate referrals to all members of the multidisciplinary team. Figure 9-3 is an example from the Gibbs Cancer Center and Research Institute, where the nurse navigator coordinates the prostate MDC, and the number of case presentations has increased 209% as highlighted by the institution's Prostate Advisory Board Committee.

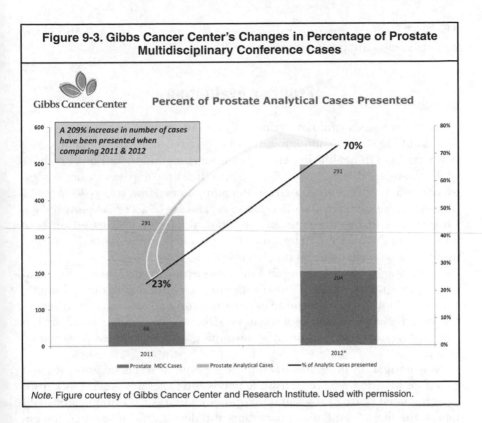

Figure 9-3. Gibbs Cancer Center's Changes in Percentage of Prostate Multidisciplinary Conference Cases

Note. Figure courtesy of Gibbs Cancer Center and Research Institute. Used with permission.

A limiting factor to the extent of navigation involvement in MDCs is the amount of preparation needed, such as securing radiology images and pathology slides for the team to review during the case presentation. These tasks detract from the navigators' time for direct patient interactions and interventions. Thus, in response to navigators' growing workload and the necessary preparations for MDCs, various innovative strategies have been implemented, such as engaging clerical staff and streamlining paperwork processes.

Summary of the Navigation Assessment Tool

The NAT is available for navigation programs, both naïve and expert, to build, strengthen, and guide growth to allow for better patient care, system viability, and sustainability. Swanson et al. (2012) proposed that periodic reevaluation with the NAT is necessary for continued growth. Establishment of appropriate quality improvement processes, including specific metrics that navigation programs can benefit from, will allow for program enhancement.

The NAT is one way to integrate the goals of programmatic growth, metric measurement, and quality improvement.

Program Evaluation

Key to any successful navigation program is ensuring that the organization is able to develop, implement, and objectively evaluate outcomes. As a new paradigm in health care emerges where competition and fiscal responsibility mandate that every dollar be spent efficiently on patient care, navigators can set a cancer center apart from competitors. However, to do so, organizations must be ready to collect, analyze, and act in accordance with data. Program leadership needs to establish meaningful metrics based on core navigation functions and determine efficient mechanisms to obtain the necessary data to evaluate program effectiveness.

Gathering baseline and ongoing data is essential for demonstrating a navigation program's economic worth. During navigation program planning, the institution should determine initial goals and outcomes to create benchmarks to focus the efforts of navigators. However, it is equally important to solicit navigators' perspectives in determining metrics to assess program efficacy.

New navigation programs need to be flexible in terms of priorities and functions in order to be responsive to needs and issues not previously known or anticipated during program development. However, it is important to establish the major emphasis of programs and define how to leverage the energies of navigators to maximum effect. For example, with the launch of a new program, in addition to navigating clinical care for patients, navigators may be expected to help develop software applications, engage in data input and extraction, and participate in program analysis and reporting. While this may be necessary because of the lack of an existing data repository that is suitable for tracking navigation outcomes, it may be helpful for new navigators to understand program priorities and the basis of each metric. Once the program has been established and perhaps supported with additional personnel, others may assume these types of clerical duties so that navigators can focus more on clinical interventions and care coordination. Early program planning should account for these often conflicting priorities in order to adjust navigator roles, responsibilities, and resources in response to emerging needs as the program evolves.

Since the conception and early success of patient navigation in a public hospital in the Harlem neighborhood of New York City in 1990, navigation efforts have expanded across the cancer care continuum, from early detection and screening efforts to survivorship and palliative care (Freeman, 2012). Cancer programs that are accredited by the ACoS CoC must comply with Standard 3.1, the Patient Navigation Process (ACoS CoC, 2012). The

Patient Protection and Affordable Care Act (ACA) includes provisions for patient navigation and is well aligned with the principles and spirit of patient navigation (Central Area Health Education Center, 2011; Freeman, 2012). As new programs are developed with the intent to improve health care, these programs must be evidence based with predictable outcomes (Byers, 2012).

The Health Services Research (HSR)-Cost work group of the American Cancer Society National Patient Navigator Leadership Summit in August 2010 proposed cost metrics to consider (Whitley et al., 2011). Cost data should be discussed at the planning stage of program development (Whitley et al., 2011). Factors such as funding, reimbursement, and sustainability may well depend on proven outcomes, so it is important for navigation programs to reflect both clinical and economic value (Whitley et al., 2011). Still, cost data alone may not reflect the benefit of navigation programs. Byers (2012) posited that greater gains from navigation programs will more than make up for program expenses, with one benefit being the detection of cancers at earlier stages, thereby reducing the cost of treating more advanced cancers.

The ACA will bring changes in how healthcare services, including oncology, will be delivered and reimbursed in the future. The legislation will change the current payment system, which rewards volume of service, to a new payment structure that rewards the delivery of quality health care with lower costs (Barkley, 2012). Accountable care organizations (ACOs) in cancer care will have implications for oncologists as well as cancer centers. ACOs will require providers to manage all health needs of the covered populations. Cost savings will be achieved by elimination of unnecessary or redundant procedures, communication of clinical information among providers, and attainment of quality targets that allow providers to keep a portion of the savings. Providers will be rewarded for keeping Medicare patients healthy and out of the hospital (Cobb & Okon, 2010). In addition to cost savings, quality measures must be satisfied. As navigators focus on eliminating barriers to care and coordinating healthcare services, they become key to the financial viability of the cancer program.

Data Collection Processes

Knowing the needs and characteristics of the patients served by navigation programs is critical, as programs should be tailored to this population (Freund et al., 2008). The specific setting in which navigation occurs should also be considered when determining program measures. To establish how navigation programs serve and benefit individuals with cancer, programs need to identify, measure, and continually report metrics. In addition to common metrics, specific challenges that populations face when seeking appropriate and timely cancer care should be reflected in the data collected (Guadagnolo, Dohan, & Raich, 2011). This will enhance navigation programs' abilities to compare and evaluate impact and overall success (Freund et al., 2008).

An important component of data management is to clearly define data elements and then adopt a standard method of data collection, such as that used by the U.S. Census Bureau and NCI for reporting of cancer data (Guadagnolo et al., 2011). Some may assume that navigators are responsible for tracking all program data; however, organizations' tumor registries also are a good resource for data and often comply with NCI's Surveillance, Epidemiology, and End Results (SEER) Program (NCI, n.d.-b). SEER program registries contain patient data information including demographics, tumor-specific information related to stage at diagnosis, timeliness of diagnosis and treatment, and survival outcomes. In addition, the SEER program collaborates with the North American Association of Central Cancer Registries to guide states in uniform data collection to allow for compatible data pooling.

Program planners must be realistic when determining program metrics and data collection methods because institutions' available resources and data capabilities, including detailed data collection and management, vary widely. Navigation programs may choose to use homegrown databases or navigation-specific software purchased through a vendor. Regardless of the data collection process, the key to tracking metrics is the ability to stratify patient-specific data for ease in data interpretation.

Data Elements

In 2005, NCI sponsored the Patient Navigation Research Program (PNRP). The PNRP's objective was to define common metrics, processes, and outcomes of navigation. This was accomplished through the establishment of a multicenter study engaging nine sites across the country that targeted vulnerable populations, such as racial and ethnic minorities and low-income individuals (Freund et al., 2008). The PNRP defined the start date of navigation as the date of the initial abnormal test with suspicion for cancer and the endpoint as the completion of treatment for patients with a diagnosis of cancer or a follow-up test that definitively ruled out cancer. The following PNRP outcomes were established: (a) elapsed time from suspicious finding to diagnostic resolution, (b) elapsed time from suspicious finding to initiation of cancer treatment, (c) patient satisfaction with care, and (d) cost-effectiveness (Freund et al., 2008). With timeliness encompassing a major focus of navigation outcomes, documentation of specific dates, such as first abnormal cancer screening examination, first navigation contact, tissue diagnosis, treatment initiation, and treatment completion, should be recorded along with specific barriers to timely care. In addition, basic demographic data such as race/ethnicity, income and educational level, marital and employment status, primary language, and family/caregiver support may be important in gaining a better understanding of the relationships of barriers the navigated population faces. Other data elements to consider collecting related to financial aspects include total case hours per navigator, missed appointments, hospital admissions, and emergency department (ED) visits during cancer treatment.

Navigation programs should incorporate and report basic characteristics of the program including setting (clinical, community, church, or other public setting), eligibility criteria (if any) for navigation, mode of navigation (including in-person or other modes of contact), time spent interacting/intervening with patients, and navigator caseloads. Documenting specific referrals generated, such as for clinical trial screening, genetic counseling, durable medical goods, dentistry, nutrition support, physical and occupational therapy, speech therapy, mental health counseling, palliative care/hospice services, pastoral care, smoking cessation programs, community transportation resources, and national organizations and foundations for treatment- or disease-related funding, allows an administration to understand what resources are needed and ensure adequate availability of such. Because many of these referrals are for revenue-generating services, navigators referring patients to these programs not only help establish loyalty within the system but also demonstrate navigation as a means for creating downstream revenue within the organization.

Although it might be desirable to have a universal set of metrics to establish and evaluate navigation programs, such a goal may not be obtainable because of program variability based on specific setting and community needs, both of which cannot be modified (Battaglia, Burhansstipanov, Murrell, Dwyer, & Caron, 2011). Rather, programs should clearly identify program features and use common data elements whenever possible so that comparisons between similar outcomes can be as relevant as possible (Battaglia et al., 2011).

Evaluation of Outcomes

Once desired program outcomes have been determined and data collection has been initiated, navigators and program administrators must regularly monitor and analyze the data to assess the impact of navigation programs. This periodic evaluation validates program activities and navigator efforts and also facilitates objective program modifications and additional resource allocations as appropriate. The following section outlines some of the most common navigation program outcomes and rationale for each.

Time-to-Treat Metrics

Established repeatedly is the relationship between navigator engagement and decreased time from abnormal finding to resolution of that finding. One retrospective Canadian study identified a statistically significant (p < 0.001) decrease in time to biopsy with the full implementation of navigation services to both screening and direct referral patients (N = 536). In 1999, median time to biopsy was 12 days for screening (navigated) patients (n = 97) and 20 days for referral (non-navigated) patients (n = 144), whereas, in 2000, when navigation services were expanded to both groups, median time to biopsy remained stable at 13 days (n = 133) for those screened and conventionally offered navigation services, and decreased to 14 days for those patients referred to the center who previously would not have received navigation services but now were offered the services of a navigator (Psooy, Schreuer, Borgaonkar, & Caines, 2004). Another study found significantly decreased time from diagnosis to oncology consultation among navigated patients older than age 60 (12 days for non-navigated patients vs. 8 days for navigated patients) but no statistically significant difference for patients ages 31–60 (10 days for non-navigated patients vs. 9 days for navigated patients) (Basu et al., 2013).

Ideally, when evaluating time-to-treat metrics, baseline data should be measured to document timeliness of care prior to navigation implementation. Although some time-to-treat benchmarks exist, these are not yet well-established and applicable targets for every navigation program. Rather, more useful comparisons have typically been found when considering incremental decreases in timeliness metrics, which ultimately provide objective evidence of a navigation program's success in eliminating barriers and facilitating timely access to care.

Emergency Department Visits

Tracking visits to the ED is necessary to demonstrate whether navigated patients who obtain targeted education on side effects along with a specific staff contact are less likely to present to the ED for care. Again, comparing pre- and postnavigation patient data provides the best assessment of the impact that navigators can have on reducing the number of ED visits, even though all variables cannot be controlled. These unplanned visits stress the healthcare system and in the future may be considered preventable. The hope is that patients will contact navigators first when questions arise, thereby allowing concerns to be managed over the telephone or facilitating immediate provider access when needed, rather than unnecessarily accessing ED services. Emergency services not only are costly and disruptive to treatment schedules but also have the potential to expose patients to hospital-acquired conditions.

Should a true emergency be impending, navigators may be able to help ED throughput by providing information to ED staff. Navigators may also be able to prevent repeated costly tests by ensuring that ED physicians have access to the most recent scans, laboratory results, and physician progress notes.

Decreased Length of Stay

Critical to the success of cancer therapy is maintaining the integrity of the treatment plan. Interruption in treatment may lead to adverse patient outcomes. Inpatient stays for treatment and non-treatment-related conditions can interrupt the therapeutic nature of cancer therapy. Although it is difficult to prevent all potential effects of treatment or cancer, navigators are well positioned to provide seamless care for patients who need hospitalization. In this respect, it is possible for navigators to actually decrease patient length of stay. Lee et al. (2011) identified a significant difference (p < 0.0001) of 8.89 days for navigated patients (n = 78) versus 18.00 days for non-navigated patients (n = 78). While a decreased length of stay results in positive outcomes for patients and the healthcare system, minimizing hospital stays for patients with cancer in active treatment can be difficult to track for the majority of cancer centers. The literature lacks consistent evidence at this time regarding the navigators' impact in decreasing length of stay or readmission rates; however, anecdotal evidence is most certainly evident at the program level and should be tracked as a cost-saving outcome of navigation services.

Cost-Effectiveness

The cost-effectiveness or ROI of navigation has been challenging to document and validate, and published literature has suggested the need for further analysis of the true cost-effectiveness of navigation programs (Whitley et al., 2011). Essential elements to include when considering navigation program costs in relation to ROI include fixed and variable costs, staff recruitment and selection, and training costs, as well as direct and indirect medical costs (Desimini et al., 2011). Results from the nine PNRP sites were released in October 2012 and hopefully will serve as a guide to develop programs that meet the needs of the intended population, provide data to determine overall cost-effectiveness, and identify areas that are working well and those requiring changes (Freund et al., 2008). Results indicated populations that benefit most from navigation are the medically underserved, which include the poor and the uninsured (Freeman, 2012).

Dudley et al. (2012) found that navigation significantly shortened the time from definitive diagnosis (57 days for navigated patients vs. 74 days for the control group, p = 0.04) to initial treatment in poor Hispanic women with an abnormal breast cancer screening examination or an untreated biopsy-proven breast cancer compared to White women in their study. In another study, patient navigation interventions were evaluated in Hispanic and Black urban women living in poor neighborhoods and undergoing screening for breast and cervical cancer. Patient navigation improved time to diagnostic resolution for patients with breast cancer. However, in patients with cervical cancer, navigation did not seem to make a difference in time to resolution for those patients who resolved within 30 days. For those women who undergo cervical cancer screening and take longer than 30 days to resolve, women who were navigated reached diagnostic resolution in a shorter time, suggesting that navigation may benefit disadvantaged women (Markossian, Darnell, & Calhoun, 2012).

As posited by Markossian and Calhoun (2011), patient navigation interventions that improve the time from abnormal screening to diagnosis in patients with breast cancer may result in offsetting program costs through survival benefits and savings in the lifetime costs of breast cancer. The cost savings of earlier breast cancer diagnosis by as much as six months would amount to $95,625 per life-year saved and are based on an increase in life-years and a decrease in lifetime cancer costs (Markossian & Calhoun, 2011). Donaldson et al. (2012) conducted an economic evaluation of a breast and colorectal navigation screening program and found that the cost-effectiveness ratio (not including the cost of cancer treatment) ranged from $511–$2,080 with breast cancer diagnoses and $1,192–$9,708 with colorectal cancer diagnoses. The authors asserted that the program only needs to prevent three or four cancer deaths annually to be cost-saving.

Resource Integration

Most navigation programs lack the ability to generate revenue solely from navigators' interactions with patients. However, navigators have the ability to generate downstream revenue by connecting patients to resources that do bill for services, such as genetic counseling, mental health services, palliative care, nutrition support, rehabilitative services, and durable medical equipment. Navigators play a critical role in introducing clinical trials to patients and can discuss the patient's possible participation in a trial as a potential opportunity in the care and treatment of cancer. Guadagnolo et al. (2011) reported clinical trial accrual rates (inclusive of both treatment and cancer control studies) among navigated American Indian patients with cancer to be 22%, compared to other published studies indicating American Indian accrual rates of less than 1%. Using nurse navigation, Holmes, Major, Lyonga, Alleyne, and Clayton (2012) found a more than twofold increase in the number of African American patients with breast cancer enrolled in clinical trials; furthermore, they identified the unavailability of trials suitable for this population as a primary limiting factor to minority accrual in clinical trials. Beyond referrals for ancillary services and clinical trial enrollment, navigators provide mechanisms for patients to access resources and services they may not otherwise have used. This is especially true with regard to free and low-cost screening programs. Screening programs facilitate an initial interaction and begin to establish loyalty to the system with patients. Both Lebwohl et al. (2011) and Elkin, Shapiro, Snow, Zauber, and Krauskopf (2012) found that navigation programs dramatically increased the number of colonoscopies performed. Elkin et al. reported that the incremental cost-effectiveness varied from $200 to $700 per additional colonoscopy. Patient navigation was associated with a 61% increase in the monthly average colonoscopy volume from 114 procedures to 184 procedures. The net revenue associated with this increase in colonoscopy volume exceeded the program cost per additional colonoscopy at two hospitals of the three, resulting in a net financial benefit to the program.

Patient-Reported Outcomes

Arguably more difficult to measure and evaluate are patient-reported outcomes. These include concepts such as QOL, patient satisfaction and experience, psychological distress, pain, and self-efficacy (Fiscella et al., 2011). Although numerous tools are available to measure the aforementioned concepts, few have been validated for navigation (Fiscella et al., 2011).

Patient Satisfaction

Navigators can improve patient satisfaction by decreasing cancer-related distress and increasing overall QOL (Campbell et al., 2010; Hook et al., 2012; Koh et al., 2011; Lee et al., 2011). Patient satisfaction surveys frequently use a Likert-scale with the ability for patients to provide additional comments. An example of a validated patient satisfaction survey used by Hook et al. (2012) is depicted in Figure 9-4. Consideration should be given for ways to encourage participation in the survey without burdening patients (for example, providing self-addressed/stamped envelopes if doing mailed surveys, using telephone surveys if feasible, and offering the opportunity to win a small gift or token of appreciation for completing the surveys). Results should be shared regularly with navigators, program directors, cancer committees, and other key stakeholders.

A number of satisfaction tools specific to navigation have been developed and validated as part of the PNRP, including the 9-item Patient Satisfaction With Navigation–Interpersonal Scale and the 10-item Perceived Navigator Similarity Scale (Fiscella et al., 2011). The PNRP also validated the Patient

Figure 9-4. Nurse Navigation Patient Satisfaction Survey

Please take a few minutes to share your comments with us. Your feedback will help to improve our services.

The following information is optional and will be used for statistical use only:
Age: _____

Race/Ethnicity:
☐ African American ☐ Asian ☐ Caucasian ☐ Hispanic ☐ Other_____

Stage of cancer:
☐ 0 ☐ I ☐ II ☐ III ☐ IV ☐ Other_____

Insurance:
☐ Private ☐ Military program ☐ Medicare ☐ Medicare + Private ☐ Medicaid
☐ Uninsured ☐ Declined

Highest level of education completed:
☐ Less than high school ☐ High school/GED ☐ College ☐ Masters ☐ Doctoral
☐ Other _____

Which best describes you:
☐ Single ☐ Married ☐ Partner ☐ Divorced ☐ Widow

Children:
☐ No ☐ Yes If "yes": ☐ Have at least one child under 18
☐ Child/children over age 18

Rank each statement by checking the number that best describes your personal experiences.

	5 Strongly agree	4 Mildly agree	3 Neutral	2 Mildly disagree	1 Strongly disagree	0 Does not apply
1. I learned new information regarding my cancer experience from my nurse navigator.	5	4	3	2	1	0
2. I feel my nurse navigator was knowledgeable about my diagnosis and treatment.	5	4	3	2	1	0
3. I feel my concerns were taken seriously and addressed by my nurse navigator.	5	4	3	2	1	0

(Continued on next page)

	5 Strongly agree	4 Mildly agree	3 Neutral	2 Mildly disagree	1 Strongly disagree	0 Does not apply
Figure 9-4. Nurse Navigation Patient Satisfaction Survey *(Continued)*						
4. The nurse navigator offered additional emotional support that helped me manage my diagnosis and treatment.	5	4	3	2	1	0
5. The personal meetings with the nurse navigator were valuable to me.	5	4	3	2	1	0
6. The follow-up calls from the nurse navigator were valuable to me.	5	4	3	2	1	0
7. My calls to the nurse navigator were returned in a timely manner.	5	4	3	2	1	0
8. I found the education binder/folder given by my nurse navigator helpful.	5	4	3	2	1	0
12*. I feel navigation service is necessary for the care of patients with cancer.	5	4	3	2	1	0
13. My overall experience with navigation services improved my cancer experience.	5	4	3	2	1	0
14. I would recommend navigation services to others.	5	4	3	2	1	0

* Survey tool reflects omission of original survey statements 9, 10, and 11, which were eliminated from the analysis.

Note. Figure copyright by Ann Hook, MSN, RN. Used with permission.

Satisfaction With Cancer Care survey; this 35-item instrument can be easily administered and has direct implications to oncology navigation (Jean-Pierre, Fiscella, et al., 2011).

Quality of Life

Hendren et al. (2012) found that patients with breast and colon cancer randomly assigned to navigation intervention or usual care showed no differences with regard to QOL scores. The researchers measured QOL at baseline and four other intervals using the validated Functional Assessment of Cancer Therapy–General (FACT-G) instrument and its breast and colorectal cancer–specific modules, the FACT-B and FACT-C. Plausible explanations for this finding may be that cancer treatment programs already have sufficient medical, nursing, and social support services in place, or, conceivably, the navigation program did not target specific populations that would benefit. Another consideration is that perhaps the patients were too overwhelmed to make a substantive effort in answering questions about navigation. This area requires further investigation.

Barriers to Care

Common barriers to care include lack of social support, financial and insurance concerns, and problems with healthcare communication. Although barriers are common among all patients with cancer, the overall effect of barriers is most keenly felt in disparate populations (i.e., racial and ethnic minorities, as well as the unemployed), who subsequently require more assistance and time in overcoming barriers to care (Hendren et al., 2011). In a small study of 50 navigated patients with breast cancer, Koh et al. (2011) found that 70% experienced two or more barriers to care. Table 9-1 shows a complete list of barriers and the average time navigators spent on resolution. Navigators can focus on resolving barriers to care, which can be assessed during interviews with patients, and gathering data on psychosocial, financial, and practical issues. Regular interaction with navigators allows periodic evaluation of the success of intervention to reduce barriers.

Distress

The initiation of therapy, as well as many other points in the cancer trajectory, has been identified as a time of increased distress (National Comprehensive Cancer Network, 2013). During the initial phase of treatment, patients must understand the implications of treatment and how they will assimilate into daily routines. Professionals are available to answer questions from a medical standpoint, but from a practical standpoint, the patient has to determine how the diagnosis and treatment will affect the family unit. Navigators should initiate this discussion with patients and maintain regular contact to determine their concerns with completing therapy. Early ac-

Table 9-1. Barriers to Care, Resolution of Barriers, and Average Time Spent by Navigator

Barrier	Total		Completely Resolved		Minutes Spent	
	n	%	n	%	x̄	SD
System Issues						
Location of healthcare facility	21	42	21	100	3.8	1.57
System problems with scheduling care	4	8	4	100	6.75	3.95
Medical and mental health comorbidity	3	6	2	67	8.33	5.77
Financial Issues						
Insurance issues	6	12	3	50	8.67	6.38
Transportation	3	6	2	67	4	1.73
Employment issues	2	4	–	–	37.5	10.61
Psychosocial Issues						
Perception or beliefs about tests or treatment	16	32	12	75	11.67	13.84
Social or practical support	12	24	7	58	8.82	8.51
Fear	10	20	4	40	5.7	2.45
Child or adult care issues	7	14	5	71	8.14	4.38
Attitudes toward providers	7	14	4	57	14.14	20.75
Out of town or country	4	8	4	100	8.75	4.79
Patient disability	4	8	2	50	6.67	2.89
Housing	1	2	1	100	5	< 0.01
Literacy	–	–	–	–	–	–
Communication Issues						
Language or interpreter	1	2	1	100	5	< 0.01
Communication concerns with medical personnel	–	–	–	–	–	–

N = 50

Note. From "Evaluation of a Patient Navigation Program," by C. Koh, J.M. Nelson, and P.F. Cook, 2011, *Clinical Journal of Oncology Nursing, 15*, p. 45. doi:10.1188/11.CJON.41-48. Copyright 2011 by the Oncology Nursing Society. Reprinted with permission.

knowledgment of the supportive role of navigation in addressing all potential concerns, not just coordination of care and side effect management, should help to alleviate distress later if issues arise.

A retrospective study (N = 55) was performed and published on the role a nurse navigator plays in cancer-related distress management (Swanson & Koch, 2010). Findings revealed that patients seen by the nurse navigator tended to have lower distress scores on dismissal (n = 33, p = 0.1046). Specifically, navigator visits had a statistically significant effect on distress scores of inpatients age 65 or younger (n = 16, p = 0.044) and those from rural settings (n = 11, p = 0.045). Data on distress management over time can be vital as an indicator of navigator impact, and in this situation, the difference was clinically significant and warranted the provision of a navigator for patient distress.

Financial Assistance

A diagnosis of cancer and the resulting financial burden can lead to overwhelming stress for patients and family members. Navigators possess a wealth of knowledge regarding resource availability, including pharmaceutical assistance. For example, a navigator may be able to contact pharmaceutical companies to obtain chemotherapy at a much-reduced rate for a patient in addition to obtaining co-pay coverage for the medication. Anecdotally, a navigator at the Gibbs Cancer Center and Research Institute was able to obtain $125,000 worth of medications for a patient with cancer undergoing treatment. Clearly, the cost of a navigator compared to the benefit was demonstrated in this situation. Thus, these types of situations, although difficult to validate in the literature, need to be tracked by individual programs because they may prove invaluable to the cancer center when tracking the ROI for navigators.

Case Example

In response to substantial delays noted in the diagnosis and treatment of non-small cell lung cancer at the Connecticut Veterans Affairs Healthcare System (CT-VAHCS), the Committee for Clinical Excellence created the Lung Nodule subcommittee to research the issue. This subcommittee examined the management of 52 lung cancer cases over a two-year period. The subcommittee documented the mean time from abnormal imaging to initiation of treatment as 136 days (median = 117, range = 12–383). Because the diagnostic process of lung cancer can involve services such as primary care, pulmonary, cardiothoracic surgery, radiology, cardiology, and oncology, the process is often time consuming and fraught with delays (Schultz, Olsson, &

Gould, 2008; Singh et al., 2010). The initial data reflected multiple delays in the process with the following intervals (Hunnibell et al., 2012).

- Abnormal chest radiography (CXR) to computed tomography (CT) scan of the thorax: 44.2 days
- Abnormal imaging to pathologic diagnosis: 131.6 days
- Abnormal imaging to bronchoscopy: 78 days
- Diagnosis to treatment: 61.8 days

The subcommittee concluded that strategic action was needed to reduce diagnostic and treatment delays. The subcommittee established a goal to create a pulmonary tumor board for the collaborative management of lung cancer from diagnosis to treatment. A new position of cancer care coordinator was requested, and after a lengthy approval and recruitment process, an oncology nurse practitioner with certification in oncology nursing was hired to fill the position. The rationale for using an oncology certified nurse practitioner in this role was to identify radiologic cases with a strong suspicion for cancer and provide patient navigation to expedite further care through recommending, ordering, and overseeing tests in the diagnostic process. The new position came under the auspices of the chief of oncology, who was appointed as the supervising physician for the cancer care coordinator.

Initially, the cancer care coordinator spent time researching what was known about navigation, as well as established benchmarks for the diagnosis and treatment of lung cancer to compare with the initial data gathered by the subcommittee, which had since disbanded. The initial data showed that the majority of the delays were from abnormal imaging to pathologic diagnosis (131.6 days). In addition, because pathologic diagnosis does not complete the diagnostic process, further staging studies to determine the extent and stage of the disease are necessary before treatment is recommended and started. This may require additional biopsies or radiologic studies to determine metastasis. The analysis revealed that once the diagnosis was determined, the interval from diagnosis to treatment was 61.8 days. This information prompted the cancer care coordinator to focus data abstraction on two intervals: first, suspicion to diagnosis, and second, diagnosis to treatment, with emphasis on the steps leading to the diagnostic process.

The cancer care coordinator reviewed the available literature regarding timeliness of lung cancer care. Most published studies found were based on European studies. Fortunately, however, studies had been conducted that identified the multifaceted and complicated processes involved with diagnosing and treating lung cancer within the Veterans Affairs (VA) system, including potential delays or barriers encountered within the system, by providers, and by patients themselves. A guiding principle gleaned from review of these early studies was an overall lack of awareness regarding responsibility for tracking and coordinating lung cancer care, lack of a sense of urgency, and poorly coordinated care within the VA system and between VA and

VA providers (Schultz et al., 2008). The cancer care coordinator used networking connections to reach out to the oncology nursing community, both within and outside of the VA system (through, for example, the Oncology Nursing Society), for advice and mentoring. Initial research revealed that a few other VA medical facilities were also working to improve the process of diagnosing lung cancer by establishing algorithms for lung nodule management and a multidisciplinary process coordinated by advanced practice nurses (Van Buskirk & Atwood, 2009). Advice from a fellow navigator emphasized the need to clearly define the point of entry. Thus, the point of entry of navigation for the CT-VAHCS's program became the initial abnormal radiology report suspicious for lung cancer.

To better understand processes, the cancer care coordinator performed a detailed analysis of services and studies leading up to a lung cancer diagnosis. This approach was advantageous because it provided an opportunity to become acquainted with processes and staff involved in diagnosing and treating cancer. In addition, it enabled the cancer care coordinator to identify bottlenecks and barriers in the existing system. Radiology was one of the first areas of focus because the first abnormality associated with lung cancer is often a suspicious CXR. One of the advantages of the VA system is the electronic medical records system, allowing extraction of data with relative ease. However, the cancer care coordinator identified a problem with the flagging or coding of abnormal radiology reports suspicious for cancer. Either codes were not being used, or radiology reports with a suspicion for lung cancer were not coded with one of the two codes designated for suspicion of lung cancer that enabled the cancer care coordinator to quickly find these reports in an electronic data search of the radiology files. Data were subsequently collected to quantify the number of radiology reports suspicious for lung cancer that were missed because of lack of or improper coding, which, not surprisingly, revealed a pattern of incomplete or improper coding. Each month thereafter, the cancer care coordinator audited radiology coding and reviewed the results with the chief of radiology, who was a strong advocate for improving the cancer care coordination process. This auditing ultimately resulted in the mandatory use of a coding field for radiology and the creation of a special "cancer alert" code to facilitate the cancer care coordinator in conducting efficient case findings for radiology reports.

Using a bottom-up approach, the cancer care coordinator examined the typical sequential steps in the diagnostic process of lung cancer. The coordinator collected the following interval data points.
- Time from abnormal CXR to CT scan
- Time from CT scan to positron-emission tomography scan
- Time to referral to specialty services
- Time from referral to specialty service to consultation appointment
- Time from suspicion of cancer to diagnostic procedure

- Time from suspicion of cancer to pathologic diagnosis
- Time from pathologic diagnosis to initiation of treatment

Engaging a collaborative approach, the nurses and staff in the supporting departments measured additional parts of the diagnostic process, including the following.

- Radiology staff: Time from consult to biopsy through interventional radiology
- Cardiothoracic surgery staff: Time from consult to surgical procedure
- Pulmonary staff: Time from referral to consultation appointment and time to bronchoscopy

The cancer care coordinator audited the timeliness of radiology examinations based on priority indicated when the orders were placed. This audit showed that a CT scan ordered as soon as possible versus routine was completed 11 days sooner. Dates and time intervals between procedures were abstracted from the electronic medical records and recorded in a database designed by the cancer care coordinator, who subsequently provided periodic reports on trends to the newly formed lung nodule task force, the cancer committee, and to the involved services. In addition, the cancer care coordinator contacted patients when there were procedure cancellations or no-shows that contributed to delays in diagnosis and treatment. This allowed the cancer care coordinator to actively identify barriers to care and intervene in real time to become part of the program's continuous quality improvement.

The lung nodule task force used the data collected to support recommended process changes. With an emphasis on improving overall timeliness and efficiency, the task force set the following interval benchmarks/goals.

- Diagnostic CT scan within seven days of a suspicious CXR
- An alert system to flag cases for the cancer care coordinator requiring further workup
- Diagnostic bronchoscopies to be done within seven days of a suspicious CT scan
- Mediastinoscopy and thoracotomy to be completed within 30 days of diagnosis
- Definitive treatment within six weeks

Many of these benchmarks were based on the Rand and British Thoracic Society guidelines (Lung Cancer Working Party of the British Thoracic Society Standards of Care Committee, 1998; Reifel, 2000).

Another process improvement included the creation of a cancer care coordinator referral, whereby a PCP could request that the cancer care coordinator oversee the diagnostic process. A service agreement was established with primary care to define patient eligibility requirements and cancer care coordinator responsibilities. A multidisciplinary pulmonary tumor board was established, which provided a mechanism for anyone, including the cancer care coordinator, to request that a particular case be presented for discussion. This was found to be especially helpful to the cancer care coordinator when challenges arose surrounding real or potential delays, as well as nonconformance with established guidelines and recommendations.

The majority of patients who had an initial abnormal screening result did not have lung cancer and were placed in a surveillance nodule-tracking program that was based on the Fleischner Society guidelines (MacMahon et al., 2005). Fleischner guidelines are established principles guiding the management and surveillance of small pulmonary nodules based on the size of the nodule and the risk factors of the individual.

The cancer care coordinator reviewed all radiology reports coded with the cancer alert and continued to track those patients with lung cancer. In some cases, the coordinator provided navigation by tracking dates and intervening to expedite appointments between the services in such a manner that the patient was never aware. For example, if a patient did not appear to be progressing through the diagnostic process, the cancer care coordinator would analyze the situation to determine what the delays were and perhaps notify the appropriate provider or request a review by the pulmonary tumor board. In other cases, such as when a cancer care coordinator referral was placed, the cancer care coordinator took a much more active role and became the point of contact for the patient and orchestrated the diagnosis and treatment planning process.

In some form, the cancer care coordinator was involved in all cases of suspicious radiology films for lung cancer, making traditional caseload measurement and reporting difficult. It was difficult to evaluate the process from the patient's perspective because some patients were not aware of the cancer care coordinator's role. Specific marketing and advertising regarding program benefits might be a solution to increase patient awareness regarding the role of the cancer care coordinator.

The process changes made at CT-VAHCS resulted in a significant reduction in the interval from suspicious finding to treatment initiation for patients with non-small cell lung cancer. Initial data revealed a median of 117 days elapsed from suspicion of lung cancer to treatment. After the cancer care coordinator was hired, the interval decreased to 64.5 days and later to 52.4 days. An unanticipated result was earlier-stage detection of non-small cell lung cancer: in the year prior to hiring of the cancer care coordinator, 33% of patients were diagnosed with stages I and II disease, but this increased to 53% within three years of implementing the cancer care coordinator's role and new processes. This stage shift can be attributed to careful tracking of incidental findings suspicious for lung cancer and the cancer care coordination process created at CT-VAHCS.

Finally, the cancer care coordination program at CT-VAHCS had strong support from administration. Regular in-services were presented to PCPs to familiarize everyone with the new role and process improvements. To further encourage primary care support, a member of the primary care team served on the lung nodule task force. The institution conducted a survey of PCPs to examine their overall satisfaction with the program. An email survey was sent to 77 PCPs who provided care or used services at CT-VAHCS, and 31% responded. Of the providers participating in the survey, 46% indicated they were "very satisfied" and an additional 29% indicated they were "satisfied" with the cancer care coordination program.

This case example demonstrates how data proved to be an invaluable and strong component of a cancer care coordination program. Being able to show metrics demonstrating positive change helped to gain institutional support and buy-in from involved services and primary care. Creating cultural change in large and well-established programs is difficult. The efforts of a dedicated team, a strong physician champion, and the resources to have a fully committed cancer care coordinator enabled the CT-VAHCS to show the benefit of investing in a navigation program to reduce time from an abnormal test suspicious for cancer to the diagnosis and initiation of treatment, as well as to report a stage shift in the diagnosis of non-small cell lung cancer.

Conclusion

Patient navigation is a developing field. With the initial planning and implementation of a navigation program, the NAT can serve as a roadmap to navigators and program administrators for systematic and strategic program growth and maturation. As evidence guides practice, it is essential for navigation programs to identify core metrics and standardize data collection in order to clearly demonstrate program outcomes. Data elements frequently collected include the start of navigation, date of abnormal screening, date of diagnosis, date treatment(s) started, patient satisfaction, and cost-effectiveness (Freund et al., 2008). Furthermore, Esparza and Calhoun (2011) recommended that navigation programs consider the unique aspects of the population served for additional culturally relevant metrics. Because programs vary in available resources and capabilities related to data collection, programs must focus on the minimum data set needed to be able to report metrics that reflect the program's overall goals and priorities.

The future of navigation programs may well rest on the ability of organizations to document reductions in time to diagnosis and treatment as a means to support the basic navigation goal of facilitating timely access to quality care (Freeman, 2012). The importance of carefully defined program metrics to document the value and validity of navigation programs cannot be understated.

References

American College of Surgeons Commission on Cancer. (2012). *Cancer program standards 2012: Ensuring patient-centered care* [v.1.2.1, released January 2014]. Retrieved from http://www.facs.org/cancer/coc/programstandards2012.pdf

Barkley, R. (2012). Where does oncology fit in the scheme of accountable care? *Journal of Oncology Practice, 8,* 71–74. doi:10.1200/JOP.2012.000550

Basu, M., Linebarger, J., Gabram, S.G., Patterson, S.G., Amin, M., & Ward, K.C. (2013). The effect of nurse navigation on timeliness of breast cancer care at an academic comprehensive cancer center. *Cancer, 119,* 2524–2531. doi:10.1002/cncr.28024

Battaglia, T.A., Burhansstipanov, L., Murrell, S.S., Dwyer, A.J., & Caron, S.E. (2011). Assessing the impact of patient navigation. *Cancer, 117,* 3553–3564. doi:10.1002/cncr.26267

Braun, K.L., Kagawa-Singer, M., Holden, A.E., Burhansstipanov, L., Tran, J.H., Seals, B.F., ... Ramirez, A.G. (2012). Cancer patient navigator tasks across the cancer care continuum. *Journal of Health Care for the Poor and Underserved, 23,* 398–413. doi:10.1353/hpu.2012.0029

Brown, C.G., Cantril, C., McMullen, L., Barkley, D.L., Dietz, M., Murphy, C.M., & Fabrey, L.J. (2012). Oncology nurse navigator role delineation study. *Clinical Journal of Oncology Nursing, 16,* 581–585. doi:10.1188/12.CJON.581-585

Byers, T. (2012). Assessing the value of patient navigation for completing cancer screening. *Cancer Epidemiology, Biomarkers and Prevention, 21,* 1618–1619. doi:10.1158/1055-9965.EPI-12-0964

Campbell, C., Craig, J., Eggert, J., & Bailey-Dorton, C. (2010). Implementing and measuring the impact of patient navigation at a comprehensive community cancer center. *Oncology Nursing Forum, 37,* 61–68. doi:10.1188/10.ONF.61-68

Case, M.A. (2011). Oncology nurse navigator: Ensuring safe passage. *Clinical Journal of Oncology Nursing, 15,* 33–40. doi:10.1188/11.CJON.33-40

Center to Reduce Cancer Health Disparities. (2013). Health disparities and CRCHD. Retrieved from http://crchd.cancer.gov/about/disparities-index.html

Centers for Disease Control and Prevention. (2013). Health disparities in cancer. Retrieved from http://www.cdc.gov/Features/cancerhealthdisparities

Central Area Health Education Center. (2011). The Affordable Care Act and patient navigation executive summary. Retrieved from http://www.centralctahec.org/downloads/Patient-Navigation-Exec-Summary.pdf

Chen, F., Mercado, C., Yermilov, I., Puig, M., Ko, C.Y., Kahn, K.L., ... Gibbons, M.M. (2010). Improving breast cancer quality of care with the use of patient navigators. *American Surgeon, 76,* 1043–1046.

Cobb, P., & Okon, T. (2010). Just "who" is the oncologist accountable to in an accountable care organization? Retrieved from http://www.oncologystat.com/viewpoints/cancer-policy-forum/Just_Who_Is_the_Oncologist_Accountable_to_in_an_Accountable_Care_Organization.html

Desimini, E.M., Kennedy, J.A., Helsley, M.F., Shiner, K., Denton, C., Rice, T.T., ... Lewis, M.G. (2011). Making the case for nurse navigators—Benefits, outcomes, and return on investment. *Oncology Issues, 26*(5), 26–33. Retrieved from http://accc-cancer.org/oncology_issues/articles/SepOct2011/SO11-Desimini.pdf

Donaldson, E.A., Holtgrave, D.R., Duffin, R.A., Feltner, F., Funderburk, W., & Freeman, H.P. (2012). Patient navigation for breast and colorectal cancer in 3 community hospital settings: An economic evaluation. *Cancer, 118,* 4851–4859. doi:10.1002/cncr.27487

Dudley, D.J., Drake, J., Quinlan, J., Holden, A., Saegert, P., Karnad, A., & Ramirez, A. (2012). Beneficial effects of a combined navigator/promotora approach for Hispanic women diagnosed with breast abnormalities. *Cancer Epidemiology, Biomarkers and Prevention, 21,* 1639–1644. doi:10.1158/1055-9965.EPI-12-0538

Elkin, E.B., Shapiro, E., Snow, J.G., Zauber, A.G., & Krauskopf, M.S. (2012). The economic impact of a patient navigator program to increase screening colonoscopy. *Cancer, 118,* 5982–5988. doi:10.1002/cncr.27595

Esparza, A., & Calhoun, E. (2011). Measuring the impact and potential of patient navigation. *Cancer, 117,* 3535–3536. doi:10.1002/cncr.26265

Fillion, L., Cook, S., Veillette, A.M., Aubin, M., de Serres, M., Rainville, F., ... Doll, R. (2012). Professional navigation framework: Elaboration and validation in a Canadian context [Online exclusive]. *Oncology Nursing Forum, 39,* E58–E69. doi:10.1188/12.ONF.E58-E69

Fiscella, K., Ransom, S., Jean-Pierre, P., Cella, D., Stein, S., Bauer, J.E., ... Walsh, K. (2011). Patient-reported outcome measures suitable to assessment of patient navigation. *Cancer, 117,* 3603–3617. doi:10.1002/cncr.26260

Francz, S., & Simpson, L. (2013). Oncology nurse navigators: A snapshot of their educational background, compensation, and day-to-day roles and responsibilities. *Oncology Issues, 28*(1), 36–43.

Freeman, H.P. (2012). The origins, evolution, and principles of patient navigation. *Cancer Epidemiology, Biomarkers and Prevention, 21,* 1614–1617. doi:10.1158/1055-9965.EPI-12-0982

Freund, K.M., Battaglia, T.A., Calhoun, E., Dudley, D.J., Fiscella, K., Paskett, E., ... Roetzheim, R.G. (2008). National Cancer Institute Patient Navigation Research Program: Methods, protocol, and measures. *Cancer, 113,* 3391–3399. doi:10.1002/cncr.23960

Gilbert, J.E., Green, E., Lankshear, S., Hughes, E., Burkoski, V., & Sawka, C. (2011). Nurses as patient navigators in cancer diagnosis: review, consultation and model design. *European Journal of Cancer Care, 20,* 228–236. doi:10.1111/j.1365-2354.2010.01231.x

Guadagnolo, B.A., Dohan, D., & Raich, P. (2011). Metrics for evaluating patient navigation during cancer diagnosis and treatment. *Cancer, 117,* 3565–3574. doi:10.1002/cncr.26269

Hendren, S., Chin, N., Fisher, S., Winters, P., Griggs, J., Mohile, S., & Fiscella, K. (2011). Patients' barriers to receipt of cancer care, and factors associated with needing more assistance from a patient navigator. *Journal of the National Medical Association, 103,* 701–710.

Hendren, S., Griggs, J.J., Epstein, R., Humiston, S., Jean-Pierre, P., Winters, P., ... Fiscella, K. (2012). Randomized controlled trial of patient navigation for newly diagnosed cancer patients: Effects on quality of life. *Cancer Epidemiology, Biomarkers and Prevention, 21,* 1682–1690. doi:10.1158/1055-9965.EPI-12-0537

Holmes, D.R., Major, J., Lyonga, D.E., Alleyne, R.S., & Clayton, S.M. (2012). Increasing minority patient participation in cancer clinical trials using oncology nurse navigation. *American Journal of Surgery, 203,* 415–422. doi:10.1016/j.amjsurg.2011.02.005

Hook, A., Ware, L., Siler, B., & Packard, A. (2012). Breast cancer navigation and patient satisfaction: Exploring a community-based patient navigation model in a rural setting. *Oncology Nursing Forum, 39,* 379–385. doi:10.1188/12.ONF.379-385

Hunnibell, L.S., Rose, M.G., Connery, D.M., Grens, C.E., Hampel, J.M., Rosa, M., & Vogel, D.C. (2012). Using nurse navigation to improve timeliness in lung cancer care at a veterans hospital. *Clinical Journal of Oncology Nursing, 16,* 29–36. doi:10.1188/12.CJON.29-36

Jean-Pierre, P., Fiscella, K., Freund, K.M., Clark, J., Darnell, J., Holden, A., ... Winters, P.C. (2011). Structural and reliability analysis of a patient satisfaction with cancer-related care measure. *Cancer, 117,* 854–861. doi:10.1002/cncr.25501

Jean-Pierre, P., Hendren, S., Fiscella, K., Loader, S., Rousseau, S., Schwartzbauer, B., ... Epstein, R. (2011). Understanding the processes of patient navigation to reduce disparities in cancer care: Perspectives of trained navigators from the field. *Journal of Cancer Education, 26,* 111–120. doi:10.1007/s13187-010-0122-x

Koh, C., Nelson, J.M., & Cook, P.F. (2011). Evaluation of a patient navigation program. *Clinical Journal of Oncology Nursing, 15,* 41–48. doi:10.1188/11.CJON.41-48

Korber, S.F., Padula, C., Gray, J., & Powell, M. (2011). A breast navigator program: Barriers, enhancers, and nursing interventions. *Oncology Nursing Forum, 38,* 44–50. doi:10.1188/11.ONF.44-50

Lebwohl, B., Neugut, A.I., Stavsky, E., Villegas, S., Meli, C., Rodriguez, O., ... Rosenberg, R. (2011). Effect of a patient navigator program on the volume and quality of colonoscopy. *Journal of Clinical Gastroenterology, 45,* e47–e53. doi:10.1097/MCG.0b013e3181f595c3

Lee, T., Ko, I., Lee, I., Kim, E., Shin, M., Roh, S., ... Chang, H. (2011). Effects of nurse navigators on health outcomes of cancer patients. *Cancer Nursing, 34,* 376–384. doi:10.1097/NCC.0b013e3182025007

Lung Cancer Working Party of the British Thoracic Society Standards of Care Committee. (1998). BTS recommendations to respiratory physicians for organizing the care of patients with lung cancer. *Thorax, 53*(Suppl. 1), S1–S8.

MacMahon, H., Austin, J.H., Gamsu, G., Herold, C.J., Jett, J.R., Naidich, D.P., ... Swensen, S.J. (2005). Guidelines for the management of small pulmonary nodules detected on CT scans: A statement from the Fleischner Society. *Radiology, 237,* 395–400.

Markossian, T.W., & Calhoun, E.A. (2011). Are breast cancer navigation programs cost-effective? Evidence from the Chicago Cancer Navigation Project. *Health Policy, 99,* 52–59. doi:10.1016/j.healthpol.2010.07.008

Markossian, T.W., Darnell, J.S., & Calhoun, E.A. (2012). Follow-up and timeliness after an abnormal cancer screening among underserved, urban women in a patient navigation program. *Cancer Epidemiology, Biomarkers and Prevention, 21,* 1691–1700. doi:10.1158/1055-9965. EPI-12-0535

National Cancer Institute. (n.d.-a). NCI Community Cancer Centers Program: About NCCCP. Retrieved from http://ncccp.cancer.gov/about/index.htm

National Cancer Institute. (n.d.-b). Surveillance, Epidemiology, and End Results Program: About the SEER registries. Retrieved from http://seer.cancer.gov/registries

National Comprehensive Cancer Network. (2013). *NCCN Clinical Practice Guidelines in Oncology: Distress management* [v.2.2013]. Retrieved from http://www.nccn.org/professionals/ physician_gls/PDF/distress.pdf

Pedersen, A., & Hack, T.F. (2010). Pilots of oncology health care: A concept analysis of the patient navigator role. *Oncology Nursing Forum, 37,* 55–60. doi:10.1188/10.ONF.55-60

Pedersen, A.E., & Hack, T.F. (2011). The British Columbia Patient Navigation Model: A critical analysis. *Oncology Nursing Forum, 38,* 200–206. doi:10.1188/11.ONF.200-206

Psooy, B.J., Schreuer, D., Borgaonkar, J., & Caines, J.S. (2004). Patient navigation: Improving timeliness in the diagnosis of breast abnormalities. *Canadian Association of Radiologists Journal, 55,* 145–150.

Reifel, J.L. (2000). Lung cancer. In S.M. Asch, E.A. Kerr, E.G. Hamilton, J.L. Reifel, & E.A. McGlynn (Eds.), *Quality of care for oncology conditions and HIV: A review of the literature and quality indicators* (pp. 133–171). Retrieved from http://www.rand.org/content/dam/rand/ pubs/monograph_reports/2007/MR1281.pdf

Robinson-White, S., Conroy, B., Slavish, K.H., & Rosenzweig, M. (2010). Patient navigation in breast cancer: A systematic review. *Cancer Nursing, 33,* 127–140. doi:10.1097/ NCC.0b013e3181c40401

Schultz, E., Olsson, J., & Gould, M. (2008). *Timeliness in lung cancer care in veterans with lung cancer.* Unpublished manuscript.

Singh, H., Hirani, K., Kadiyala, H., Rudomiotov, O., Davis, T., Khan, M.M., & Wahls, T.L. (2010). Characteristics and predictors of missed opportunities in lung cancer diagnosis: An electronic health record-based study. *Journal of Clinical Oncology, 28,* 3307–3315. doi:10.1200/ JCO.2009.25.6636

Swanson, J., & Koch, L. (2010). The role of the oncology nurse navigator in distress management of adult inpatients with cancer: A retrospective study. *Oncology Nursing Forum, 37,* 69–76. doi:10.1188/10.ONF.69-76

Swanson, J.R., Strusowski, P., Mack, N., & Degroot, J. (2012). Growing a navigation program: Using the NCCCP Navigation Assessment Tool. *Oncology Issues, 27*(4), 36–45. Retrieved from http://www.nxtbook.com/nxtbooks/accc/oncologyissues_20120708/index.php

Thygesen, M.K., Pedersen, B.D., Kragstrup, J., Wagner, L., & Mogensen, O. (2011). Benefits and challenges perceived by patients with cancer when offered a nurse navigator. *International Journal of Integrated Care, 11,* e130. Retrieved from https://www.ijic.org/index.php/ ijic/article/viewFile/URN%3ANBN%3ANL%3AUI%3A10-1-101627/1481

Thygesen, M.K., Pedersen, B.D., Kragstrup, J., Wagner, L., & Mogensen, O. (2012). Gynecological cancer patients' differentiated use of help from a nurse navigator: A qualitative study. *BMC Health Services Research, 12,* 168. doi:10.1186/1472-6963-12-168

Van Buskirk, M.C., & Atwood, C.W. (2009). Expediting lung nodule evaluations: Experience from the VA Pittsburgh Healthcare System. *Federal Practitioner, 26*(3), 14–16, 19–23.

Weber, J.J., Mascarenhas, D.C., Bellin, L.S., Raab, R.E., & Wong, J.H. (2012). Patient navigation and the quality of breast cancer care: An analysis of the breast cancer care quality indicators. *Annals of Surgical Oncology, 19,* 3251–3256. doi:10.1245/s10434-012-2527-8

Whitley, E., Valverde, P., Wells, K., Williams, L., Teschner, T., & Shih, Y.C. (2011). Establishing common cost measures to evaluate the economic value of patient navigation programs. *Cancer, 117,* 3616–3623. doi:10.1002/cncr.26268

Yosha, A.M., Carroll, J.K., Hendren, S., Salamone, C.M., Sanders, M., Fiscella, K., & Epstein, R.M. (2011). Patient navigation from the paired perspectives of cancer patients and navigators: A qualitative analysis. *Patient Education and Counseling, 82,* 396–401. doi:10.1016/j.pec.2010.12.019

CHAPTER 10

Documentation and Patient Navigation Software

Kathleen A. Gamblin, RN, BSN, OCN®, and Karyl D. Blaseg, RN, MSN, OCN®

Introduction

Documentation of patient assessments, interactions, multidisciplinary team communications, and referrals to resources is essential for oncology nurse navigators. The documentation process must be considered to be of primary importance in the development of a navigation program. The lack of a national standardized electronic medical record (EMR), or in many cases even a standardized institutional EMR, has led to much discussion and confusion, as programs and nurse navigators struggle with the issue of documentation processes and the selection of a documentation system.

Documentation and Nursing Practice

Oncology nurse navigators must recognize and understand the role of documentation and its importance. Anecdotally, nurse navigators have indicated that precise and timely documentation of actions and interventions is often viewed as insignificant when compared to the multiple patient care priorities associated with juggling a full caseload. Although oncology nurse navigators may not provide direct clinical care, key nursing roles and functions are still performed; therefore, nurse navigators are required by law and institutional policies and procedures to adhere to documentation requirements (Campos, 2010).

State boards of nursing are governmental agencies charged with the regulation of nursing practice. These boards of nursing protect patients by ensuring that standards of practice in nursing care are met (American Nurses Association, 2012). Each state and territory has a law called the Nurse Practice Act, which is enforced by the board (National Council of State Boards of Nursing, 2013). The objective of the different states' nurse practice acts in regard to documentation is not specific but broad; documentation, in general, needs to provide an accurate and understandable account of patient care that the healthcare team provided (Campos, 2010). Individual state nurse practice acts define more specific guidelines regarding required details of documentation, whereas healthcare institutions further establish policies and procedures on standard mechanisms for documentation.

Before development of the navigation documentation processes and implementation of the documentation system, nurse navigators must understand the state nurse practice acts governing documentation in the state where they practice. Such information can be accessed at the National Council of State Boards of Nursing website, which provides links to the state and territory member boards (National Council of State Boards of Nursing, 2013). Navigators must also be familiar with their healthcare institution's documentation policies and procedures.

Navigation Documentation Considerations

Before a documentation system can be selected, navigation program administrators must contemplate some fundamental considerations. This includes determining the elements of utmost importance for navigators to capture within the medical record, as well as defining expectations related to timeliness of the documentation. Furthermore, programs must decide the mechanism for navigation documentation, whether this involves basic paper documentation methods or more sophisticated integration of software packages that interface with the EMR.

Essential Elements of Documentation

The process for navigation documentation should be determined during program planning and should be clearly outlined from the outset. The navigation program, guided by institutional policies and procedures, must determine what is essential for navigators to document not only to depict an accurate portrayal of the care provided but also to provide metrics for outcome measures.

Examples of basic elements that oncology nurse navigators might consider incorporating into documentation processes include (a) demographics and contact information, (b) referral source, (c) diagnosis, (d) barriers to care, and (e) referrals initiated. In addition, dates of biopsies, diagnostic evaluations, consultations, and treatment initiation and completion may be beneficial, depending on the scope of the navigator's roles and responsibilities. These elements often are necessary to capture for various program metrics. Most significant, however, is the need for nurse navigators to document navigation actions and interventions relevant to the coordination of care, education, and support of patients. This information not only provides an accurate account of navigator activities but, more importantly, keeps other members of the healthcare team apprised of current issues and concerns, as well as the nurse navigator's involvement in facilitating the patient's experience.

When considering essential elements of navigation documentation, the time spent on documentation tasks should be weighed against other responsibilities of the navigators. Because the primary objective of navigation programs is typically to optimize care by eliminating barriers that patients may encounter, it is imperative that the majority of the navigators' time be spent interacting with patients rather than being taxed with collecting volumes of outcomes data. Programs must carefully consider the value of specific data elements to be extracted from navigators' documentation and then strategize the most efficient mechanisms for data collection. Many navigation programs have created patient intake and assessment tools to provide a relatively quick way to assess patients and document needs. An example is shown in Figure 10-1.

Another strategy to minimize the time spent by navigators on documentation is to develop documentation notes using a template with prebuilt key phrases. Figure 10-2 depicts one navigation program's EMR progress note template. This template allows navigators to select only those phrases and elements pertinent to a given situation. In addition, navigators are able to enter information not covered by the prebuilt phrases.

Timeliness of Documentation

In the clinical care of patients, in both the inpatient and outpatient settings, documentation must occur in a timely manner. This is no less important for navigation documentation, especially given that the role of navigators is often to bridge communication among team members. Realistic expectations must be set in order to prevent navigation documentation from becoming a task that can be set aside for later. The development of a policy and procedure for navigation documentation establishes expectations and can help guide the process (see Figure 10-3). Anecdotally, most navigation documentation policies require that documentation occur within 24–48 hours of patient encounters, which tends to coincide with expectations placed upon other members of the healthcare team (e.g., physicians and ancillary staff).

Paper Documentation Systems

Perhaps one of the simplest ways in which to document navigation interactions and interventions, as well as track patient encounters, is to use a paper

Figure 10-1. Northside Hospital Cancer Institute's Navigation Intake and Assessment Form

NH
NORTHSIDE HOSPITAL
CANCER INSTITUTE

Date: _____ **Priority:** STAT __ ASAP __ TIMED __   **INPT __ OUTPT __**

Navigator Site/Reason for Referral
Breast: _____
GI: _____
GYN: _____
Other: _____
Disparities: _____

Referred By:
Patient Navigation: _____
Physician's Office: _____

Diagnosis: _____
Physician Name: _____
Preferred Language: _____
Patient Name: _____ **DOB:** _____
Address: _____ **City/State:** _____ **Zip:** _____
Phone Number(s): HOME _____ CELL _____ WORK _____
Email Address: _____
Preferred Contact Time: _____
Additional Comments: _____
_____
_____

Date/Time Reviewed: _____ **Date/Time of Initial Patient Contact:** _____

American Cancer Society (ACS) Navigator
☐ Transportation issues (difficulty getting to appointments, Medicaid van scheduling)
☐ Lodging assistance (for those with a home residence more than 40 miles away)
☐ Difficulty in meeting rent
☐ Prescription assistance
☐ General nutrition questions (phone consult only)
☐ Caregiver support
☐ Female oncology patient—Look Good Feel Better Referral
☐ Referral to disparity nurse navigator (automatic referral to ACS Navigator)
☐ _____
_____
_____

(Continued on next page)

Figure 10-1. Northside Hospital Cancer Institute's Navigation Intake and Assessment Form *(Continued)*

Behavioral Health
☐ Referral to Northside Mental Health Center
☐ Referral to Cancer Support Community for general support
☐ Referral to State Line Number

Cancer Support Community
☐ Support group interest
☐ Exercise and fitness interest
☐ Class interest_____
☐ General referral
☐ Other _____
_____

Clinical Trials
☐ General interest in clinical trials
☐ Specific trial_____

Disparities Navigator (Any referral to Disparities Navigator will result in automatic referral to ACS Navigator)
☐ Inadequate or lack of insurance coverage
☐ Cultural barriers to care
☐ Poor health literacy, Inability to read or write
☐ Need for financial assistance from Medicaid/Medicare

Genetic Counseling
☐ Information requested by patient
☐ Patient meets screening criteria
☐ Physician request to coordinate appointment _____

Interpretative Services
☐ Primary language other than English _____

Network of Hope
☐ Coordinator

Nutritional Services
☐ General nutrition questions (phone consult with ACS Navigator)
☐ One-on-one nutritional consult (Cancer Support Community)

Note. Figure courtesy of Northside Hospital Cancer Institute. Used with permission.

Figure 10-2. Billings Clinic's Navigation Progress Note Template

Billings Clinic

Patient Navigation Documentation Template for EMR

Patient:_____ MRN:_____ FIN:_____

Age: _____ Gender:_____ DOB:_____

Author: _____

Visit Information

SITUATION
☐ This is an initial Cancer Care Navigation visit for introduction, education and support.
☐ This is a follow-up visit.
☐ This is a phone note.
☐ This is an email note.
☐ This is a family meeting with *(free text)* _____ present.
☐ Referral received from *(free text)* _____ for *(free text)* _____.
☐ I met with the *(choose from the following options)* to offer support and assess needs and/or concerns.
    ☐ patient
    ☐ patient and family member(s)
    ☐ patient and spouse
    ☐ patient and significant other
    ☐ patient and support person
    ☐ *(Free text)* _____.

BACKGROUND
☐ Patient has been recently diagnosed with *(free text)*_____.
☐ Patient is receiving treatment for *(free text)*_____.
☐ Patient is being discharged from the hospital after an inpatient stay for *(free text)*
_____.
☐ Patient has a diagnosis of *(free text)*_____.
☐ *(Free text)* _____.

ASSESSMENT
☐ Further education is needed regarding *(free text)* _____.
☐ There are concerns about coordination of services, specifically related to:
    ☐ appointments
    ☐ diagnostic imaging
    ☐ diagnostic labs
    ☐ infusion schedule
    ☐ surgery
    ☐ venous access device placement
    ☐ venous access device removal
    ☐ transportation
    ☐ housing
    ☐ *(Free text)* _____.

(Continued on next page)

Figure 10-2. Billings Clinic's Navigation Progress Note Template *(Continued)*

☐ There are concerns regarding dependent care, specifically related to *(free text)*

_____ .

☐ There are concerns about drug interactions, specifically related to *(free text)*

_____ .

☐ There are end-of-life concerns, specifically related to:
   ☐ POLST
   ☐ Five Wishes
   ☐ *(Free text)* _____ .
☐ There are financial concerns, specifically related to:
   ☐ loss of employment
   ☐ loss of income
   ☐ loss of insurance
   ☐ application for Social Security/Disability Insurance
   ☐ cost of housing
   ☐ cost of transportation
   ☐ determination of insurance coverage
   ☐ *(Free text)* _____ .
☐ There are concerns about home health, specifically related to:
   ☐ safety
   ☐ wound care
   ☐ home oxygen needs
   ☐ durable medical equipment
   ☐ medication management
   ☐ home IV antibiotics
   ☐ home IV fluids
   ☐ PT/OT
   ☐ blood draws
   ☐ symptom management
   ☐ *(Free text)* _____ .
☐ There are concerns about hospice, specifically related to *(free text)* _____ .
☐ There are housing concerns, specifically related to:
   ☐ living out of the area
   ☐ homelessness
   ☐ long-term care residence
   ☐ *(Free text)* _____ .
☐ There are insurance concerns, specifically related to:
   ☐ no insurance coverage
   ☐ need for preauthorization of chemotherapy
   ☐ no prescription drug benefit
   ☐ amount of deductible
   ☐ treatment costs
   ☐ amount of prescription co-pay(s)
   ☐ cost of COBRA insurance
   ☐ long-term care residency
   ☐ *(Free text)* _____ .
☐ There are integrative medicine concerns, specifically related to *(free text)*_____ .
☐ There are concerns about meals/nutrition, specifically related to:
   ☐ weight loss

(Continued on next page)

Figure 10-2. Billings Clinic's Navigation Progress Note Template *(Continued)*

☐ anorexia
☐ nausea/vomiting
☐ difficulty chewing
☐ dysphagia
☐ parenteral nutrition
☐ enteral nutrition/tube feedings
☐ mucositis
☐ stomatitis
☐ esophagitis
☐ diabetes
☐ wound/pressure ulcer(s)
☐ healthy eating habits
☐ potential need for feeding tube
☐ potential effects of chemotherapy on nutrition status
☐ potential effects of radiation therapy on nutrition status
☐ *(Free text)* _____ .
☐ Medical records are needed for *(free text)*_____ .
☐ There are pain management concerns, specifically related to *(free text)* _____ .
☐ There are concerns about palliative care, specifically related to *(free text)*_____ .
☐ There are psychosocial concerns, specifically related to:
  ☐ cultural considerations
  ☐ ethnic considerations
  ☐ spiritual issues
  ☐ emotional well-being
  ☐ anxiety
  ☐ mood changes
  ☐ behavior changes
  ☐ coping
  ☐ family coping
  ☐ lack of support
  ☐ relationships
  ☐ dependencies
  ☐ cognitive deficits
  ☐ body image
  ☐ potential effects of chemotherapy on overall well-being
  ☐ potential effects of radiation therapy on overall well-being
  ☐ potential effects of new diagnosis and treatment
  ☐ potential diagnosis and treatment on overall well-being
  ☐ *(Free text)* _____ .
☐ Tobacco dependency:
  ☐ Currently smokes
  ☐ Stopped smoking
  ☐ Currently uses smokeless tobacco
  ☐ *(Free text)* _____ .
☐ There are rehabilitation concerns, specifically related to:
  ☐ activities of daily living
  ☐ lymphedema
  ☐ speech deficits

(Continued on next page)

Figure 10-2. Billings Clinic's Navigation Progress Note Template *(Continued)*

☐ swallowing difficulties
☐ pulmonary rehabilitation
☐ *(Free text)* _____.
☐ There are concerns about sleep disturbances, specifically related to:
   ☐ insomnia
   ☐ sleep apnea
   ☐ nightmares
   ☐ positioning
   ☐ *(Free text)* _____.
☐ There are symptom management concerns, specifically related to:
   ☐ anemia
   ☐ bleeding
   ☐ breathing problems
   ☐ constipation
   ☐ dehydration
   ☐ diarrhea
   ☐ dizziness
   ☐ edema
   ☐ fatigue
   ☐ fever/infection
   ☐ hand-foot syndrome
   ☐ headache
   ☐ memory and concentration
   ☐ mucositis
   ☐ nausea
   ☐ neuropathy
   ☐ neutropenia
   ☐ rash
   ☐ sexuality
   ☐ side effects from radiation
   ☐ vomiting
   ☐ *(Free text)* _____.
☐ There are tracheostomy concerns, specifically related to *(free text)* _____.
☐ There are transportation concerns, specifically related to:
   ☐ living out of the area
   ☐ weather
   ☐ driving limitations
   ☐ cost of transportation
   ☐ lack of transportation options
   ☐ obtaining a handicap parking sticker
   ☐ long-term care transportation schedule and/or abilities
   ☐ *(Free text)* _____.
☐ There are treatment adherence concerns, specifically related to *(free text)* _____.
☐ There are treatment/staging concerns, specifically related to *(free text)*_____.
☐ *(Free text)* _____.

(Continued on next page)

Figure 10-2. Billings Clinic's Navigation Progress Note Template *(Continued)*

RESPONSE
☐ *(Free text)* _____ .
☐ We discussed:
    ☐ coordination of care *(free text)*_____ .
    ☐ available services (*(free text)*_____ .
    ☐ education resources *(free text)* _____ .
    ☐ integrative care *(free text)* _____ .
    ☐ support groups *(free text)* _____ .
    ☐ symptom management *(free text)* _____ .
    ☐ side effects of:
        ☐ chemotherapy (free text) _____ .
        ☐ radiation therapy (free text) _____ .
        ☐ surgery (free text) _____ .
☐ I reinforced treatment options presented by the physician.
☐ I reinforced staging studies presented by the physician.
☐ The Patient Guidebook was reviewed and given to the:
    ☐ patient
    ☐ family member
    ☐ spouse
    ☐ significant other
    ☐ support
    ☐ *(Free text)* _____ .
☐ Information was given regarding *(free text)* _____ .
☐ I encouraged the *(choose from the following options)* to contact insurance company(s) regarding diagnosis and treatment plan.
    ☐ patient
    ☐ family member
    ☐ spouse
    ☐ significant other
    ☐ support person
    ☐ *(Free text)* _____ .
☐ Referral to:
    ☐ ACS *(free text)*_____ .
    ☐ the diabetes educator *(free text)* _____ .
    ☐ the dietitian
        ☐ for initial assessment of nutrition status
        ☐ *(Free text)* _____ .
    ☐ the financial counselor
        ☐ for preauthorization of chemotherapy
        ☐ for assessment of insurance coverage
        ☐ to address financial concerns
        ☐ *(Free text)* _____ .
    ☐ the genetic counselor *(free text)* _____ .
    ☐ hospice *(free text)* _____ .
    ☐ integrative medicine *(free text)* _____ .
    ☐ inpatient care management *(free text)*_____ .
    ☐ MAP (Medication Assistance Program) *(free text)* _____ .

(Continued on next page)

Figure 10-2. Billings Clinic's Navigation Progress Note Template *(Continued)*

- ☐ the oncology social worker
  - ☐ for assessment of psychosocial needs
  - ☐ for transportation/lodging
  - ☐ related to diagnosis and treatment
  - ☐ *(Free text)* _____.
- ☐ the pharmacist *(free text)* _____.
- ☐ radiation oncology *(free text)* _____.
- ☐ rehabilitation *(free text)* _____.
- ☐ the research division
  - ☐ for assessment of available trials and patient's eligibility status
  - ☐ *(Free text)* _____.
- ☐ Senior Life Partners *(free text)* _____.
- ☐ smoking cessation *(free text)* _____.
- ☐ speech and swallow therapy *(free text)* _____.
- ☐ multidisciplinary conference for case presentation on *(date) (free text)* _____.
- ☐ wound care *(free text)* _____.
- ☐ *(Free text)* _____.
- ☐ I explained my role, gave my contact information, and encouraged the patient to call if there are further questions.
- ☐ Medical records provided to *(free text)* _____ via
  - ☐ fax at *(free text)* _____.
  - ☐ *(Free text)* _____.
  - ☐ Notified file room of needed scans *(free text)* _____.
- ☐ Appointment scheduled for
  - ☐ imaging on *(free text)* _____.
  - ☐ labs on *(free text)* _____.
  - ☐ PET scan on *((free text)* _____.
  - ☐ vascular access device on *(free text)* _____.
  - ☐ consult on *(free text)* _____.
  - ☐ return visit on *(free text)* _____.
  - ☐ *(Free text)* _____.
- ☐ A PET scan is in the process of being scheduled.
- ☐ A vascular access device is in the process of being scheduled.
- ☐ A breast MRI is in the process of being scheduled.
- ☐ A dental appointment is in the process of being scheduled.
- ☐ I will follow-up with the patient during physician visits and/or as needed.
- ☐ *(Choose Care Navigator Name)* will follow the patient for subsequent visits.
- ☐ The *(choose from the following options)* verbalized understanding of today's discussion.
  - ☐ patient
  - ☐ patient and support person(s)
  - ☐ support person(s)
- ☐ A total of *(free text)* _____ minutes was spent today:
  - ☐ answering questions
  - ☐ offering support
  - ☐ providing education
  - ☐ *(Free text)* _____.

ACS—American Cancer Society; COBRA—Consolidated Omnibus Budget Reconciliation Act; EMR—electronic medical record; IV—intravenous; MRI—magnetic resonance imaging; OT—occupational therapy; PET—positron-emission tomography; POLST—physician orders for life-sustaining treatment; PT—physical therapy

Note. Figure courtesy of Billings Clinic. Used with permission.

Figure 10-3. Northside Hospital Cancer Institute's Policy Regarding Oncology Patient Navigation Documentation

NH
NORTHSIDE HOSPITAL
CANCER INSTITUTE

Northside Hospital
Oncology Patient Navigation Documentation
Oncology Navigation General Policies

Purpose
To provide the navigation program of Northside Hospital Cancer Institute with clear guidelines regarding timely documentation.

Policy
All navigation assessments and interactions will be documented in Morrisey Concurrent Care Manager (MCCM) in a timely manner.

Personnel
Oncology Nurse Navigators, American Cancer Society (ACS) Resource Navigator.

Procedures
1. The navigation assessment and all patient interactions will be documented in MCCM and according to policy set forth in MCCM guidelines.
2. All documentation will be completed as soon as possible after interaction with the patient but will occur no later than 24 hours after encounter.
3. If the Oncology Nurse Navigator is unable to document within the 24 hour time period, the Oncology Navigation Coordinator must be notified and a plan given for completing documentation.

Note. Figure courtesy of Northside Hospital Cancer Institute. Used with permission.

---

documentation system. The Association of Community Cancer Centers (2012) offers tools to help guide the implementation of a navigation program, including various templates that healthcare institutions can adapt. If navigators use paper documentation, they must consider the following.

• Will paper charts be made for each patient?
• What information will be included in these charts?
• Where will the chart be stored to allow easy access for the navigator while maintaining security?
• How will information be made available to other members of the healthcare team and to other departments within the institution?

Ultimately, although paper documentation may appear relatively straightforward, input from key stakeholders, including physicians, inpatient and outpatient departments, and the medical records department, is essential during initial development and implementation. In particular, the medical records department is able to advise on institutional policies regarding documentation and privacy of information, including what can and cannot be maintained in individual departments.

Electronic Documentation Systems

In a 2010 survey of approximately 1,000 members of the National Coalition of Oncology Nurse Navigators, one of the greatest challenges noted to establishing effective navigation programs included obsolete documentation processes (Francz, 2012). This frustration leads many oncology nurse navigators and navigation programs to explore electronic documentation systems. Electronic documentation systems used for navigation can be divided into three categories: facility-developed programs, general medical commercial off-the-shelf (COTS) programs, and navigation-specific programs.

Facility-Developed Programs

Facility-developed programs are designed in-house specifically for the purpose of collecting and tracking data for navigation outcomes. Commonly, these programs are built using a Microsoft® Access database or Excel spreadsheet. Advantages to using this type of system include design simplicity, ease of use, and minimal cost, from both a design and maintenance perspective. The chief disadvantage to using this type of system is the limitations to what information can be gathered and subsequently extrapolated for program metrics and outcomes.

It is important to note that any system developed for gathering patient information must be designed to ensure protection of patient privacy. This would preclude the system from being maintained on a data source accessible to unauthorized individuals in or outside the institution. Each institution has a privacy official responsible for the development of the institution's privacy policies and procedures as mandated by the Health Insurance Portability and Accountability Act of 1996 (HIPAA) (U.S. Department of Health and Human Services, n.d.), and this person should be used as a resource to validate that appropriate precautions have been taken to protect patient information when a facility-developed system is used.

Commercial Off-the-Shelf Programs

Multiple COTS systems can be used for navigation documentation and tracking of program outcomes. These systems often are used for case management and other comprehensive systems documenting the care of individuals across the continuum; a few examples include Morrisey® Concurrent Care Manager, MIDAS+™ Care Management, and ARIA® oncology information system. Key functionality often embedded within COTS programs involves a direct feed from other software programs within the institution to populate various information fields (for example, patient demographics) and the ability to customize electronic forms for specific data collection needs. Benefits of a COTS system include (a) using a system that may already be in use by other departments within the organization (leading to potentially lower usage costs), (b) capability for a direct feed from registration systems (resulting in decreased time entering data), and (c) increased communication among the healthcare team members using the system. However, because these systems are not developed exclusively for navigation programs, the healthcare institution's information technology (IT) department may be needed to significantly customize the system to meet the navigators' needs of capturing certain patient information and metrics.

Navigation-Specific Programs

Navigation-specific systems have captured the majority of interest for those navigation programs looking to move to an electronic documentation system. Cantril and Haylock (2013) identified Nursenav® Oncology, OncoNav, and Priority Consult® as three commercially available navigation software programs, although an increasing number of systems are being developed. These systems are built specifically for documentation of patient navigation activities and tracking of metrics; in fact, many were developed by or in consultation with oncology nurse navigators.

When considering a navigation-specific program, the navigators and program administrator must work closely with the healthcare institution's IT department in selecting a system because, ultimately, the IT department will be supporting the system implementation and maintenance. Often, interfaces, which allow information to be relayed between different information systems, must be built. Such interfaces can be costly and time consuming to maintain when upgrading either the navigation software or the information systems with which the navigation software interfaces.

With the increasing demand for patient navigation and the addition of patient navigation requirements for accreditation by the American College of Surgeons Commission on Cancer, more navigation-specific software systems will likely be brought to the market. An expanded listing of current (at the time of publishing) electronic navigation documentation systems and corresponding websites is included in Chapter 11.

Evaluation of a Navigation Documentation Software System

Although researching and selecting a documentation system for navigation may seem overwhelming, having more information obtained and considered up front will lead to better informed decision making and a greater likelihood of successful implementation of the chosen system. Because each navigation program is distinct and unique, what works for one program may not work for another. Navigators and program administrators may find it helpful to use a checklist when evaluating potential software systems. Figure 10-4 depicts a checklist containing key areas that require careful consideration and are explained in more detail in the following text.

Web-Based or Server-Based Systems

Choosing between a web-based and server-based software system has implications on use and cost. Web-based systems have become known for easy accessibility wherever a standard browser with Internet access is available. This is particularly appealing to navigators who may see patients in multiple locations and who have the ability to access the Internet in those places. It does, however, make navigators dependent on having Internet access, which may not always be available. In contrast, server-based systems must be

---

Figure 10-4. Navigation Documentation Software Checklist

- Is the system web-based or server-based?
- Is the system disease site–specific or made for general use?
- Is customization of the system available? If so, can it be customized by the user or only by the vendor?
- Does the system interface with other systems? If so, what electronic medical record systems has the software already been successfully interfaced with?
- Does the system allow importation of data from other sources?
- Is a patient portal for contact with the navigation team available?
- Does the system have calendars and allow scheduling of future reminders and appointments?
- Does the system allow for the creation of work lists?
- Does the system allow for the sharing of patients and/or viewing by other navigators?
- Is the system set up to print summary reports for physicians?
- Does the system come with standard reports?
- Are customizable reports available?
- Can the user create a queried report?
- Can letters be printed from the system?
- Can navigation notes be printed from the system?
- Can treatment summaries be generated in the system?
- Is there a limit to the number of users on the system?
- What is the initial cost and yearly cost?
- Is there a per person usage charge?
- Is there help desk support, and if so, what are the hours of availability?
- Is training done on site by a vendor representative or via online methods?
- Is a training manual available?

accessed through a local network and might not be available in every setting navigators encounter. However, being on the network creates reasonably quick response times and allows autonomy from the Internet.

With regard to cost, web-based systems usually charge a monthly subscription or usage fee, which allows for cost control in the beginning and may equate to a less expensive program start-up. However, consideration must be given to the cost over the many months and years a system may be in place because, in the long run, web-based systems tend to be more expensive. Server-based systems are generally paid for up front, resulting in higher initial system costs; however, the user is in control of the system and can decline upgrades, as well as dissolve the relationship with the system provider if desired while still maintaining ownership and the ability to use the system initially purchased.

System Interfaces

As the field of patient navigation has grown and oncology nurse navigators have become accepted members of the healthcare team, navigation documentation systems ideally would be able to interface with other information systems to allow for data importation and exportation.

An example of the value of an importation interface relates to entering patient demographic information. Although this may seem like a relatively quick and easy process, when considering the time it takes to key in this information for one patient and then multiplying this by the number of patients navigated, it can actually be a time-consuming task that takes the valuable navigator resource away from more critical activities. Another area of concern pertains to the potential for patient information to be entered incorrectly. One wrong keystroke can make it difficult to locate the patient within the system. Having an importation system interface allows the institution's registration system to link with the navigation system and to automatically populate the demographics section. This decreases the navigator's workload and decreases the likelihood of keystroke errors.

The exportation interface is also an important consideration. Navigators should be documenting all actions and interventions related to patient encounters and coordination of care. This not only provides a record of the care provided from a legal perspective but also is crucial information for other members of the healthcare team in order to avoid duplication of effort. Oncology nurse navigators often document information that is useful for compiling treatment plans or summaries; therefore, navigators and program administrators must contemplate systems' abilities to extract information from the navigation documentation software to be used for other purposes.

System interfaces can be costly and time consuming. Therefore, it is important to discuss the institution's specific desires for data importation and exportation with the software vendor. Often the vendor is eager to provide information about other institutions that have successfully integrated similar software systems as a mechanism for demonstrating the ease with which interfacing can be accomplished.

Reporting Capabilities

Outcome metrics are critical to proving the value and success of a navigation program. Navigators and program administrators should determine the key metrics important to demonstrating program accomplishments. When researching documentation software, it is essential to first determine what standard reports are available within the system and compare these to the desired reports needed for navigation program outcomes. Although metric overlap may occur with many of the reports, other metrics may not be captured in the standard reports. In these cases, it is important to determine how this information will be obtained and whether the system allows for customized reports. If customized reports can be built, it should be determined whether this can be designed by the institution's IT department or whether the software vendor needs to do the report build, which can again involve additional costs. These additional expenses must be taken into account when considering the cost of a particular navigation documentation system.

Scheduling and Alert Systems

Over time, most navigators have come to appreciate the value of an organized way to track patients through the healthcare system. Initially, many navigators used manual methods consisting of a calendar to track patient appointments, future telephone calls, and necessary follow-up. This evolved to using Excel spreadsheets to maintain information for program metrics. However, this method has proved to be problematic in a few ways. First, Excel spreadsheets offer no alert system capability. Rather, navigators need to continually go into the spreadsheet to look for upcoming appointments, testing, or follow-up telephone calls. Additionally, often not enough attention was given to the issue of patient privacy. When using a basic spreadsheet, patients' names and other identifying information potentially can be stored in an unsecure manner, thereby violating HIPAA requirements. Many software systems now use calendars that enable navigators to see at a glance active patients and upcoming events. Several systems also contain the ability for navigators to schedule reminders and other triggers to ensure timely and appropriate follow-up.

System Costs

Several factors should be considered when determining the cost of a software system. Foremost is the expense of the software system or application; the actual cost of this may vary greatly depending on whether an institution chooses a web-based or server-based application. Additionally, individual license fees, maintenance dues, technical support charges, and expenses associated with system upgrades also need to be determined and included in the overall system costs. Furthermore, hardware costs for servers and networks need to be considered based on the requirements of the chosen system. When calculating and analyzing system costs, it may be helpful to create a spreadsheet to itemize these expenses, as well as system specifications and features, for each of the software systems an institution is considering. This strategy can provide an objective basis to systematically evaluate software programs based on design features and overall expenditures.

The choice of a software system should not be made in haste or without careful consideration. Selecting the right navigation software can be the difference between a successful documentation system and a navigation program that struggles to effectively and efficiently demonstrate program outcomes. Each navigation program has its own unique needs to be considered prior to deciding on a specific navigation software system.

Case Example

Northside Hospital is a nonacademic, community-based hospital system with a comprehensive cancer program that incorporates medical, surgical, and radiation oncology under a single administrative, financial, and medical structure. Its market service area covers 13 counties, with just less than three million residents—representing roughly 33% of Georgia's total population (9.3 million). Northside Hospital is committed to providing a full spectrum of multidisciplinary services (prevention and education, diagnosis, clinical research, treatment, support and rehabilitation, and survivorship) to the community, including those who are uninsured, underrepresented, and disadvantaged. In 2010, Northside Hospital began a formalized navigation program and hired an oncology navigation coordinator and six oncology nurse navigators in an effort to accelerate and improve care for patients with cancer, with an emphasis on care to those experiencing healthcare disparities. Key roles and responsibilities of the navigators include (a) providing clinical education to patients, (b) offering assistance and support across the continuum of care, (c) connecting patients to the hospital's cancer support services, (d) participating in multidisciplinary tumor site conferences, and (e) coordinating care for patients as needed. Given the scope of services provided by the navigators, it was of utmost importance to develop a standardized documentation process.

The first step in the documentation process was the development of a paper navigation intake form (see Figure 10-1). This form was developed by assessing other institutions' forms and adapting these to the needs of Northside Hospital. During the navigators' implementation of the navigation intake form, questions quickly arose, including

- Where will documentation of continued interactions with patients be captured?
- Where will documentation be stored?
- How will documentation be shared with other departments that the navigators interacted with in caring for the patient?

It was readily apparent that the initial process necessitated expansion beyond the navigation intake form and that a paper documentation process would not be sufficient for the navigators' needs. From here, consideration of an electronic documentation system began. The navigation team was seeking a system that would track patients and treatment information throughout the continuum (from postscreening to survivorship), as well as capture referrals to connect patients to appropriate resources (Northside Hospital, 2011). The initial desire of the navigation team was to evaluate navigation-specific software programs, with the ultimate intention of determining the optimal system for purchase and implementation at the hospital.

At this point, the IT department became involved and a steering committee was formed that consisted of an IT coordinator, the oncology navigation coordinator, and an oncology program coordinator. Further along in the process, ad hoc members from supportive services (e.g., genetics, palliative care, clinical trials) were added to the steering committee. This team, led by the IT coordinator, began to explore and evaluate electronic documentation systems, both COTS and navigation-specific systems. They looked at new systems as well as those already in use at Northside Hospital. The steering committee's objective was to identify a software solution for the navigators that appropriately captured coordination of care, multidisciplinary teamwork, and program outcomes (Northside Hospital, 2011).

To better guide selection of a system, the IT coordinator spent considerable time meeting with the navigators to understand workflow patterns, information needed to navigate patients, and potential metrics the navigation program wished to monitor. The IT coordinator also met with the American Cancer Society resource navigator and ancillary staff from clinical trials, genetics, survivorship, community outreach, palliative care, and psychosocial care to generate workflow patterns along with a needs list and a goals and outcomes list to help guide the selection process.

Allowing the IT coordinator to lead the team facilitated a broader perspective, looking beyond the individual needs of the oncology nurse navigators. Instead, the concept of choosing a system that would link all areas began to emerge and take shape, whereby documentation and communication would be enhanced for larger purposes beyond navigation.

The steering committee identified two programs for consideration, both of which were COTS. One consisted of a module to the existing case management system used by Northside Hospital, whereas the other was a healthcare management system with the ability to be used across all areas of the institution. After careful consideration of the needs of the oncology nurse navigators and other steering committee stakeholders at Northside Hospital, as well as the advantages and disadvantages of the two systems, the steering committee chose to proceed with the COTS module associated with the existing case management system.

This system was by no means a "turnkey" system for navigation or the ancillary departments after purchase. Training revealed that necessary elements were not intrinsic. An example of one of these features was the ability to capture race and ethnicity of patients. The IT department worked with the vendor to build an interface from Northside Hospital's registration system to resolve this issue. Other areas within the COTS software program that required further development included

- The navigation assessment
- Physician lists
- Disease site–specific program screens
- Navigation activities/interventions
- Acuity scales
- Work lists for both referrals and patients currently undergoing navigation.

The time spent developing the system to make it applicable for navigation was considerable and required the efforts of the oncology navigation coordinator and the IT coordinator to work on the design and flow of the software program. The upside to this work is the ability to customize the system to capture the necessary information and activities to fit within the current patient navigation program. The IT department provided customization as requested and continues to offer the navigation department support with a dedicated IT resource for upgrades and changes.

Although the chosen COTS software system has met the basic needs of the Northside Hospital navigation team and ancillary departments, one of the system's limitations is the inability of the navigation team to access and query data. To do so requires a Crystal report to be written by a trained person within the IT department; however, integration of the software into the organization is currently under development.

Conclusion

Establishing a comprehensive and efficient documentation process can be a time-consuming and somewhat overwhelming task for navigators to consider, but it is imperative that documentation is recorded according to nurse practice acts and institutional policy while protecting patient privacy. Due diligence and careful consideration must be given to the selection of a system and input must be gathered from all key stakeholders to ensure the system will meet the institution's needs and requirements. Chapter 11 includes a listing of navigation-specific systems available at the time of publishing and corresponding websites.

References

American Nurses Association. (2012). Frequently asked questions: Roles of state boards of nursing: Licensure, regulation and complaint investigation. Retrieved from http://www.nursingworld.org/MainMenuCategories/Tools/State-Boards-of-Nursing-FAQ.pdf

Association of Community Cancer Centers. (n.d.). Cancer care patient navigation: Overview. Retrieved from http://accc-cancer.org/education/patientnavigation.asp

Campos, N.K. (2010). The legalities of nursing documentation. *Nursing Management, 40*(8), 16–19. doi:10.1097/01.NUMA.0000359202.59952.d2

Cantril, C., & Haylock, P.J. (2013). Patient navigation in the oncology care setting. *Seminars in Oncology Nursing, 29,* 76–90. doi:10.1016/j.soncn.2013.02.003

Francz, S. (2012). Today's nurse navigator: Educating and advocating for cancer patients. *Oncology Nursing News.* Retrieved from http://nursing.onclive.com/publications/oncology-nurse/2012/October-2012/Todays-Nurse-Navigator-Educating-and-Advocating-for-Cancer-Patients

National Council of State Boards of Nursing. (2013). Member boards. Retrieved from https://www.ncsbn.org/521.htm

Northside Hospital. (2011). *NSH NCCCP system selection decision: Nurse navigation decision paper.* Atlanta, GA: Author.

U.S. Department of Health and Human Services. (n.d.). Understanding health information privacy: For covered entities and business associates. Retrieved from http://www.hhs.gov/ocr/privacy/hipaa/understanding/coveredentities/index.html

CHAPTER 11

Navigation Resources

Karyl D. Blaseg, RN, MSN, OCN®, and Kathleen A. Gamblin, RN, BSN, OCN®

Introduction

One of the core functions of oncology nurse navigators is to connect patients with cancer and their families to available resources to reduce barriers and facilitate access to care. To do this, navigators must be thoroughly familiar with associations, organizations, and agencies committed to supporting the needs of the oncology community. This starts with actively researching what exists for the defined needs of the populations that navigators are serving. Once available resources are identified, it then becomes important for navigators to continually monitor for changes to eligibility criteria and program closures, as well as for new programs that emerge, for such resources are constantly evolving.

Many healthcare institutions have outreach departments, which have established relationships with various community organizations and local chapters of larger national organizations offering supportive services to patients with cancer and their families. Accessing the outreach department's knowledge and previous partnerships with these organizations may greatly benefit navigators in furthering relationship-building efforts. Another important consideration is an understanding of the organizations' goals beyond the assistance provided to patients, so that navigators can offer additional assistance to organizations that are beneficial in meeting such goals. This might be as simple as referring patients to community events, participating in a health fair, or assisting with a fund-raising activity. Understanding the needs and goals of other organizations has great potential to enlist higher levels of cooperation between groups, thereby creating synergy among organizations.

The Internet offers a seemingly endless array of websites and nonprofit entities dedicated to promoting awareness of cancer, advancing research, and offering psychosocial support. Because of the sheer abundance of websites and nonprofit entities, as well as the frequency with which resources change, it is important for navigators to be familiar with how to search for and identify reputable sites that offer education and psychosocial support. For example, an oncology nurse navigator looking to provide information to a 32-year-old woman with hereditary breast cancer might enter search terms such as *breast cancer, patient education, cancer genetics,* and *young adult cancer support* (or any combination of these and similar terms) to identify sites that might be appropriate for this patient.

One of the biggest advantages of using the Internet is the incredible opportunity it provides to not only gather information but also to share knowledge and experiences as well. However, one of the downsides is that anyone can offer advice or information, thereby creating issues and concerns related to reliability and accuracy of content. Thus, it is helpful to identify content *sources* and evaluate websites before providing these as potential resources to patients. The following considerations might be useful to navigators for evaluating patient resource websites.

- Who is responsible for writing, sponsoring, or publishing the site?
  - This information can be obtained by reading the section commonly found on websites devoted to information about the organization, determining who the publisher is (which is often found by the copyright date at the bottom of the page), or looking at author names or individual articles found on the website. Further information can be found by doing an Internet search on the publisher and authors.
- When was the site last updated, or when were site materials copyrighted?
  - It is important that information be current and not outdated, especially when dealing with medical information. Dates are commonly found at the bottom of the webpage.
- Who is the information intended for?
  - By reading the sections on the website devoted to information about the organization, one should be able to get a sense of the audience for which the information is intended. It is important to recognize whether the site and information is targeted for healthcare professionals or for patients and families.
- What is the site's domain?
  - The domain name of the site (for example, .com, .net, .org) indicates who is sponsoring the site and can be indicative of the site's reliability. Sites with *.gov* are sponsored by the government, *.edu* sites are sponsored by education entities, *.org* sites are sponsored by nonprofits, and those with *.com* and *.net* are used by a variety of businesses and entities. Websites should not be evaluated by the domain name alone, but this information is helpful in conjunction with other criteria.
- Where does the site's information come from?
  - Are references and citations provided on the site to indicate where information was obtained? Is the writing balanced, or is there a particular bias in the writing?
- What links are contained on the site?

– Follow the links provided to other sites. Are these sites reliable and reputable?

A number of navigation resources with corresponding websites are presented herein. The sites included merely represent a sample of the sources available and should not be considered an inclusive list. The focus of the organizations and websites identified is intended to assist navigators in gaining the knowledge and expertise needed to guide patients with cancer and their families through the complex cancer journey.

In addition to websites dedicated to patient education, support, and financial assistance, various healthcare professional associations and societies, as well as governmental agencies, are identified. These organizations often establish evidence-based guidelines, which oncology nurse navigators must be familiar with to ensure that care is progressing according to practice standards. Many of these organizations lead ground-breaking research and initiatives related to patient-centered care that are essential for oncology nurse navigators to be informed of. Navigation training programs and other resources to aid in navigation program development are also included, as are documentation software and textbooks that are pertinent to navigation roles and responsibilities.

Professional Associations for the Oncology Nurse Navigator

Academy of Oncology Nurse and Patient Navigators (AONN+): www.aonnonline.org
National Coalition of Oncology Nurse Navigators (NCONN): www.nconn.org
Oncology Nursing Society Nurse Navigator Special Interest Group: http://navigator.vc.ons.org

Other Professional Associations and Societies

American Cancer Society (ACS): www.cancer.org
American College of Surgeons (ACoS) Commission on Cancer (CoC): www.facs.org/cancer
American Society for Radiation Oncology (ASTRO): www.astro.org
American Society of Clinical Oncology (ASCO): www.asco.org
Association of Community Cancer Centers (ACCC): www.accc-cancer.org
Association of Oncology Social Work (AOSW): http://aosw.org
Association of Pediatric Hematology/Oncology Nurses (APHON): www.aphon.org

C-Change: http://c-changetogether.org
National Association of Social Workers (NASW): www.socialworkers.org
National Coalition for Cancer Survivorship (NCCS): www.canceradvocacy.org
National Comprehensive Cancer Network (NCCN): www.nccn.org/index.asp
North American Association of Central Cancer Registries (NAACCR): www.naaccr.org
Oncology Nursing Society (ONS): www.ons.org
National Consortium of Breast Centers (NCBC): www2.breastcare.org
Society of Gynecologic Oncology (SGO): www.sgo.org

Governmental Websites

Centers for Disease Control and Prevention (CDC): www.cdc.gov
Centers for Medicare and Medicaid Services (CMS): www.cms.gov
Medicaid and CHIP Services: www.medicaid.gov
Medicare: www.medicare.gov
National Cancer Institute (NCI): www.cancer.gov
National Center for Complementary and Alternative Medicine (NCCAM): http://nccam.nih.gov
National Institutes of Health ClinicalTrials.gov: www.clinicaltrials.gov
U.S. Department of Health and Human Services: www.hhs.gov
U.S. Department of Veterans Affairs: www.va.gov
U.S. Social Security Administration: www.ssa.gov

Training Programs and Program Development Resources

Association of Community Cancer Centers: Patient Navigation Resources and Tools for the Multidisciplinary Team: www.accc-cancer.org/resources/patientnavigation.asp
EduCare: www.breasthealthcare.com/training.php
George Washington University Cancer Institute's Center for the Advancement of Cancer Survivorship, Navigation and Policy: http://smhs.gwu.edu/gwci/education
Harold P. Freeman Patient Navigation Institute: www.hpfreemanpni.org
Northwest Georgia Regional Cancer Coalition Cancer Navigator Program: http://cancernavigatorprogram.org
Patient Navigation in Cancer Care (Pfizer Inc.): www.patientnavigation.com
Patient Navigator Training Collaborative, University of Colorado Cancer Center: http://patientnavigatortraining.org
Smith Center for Healing and the Arts: www.smithcenter.org/integrative-patient-navigation.html

Sonoma State University: www.sonoma.edu/exed/patient-navigator

Textbooks and Chapters

Sein, E. (2011). Building breast centers of excellence through patient navigation and care coordination. In S.M. Mahon (Ed.), *Site-specific cancer series: Breast cancer* (2nd ed., pp. 213–229). Pittsburgh, PA: Oncology Nursing Society.

Shockney, L. (2010). *Becoming a breast cancer nurse navigator.* Burlington, MA: Jones and Bartlett.

Documentation Software

General Navigation

MagView: www.magview.com/navigators
Medical Concierge: Navigator: www.healthcareoss.com/medical_concierge.php
Navigation Tracker: www.navigationtracker.com
Nursnav Oncology: www.nursenav.com
Oncology OnTrack: www.oncology.priorityconsult.com
OncoNav: www.onco-nav.com

Survivorship Navigation

Equicare CS: www.varian.com/us/oncology/radiation_oncology/aria/survivorship.html

Websites Offering Patient Education, Support, or Financial Assistance

Air Travel

Air Charity Network: http://aircharitynetwork.org
Angel Flight at National Institutes of Health: www.angelflightatnih.org
Corporate Angel Network: www.corpangelnetwork.org
LifeLine Pilots: www.lifelinepilots.org

Mercy Medical Airlift: www.mercymedical.org
National Patient Travel Center: www.patienttravel.org

Career/Workplace

Cancer and Careers: www.cancerandcareers.org

Children

Locks of Love: www.locksoflove.org
National Children's Cancer Society: www.thenccs.org

College Scholarships

Aplastic Anemia and MDS International Foundation College Scholarships: www.aamds.org/support-and-community/scholarships
Cancer for College: www.cancerforcollege.org
Patient Advocate Foundation Scholarships for Survivors: www.patient advocate.org/index.php?p=69

Fertility

Fertile Hope: www.fertilehope.org

General

Cancer*Care*: www.cancercare.org
Cancer Financial Assistance Coalition: www.cancerfac.org
CancerQuest: www.cancerquest.org
Chronic Disease Fund: www.cdfund.org
Friends of Man: www.friendsofman.org
Patient Advocate Foundation: www.patientadvocate.org
Patient Access Network Foundation: www.panfoundation.org
Patient Services, Inc.: www.patientservicesinc.org

Housing

Healthcare Hospitality Network: www.hhnetwork.org
Ronald McDonald House Charities: www.rmhc.org

Legal

Disability Rights Legal Center Cancer Legal Resource Center: www
.disabilityrightslegalcenter.org/cancer-legal-resource-center
Legal Services Corporation: www.lsc.gov
National Cancer Legal Services Network: www.nclsn.org

Prescription Programs

Free Medicine Program: www.freemedicineprogram.org
HealthWell Foundation: www.healthwellfoundation.org
The Medicine Program: www.themedicineprogram.com
NeedyMeds: www.needymeds.org
Partnership for Prescription Assistance: www.pparx.org
Patient Advocate Foundation Co-Pay Relief: www.copays.org
RxAssist: www.rxassist.org
RxHope: www.rxhope.com
Rx Outreach: http://rxoutreach.org

Prosthetics

Limbs for Life Foundation: http://limbsforlife.org

Site-Specific

Bladder Cancer
Bladder Cancer Advocacy Network: www.bcan.org

Brain Tumors
Brain Tumor Foundation for Children: www.braintumorkids.org
National Brain Tumor Society: www.braintumor.org

Breast Cancer
Breast Cancer Research Foundation: www.bcrfcure.org
National Breast Cancer Foundation: www.nationalbreastcancer.org
Susan G. Komen: http://ww5.komen.org

Cervical Cancer
National Cervical Cancer Coalition: www.nccc-online.org

Colorectal Cancer and Gastrointestinal Stromal Tumor

Colon Cancer Alliance: www.ccalliance.org
Fight Colorectal Cancer: http://fightcolorectalcancer.org
GIST Support International: www.gistsupport.org

Esophageal Cancer

Esophageal Cancer Awareness Association: www.ecaware.org

Kidney Cancer

Kidney Cancer Association: www.kidneycancer.org

Leukemia and Lymphoma

Aplastic Anemia and MDS International Foundation: www.aamds.org
Bone Marrow Foundation: http://bonemarrow.org
Cutaneous Lymphoma Foundation: www.clfoundation.org
International Myeloma Foundation: http://myeloma.org/Main.action
Leukemia & Lymphoma Society: www.lls.org
Lymphoma Research Foundation: www.lymphoma.org
Myelodysplastic Syndromes Foundation: www.mds-foundation.org

Liver Cancer

American Liver Foundation: www.liverfoundation.org

Lung Cancer

American Lung Association: www.lung.org
Lung Cancer Alliance: www.lungcanceralliance.org
LUNGevity Foundation: www.lungevity.org

Melanoma and Skin Cancer

AIM at Melanoma Foundation: www.aimatmelanoma.org
Melanoma Research Foundation: www.melanoma.org
Skin Cancer Foundation: www.skincancer.org

Oral/Head and Neck Cancer

Oral Cancer Foundation: http://oralcancerfoundation.org
Support for People With Oral and Head and Neck Cancer: www.spohnc.org
ThyCa: Thyroid Cancer Survivors' Association: www.thyca.org

Ovarian Cancer

Ovarian Cancer National Alliance: www.ovariancancer.org

Pancreatic Cancer

Lustgarten Foundation: www.lustgarten.org
Pancreatic Cancer Action Network: www.pancan.org

Prostate Cancer

Prostate Cancer Foundation: www.pcf.org

Sarcoma

Sarcoma Alliance: http://sarcomaalliance.org

Testicular Cancer

Testicular Cancer Resource Center: http://tcrc.acor.org
Testicular Cancer Society: www.testicularcancersociety.org
TesticularCancer.com: www.tc-cancer.com

Tobacco Cessation

North American Quitline Consortium: www.naquitline.org

Young Adults

Brenda Mehling Cancer Fund: www.bmcf.net
Cameron Siemers Foundation for Hope: www.cameronsiemers.org
Cancer Survivors' Fund: www.cancersurvivorsfund.org
Planet Cancer: http://myplanet.planetcancer.org
The SAMFund for Young Adult Survivors of Cancer: www.thesamfund.org
   /who-we-are
Stupid Cancer: www.stupidcancer.org
Ulman Cancer Fund for Young Adults: www.ulmanfund.org

Index

The letter f *after a page number indicates that relevant text appears in a figure; the letter* t, *in a table.*

A

Academy of Oncology Nurse and Patient Navigators (AONN+), 6t, 8, 30, 299
accessibility, for patients with disabilities, 85–87
accreditation standards, 10–11, 43–44
acuity scales, 101, 102t, 245–246
advance directives, 130, 159
Agency for Healthcare Research and Quality, 98–99
AIM at Melanoma Foundation, 304
Air Charity Network, 301
air travel, 301–302
alcohol counseling, 164
American Cancer Society (ACS), 2, 299
  Cancer in the Poor report, 3, 5t, 47
  Patient Navigator Program, 29
  survivorship care guidelines, 198
American College of Surgeons Commission on Cancer (ACoS CoC), 299
  accreditation standards, 10–11, 43–44, 72–73, 94, 106, 176, 178

Survivorship Care Plan standard, 111, 188
American Liver Foundation, 304
American Lung Association, 304
American Society for Radiation Oncology (ASTRO), 299
American Society for the Control of Cancer (ASCC), 2
American Society of Clinical Oncology (ASCO), 97, 199, 299
  Quality Oncology Practice Initiative (QOPI), 188
Americans With Disabilities Act, 87
Angel Flight, 301
ANGEL Network, 183
anxiety, 107. *See also* psychosocial distress
Aplastic Anemia and MDS International Foundation, 302, 304
ARIA system, 287
assessment/evaluation
  of documentation systems, 288–292, 289f
  of navigation program, 66f, 67–69, 68f, 252–255, 264–269. *See also* program metrics

of patient distress, 106–110, 157, 162
Association of Community Cancer Centers (ACCC), 6t, 286, 299–300
Association of Oncology Social Work (AOSW), 299
  joint position with ONS/NASW, 6t, 8, 9f, 16, 24
Association of Pediatric Hematology/Oncology Nurses (APHON), 299

B

barriers, 262–264, 263t
  at end of life, 112. *See also* end-of-life care
  identification/resolution of, 16–17
  to palliative care, 97
  patient-centered, 104–105
  to survivorship care, 196–198
Billings Clinic
  acuity scale, 101, 102t
  progress note template, 280f–285f
  workflow, 78, 79f–80f
Bladder Cancer Advocacy Network, 303

D

decision making, for treatment planning, 125–126, 145–146, 147*f*–151*f*, 170. *See also specific cancer sites;* treatment phase
decision-making tasks, for patients, 48
decreased length of stay, tracking of, 257
depression, 107. *See also* psychosocial distress
Design for Six Sigma methodology, 49
development resources, 66*f*, 300–301
diagnosis, as navigation entry point, 88–89. *See also specific cancer sites*
diet modifications, 93–94, 196
disabilities, patients with, 85–87
Disability Rights Legal Center, 303
disease-specific model, of survivorship care, 191
distress. *See* psychosocial distress
documentation systems
case example of, 292–294
costs of, 292
electronic/software-based, 287–288, 301
essential elements of, 178*f*–185*f*, 276–277
evaluation of, 288–292, 289*f*
of nurse navigation, 275–276
paper-based, 277–286
reporting capabilities of, 291
scheduling/alert features in, 291
of survivorship care, 194, 200–201
system interfaces for, 288, 290–291
timeliness of use, 277, 286*f*
time spent using, 277
web-based vs. server-based, 289–290
due diligence, 146, 170. *See also* decision making, for treatment planning; treatment phase
dysphagia, 168

E

economic costs
of cancer, 189
of documentation systems, 292
EduCare, 30, 300
education/experience, for nurse navigators, 23–24, 25*f*
Education in Palliative and End-of-Life Care (EPEC) curriculum, 97
Education in Palliative and End-of-Life Care for Oncology (EPEC-O) training, 97
80/20 rule, 101
electronic medical record (EMR), 197, 199, 275. *See also* documentation systems
emergency department visits, tracking of, 256–257
emotional support, provided by navigators, 18–19
"Encrucijada" ("Crossroads") program, 181–182
end-of-life care
with breast cancer, 130
with head and neck cancer, 166
navigation in, 111–112
with prostate cancer, 151
entry points, into navigation system, 71, 74, 87–88, 161–162, 169–171. *See also specific cancer sites*
Equicare CS, 301
Esophageal Cancer Awareness Association, 304
exercise, 95, 196

F

facility-developed programs, for documentation, 287
FACIT-Pal-14 (QOL assessment), 108–109
Fertile Hope, 302
fertility, resources on, 302
Fight Colorectal Cancer, 304
financial assistance, 264, 301–305
fine needle aspiration, 161
fishbone diagram, 78, 80*f*
Fisher, Bernard, 124
fitness programs, 95, 196
Fletcher Allen Health Care Upper GI Clinic, 138–139
flow diagrams, 56*f*–58*f*, 78*f*, 78–83, 80*f*–83*f*
for GI navigation, 142*f*–143*f*
focus group interviews, 50, 52*f*, 154
formal partnerships, in outreach navigation, 182
Freeman, Harold P., MD, 3, 15, 47, 71, 74, 75*f*, 121, 175–176
Free Medicine Program, 303
Friends of Man, 302
From Cancer Patient to Cancer Survivor: Lost in Transition (IOM), 111, 188
Functional Assessment of Cancer Therapy–General (FACT-G), 108, 262